Mental Retardation and Developmental Delay

Mental Retardation and Developmental Delay

Genetic and Epigenetic Factors

MOYRA SMITH, MD, PHD, MFA

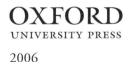

OXFORD
UNIVERSITY PRESS

2006

OXFORD
UNIVERSITY PRESS

Oxford University Press, Inc., publishes works that further
Oxford University's objective of excellence
in research, scholarship, and education.

Oxford   New York
Auckland   Cape Town   Dar es Salaam   Hong Kong   Karachi
Kuala Lumpur   Madrid   Melbourne   Mexico City   Nairobi
New Delhi   Shanghai   Taipei   Toronto

With offices in
Argentina   Austria   Brazil   Chile   Czech Republic   France   Greece
Guatemala   Hungary   Italy   Japan   Poland   Portugal   Singapore
South Korea   Switzerland   Thailand   Turkey   Ukraine   Vietnam

Copyright © 2006 by Oxford University Press, Inc.

Published by Oxford University Press, Inc.
198 Madison Avenue, New York, New York 10016

www.oup.com

Oxford is a registered trademark of Oxford University Press

Library of Congress Cataloging-in-Publication Data
Smith, Moyra.
Mental retardation and developmental delay : genetic and epigenetic factors / Moyra
Smith ; with Stuart M. Arfin and Ira T. Lott.
p. ; cm.
Includes bibliographical references and index.
ISBN-13 978-0-19-517432-8
ISBN 0-19-517432-1
1. Mental retardation—Etiology.   2. Mental retardation—Genetic aspects.   3.
Developmental disabilities—Etiology.   4. Developmental disabilities—Genetic aspects.
[DNLM: 1. Mental Retardation—genetics—Child.   2. Mental Retardation—genetics—
Infant.   3. Developmental Disabilities—etiology—Child.   4. Developmental Disabilities—
etiology—Infant.   5. Developmental Disabilities—genetics—Child.   6. Developmental
Disabilities—genetics—Infant.   7. Mental Retardation—etiology—Child.   8. Mental
Retardation—etiology—Infant.   WS 107.5.B4 S655m 2006]   I. Arfin, Stuart M.   II. Lott, Ira
T.   III. Title.
RC570.S64 2006
616. 85'88042—dc22   2005013749

9 8 7 6 5 4 3 2 1

Printed in the United States of America
on acid-free paper

"Understanding is always a journey, never a destination."
—Richard Fortey, 2004

Preface

My motivation to study human genetics and birth defects grew out of the overwhelming sense of tragedy I felt when, in 1962, as a medical student I visited a home for severely retarded children and adults. There I saw children who sat rocking back and forth, banging their heads against the wall, apparently oblivious to their surroundings. From time to time, they shrieked in frustration or anger. As I entered a room where adult males lived, a man crawled along the floor and grabbed my ankles. He looked up at me with a strange expression, his features contorted into a grimace; perhaps it was a smile. I tried not to show my fear; somehow though I felt he sensed it.

For days and weeks after that visit, I could not dispel from my mind the images of the inhabitants of that home, enclosed as they were in a sensually deprived environment. They were housed, fed, and observed so that they did not seriously harm themselves or others; otherwise, they were left to their own torturous thoughts and frustrations. I resolved to search for information about mental retardation.

In our medical school library, I found Lionel Penrose's book *The Biology of Mental Defect*. In the 1954 edition of this book, Penrose reviewed the classification of mental retardation, biological and social aspects, and its few known genetic causes; these included the rare recessive disorder phenylketonuria (PKU) and the rare dominant disorder epiloia (now known as tuberous sclerosis). Most remarkable was the fact that Penrose was grappling with the biological aspects of mental retardation, trying to understand root causes.

I knew then that I wanted to be involved in studies on the causes of mental handicap.

A few years later, I wrote from South Africa to Professor Penrose and asked him how one became a human geneticist. He replied kindly and recommended graduate studies in Great Britain. He had just retired from University College London and referred me to his successor, Harry Harris. Thus began my journey.

Now, after 40 years spent in genetic and inborn errors of metabolism clinics and in the laboratory studying biochemical variation, developmental changes in gene expression, and the mapping and cloning of genes, I find my-self striving to write a book that has a title very similar to the one that Lionel Penrose wrote.

Perhaps at last I understand the verse from T. S. Eliot:

> We shall not cease from exploration
> And the end of all our exploring
> Will be to arrive where we started
> And know the place for the first time.
>
> T. S. Eliot, "Little Gidding in Four Quartets"

Acknowledgments

Stuart Arfin read through each chapter and provided the expert opinions of a biochemist and molecular biologist. Any errors in the text are, of course, mine. Stuart Arfin contributed a section on the ubiquitin pathway of protein degradation, one area of his specialization. Ira Lott, pediatric neurologist, read material in Chapters 2, 3, and 9. I took his expert opinion into account as I revised those chapters; again, any errors or misconceptions that remain are my responsibility.

I wish to express my gratitude to Michelle Sands-Kidner, who read each chapter and provided feedback from the point of view of a genetic counselor. I am grateful for the assistance of Rebekah Smith and Andy Fedak, who prepared many of the illustrations, and Michele Hinojosa, who helped assemble the references.

I thank the editors at Oxford University Press, Jeff House, William Lamsback, Nancy Wolitzer, and Andrew Pachuta. Jeff House guided me through several iterations of the proposal for this book. William Lamsback provided guidance for preparation of the manuscript and illustrations.

The Wellcome Library for the History and Understanding of Medicine in London, England, and the Centre for the Study of the History of Medicine at University College London provided resources and inspiration as I set out on this writing adventure. I have also benefited enormously from the resources available through the University of California Library system, and I am grateful for these.

Finally, I wish to pay tribute to my mentors, patients, students, and family and to thank them for teaching me and enriching my life.

Contents

Contributors

Stuart M. Arfin, Ph.D.
Emeritus Professor of Biological Chemistry
College of Medicine
University of California, Irvine

Ira T. Lott, M.D.
Professor of Pediatrics and Neurology
Associate Dean, Clinical Neurosciences
Director, Child Neurology
College of Medicine
University of California, Irvine

Introduction

In this book, we start with the premise that developmental delay and mental retardation are symptoms. The underlying causes of these symptoms may be primarily genetic or primarily environmental in origin. Defining the etiology as well as the pathophysiology in a given case may enable us to design therapies to counteract some of the consequences of underlying problems. Furthermore, we may be able to consider aspects of prevention.

Developmental disabilities occur in 5%–10% of the pediatric population (Shevell et al. 2000). Deficits may exist in a single domain or across several domains. Included within the spectrum of developmental disabilities are global developmental delay, isolated speech and language delay, motor delay, cerebral palsy, pervasive developmental disabilities, and profound primary and sensory impairments, such as deafness and blindness.

The American Association on Mental Retardation (AAMR) and the American Psychiatric Association (*Diagnostic and Statistical Manual of Mental Disorders*, DSM-IV) define *mental retardation* as a significantly subaverage intellectual function with limitations of adaptive skills. Adaptive skills include communication, self-care, social and interpersonal skills, health and safety, functional academic skills, use of community resources, work, and leisure. Determination of mental retardation according to DSM-IV criteria requires intelligence quotient (IQ) testing. Categories of mental retardation are defined in the DSM-IV criteria as mild, 2–3 standard deviations below the mean (IQ 50–70); moderate, 3–4 standard deviations below the mean (IQ 40–55); severe, 4–5 standard deviations below the mean (IQ 25–40); and profound, at least 5 standard deviations below the mean (IQ <25). The classification criteria of the AAMR focus primarily on the functional abilities of individuals and on the level of support they require (Bodensteiner et al. 2002).

The overall prevalence of mental retardation is 1%–3% (World Health Organization 2002). Severe mental retardation occurs in 0.3% of the world's population, and genetic factors are thought to play a role in 50% of such cases.

There can be no doubt that through elucidation of the underlying causes of developmental delay and mental retardation we are able, at least in a small but growing number of cases, to make a positive impact on the lives of individual patients. This is especially the case with environmental causes of delay, though in many cases sociopolitical factors present major obstacles. With respect to developmental delay due to genetic causes, we are sometimes also able to have an impact. This is particularly the case in certain inborn errors of metabolism. Following accurate diagnosis, treatment can be initiated. In cases where diagnosis is made early through biochemical or molecular studies in the newborn period or early infancy, treatment may be initiated before the onset of symptoms. In certain inborn errors of amino acid or organic acidic metabolism, correct diagnosis can make an impact even when this takes place only after the onset of symptoms. In situations where correct diagnosis is not likely to improve the outcome for the patient, it may still be of value to the family. Accurate diagnosis in an affected individual may empower family members as they seek counseling and embark on family planning. Accurate diagnosis and a team approach to individuals with developmental delay or mental retardation facilitate management of health issues, exploration of educational options, and development of a support system for the family.

Wise physicians have stressed the individuality of patients. A patient with a disorder due to defects or deficiency of a specific gene has other genes in his or her makeup that impact on the phenotype. Environmental factors also play a role in the long-term outcome. David Weatherall (2004) has emphasized that every disorder due to a single gene defect is in a sense a complex genetic disorder since other genes and the environment impact the phenotype.

Mutant genes may be passed on through generations. It is important to emphasize, however, that gene mutations and chromosomal changes may arise de novo during oogenesis or spermatogenesis or following fertilization. These changes often arise as a de novo event in a specific pregnancy.

Gene mutations that lead to mental retardation may manifest in the neonatal period. This is particularly the case if defective function affects multiple body functions or leads to physical abnormalities. Evidence of delayed development, or indeed of regression in behavior, may first occur later in childhood. Such is the case, for example, in disorders where defects in gene function lead to accumulation of metabolites or breakdown products that progressively damage the nervous system.

We will confine discussion to forms of mental retardation that occur during childhood. We will not consider loss of intellectual function that occurs in adults and that frequently falls into the category of dementia. We concentrate primarily on genetic causes of developmental delay and mental retardation. However, it is always important to consider the role of environmental factors; and we review several of these, particularly in the context of cognitive impairment that develops later in childhood. Obviously, we have selected a subset of genetic conditions for discussion. We discuss conditions where the specific gene defects that lead to particular cognitive impairments have been defined. We also discuss developments in the emerging field of epigenetic disorders, defining *epigenetics* as altered expression of a gene in the absence of DNA sequence mutations in that specific gene.

What degree of mental retardation is consistent with a meaningful life and some degree of happiness? To even approach an answer to this difficult question, it is important to have a comprehensive insight into the various complications that may result from a gene defect; in many cases, mental retardation is but one of the consequences. Mentally handicapped persons were in the past further disabled by understimulating environments and low expectations. The answer to the question lies not only in scientific and medical studies. It depends in part on the resources that societies are willing to make available for the care of individuals who show some level of compromise.

Mental Retardation and
Developmental Delay

1

Science, Society, and Mental Retardation: A History

In this chapter, we trace a history of societal attitudes to mental retardation during the period when it was becoming evident that mental retardation is due to biological factors. We will discuss the history of the study of mental retardation beginning in the second half of the nineteenth century, when interest in brain structure and function intensified. In addition, we will consider a number of scientific developments in the fields of biochemistry and genetics that were, in due course, to impact our understanding of the causes of mental retardation.

Societal Attitudes and Biological Concepts of Mental Retardation: 1860–1980

In the latter half of the nineteenth century, neuroanatomists used clinical observations in humans and studies in other animals to define the functional roles of different parts of the brain. Knowledge of the histology of cells of the central and peripheral nervous systems was greatly enhanced by the work of Santiago Ramon y Cajal, Vladimir Betz, Jan Purkinje, and Theodor Meynert. By 1891 the neuron doctrine was firmly established. Marshall and Magoun published a detailed history of this period in the development of the fields of neuroanatomy and neurohistology in 1998.

Recognition of the Roles of Congenital, Developmental, and Environmental Factors in Developmental Delay and Mental Retardation

Between 1860 and 1900, advances in neurology and pathology led to the recognition that mental retardation has many different causes. In Britain, John Langdon Down (1866, 1876, 1887) and William W. Ireland began to promote a classification of mental retardation (unfortunately termed *idiocy* at that time) based on etiology rather than solely on quantitation of degree of impairment. Down distinguished three different forms of idiocy: *congenital idiocy*, where subjects never possessed ordinary mental powers; *developmental idiocy*, where deterioration occurred after a satisfactory start; and *accidental idiocy*, which resulted from injury or infection.

In 1866, Down recognized the syndrome that he defined as "mongolism." This syndrome now bears his name. He wrote "A very large number of congenital idiots are typical Mongols. So marked is this that when placed side by side it is difficult to believe that the specimens compared are not children of the same parents."

Ireland (1877, 1898) recognized that in some patients mental defect was but one of the disease manifestations. In 1898 he reported that this was the case in tuberous sclerosis, and Pelizaeus-Merzbacher disease. It was also true in a disorder characterized by cerebro-macular degeneration and mental defect beginning in early childhood and named Tay-Sachs disease, for the New York physicians who described it (Sachs 1887; Tay 1891). Ireland recognized that lesions affecting the growth of the brain in early life had an effect on mental power. In this category he included hydrocephalus and epilepsy, "the predisposition to take fits." He noted that a child deprived of hearing or sight was oftentimes incorrectly classified as an "idiot."

Ireland (1898) drew attention to the fact that unusual facial appearance and congenital malformations were frequent, though not inevitable, features in patients who were retarded:

> The dyscrasy which accompanies genetous [congenital] idiocy affects both the constitutional vigour and the symmetrical growth of the frame, though not equally in every part. Nature works like a bad sculptor, who fails to give the proper form, sometimes to one member of the body and sometimes to another. There are errors, now here and now there; and some parts are more happily shaped than others. Occasionally, however, genetous idiots are strong and good looking, with well formed heads good teeth, and no deformities whatever. (p. 54)

Cretinism and Goiter: Mental Retardation Primarily Due to Environmental Factors but Due in Some Cases to Genetic Factors

One of the most important medical and scientific breakthroughs of the mid-nineteenth century was the recognition of the role of iodine deficiency in the etiology of endemic goiter and the recognition that goiter, myxedema, and cretinism were associated. Cretinism, with its accompanying disabilities including growth and developmental retardation as well as deaf mutism, was recognized for centuries in Europe; paintings, woodcarvings, and sculptures frequently depicted dwarfed cretins with apathetic expression, puffy features, large tongues, and goiters. Cretinism was sometimes referred to as "pachydermic idiocy." In 1984, F. Merke compiled his *History and Iconography of Endemic Goiter and Cretinism*. Goitrous cretinism was endemic in the mountainous regions of Switzerland and in the villages of the Pyrenees, the Andes, and the Himalayas.

Writings from the twelfth through fourteenth centuries indicate that cretinism was recognized as a disease of people who lived far from the ocean. It was sometimes treated with ash derived from seaweed and sponges. A Frenchman, J. Boussingault, who worked in South America, learned from the people of Colombia that salt obtained from an abandoned mine cured goiters. He analyzed the salt and found it had high iodine content. In 1825, he documented the fact that iodine cured goiter. In 1873, Cesar Lombroso promoted the practice of iodine administration to goitrous persons. Switzerland was the first country to vigorously implement administration of iodine.

Fagge in 1871 reported the occurrence of sporadic cretinism in England, a country where endemic cretinism was not present.

Later in the nineteenth century, physicians began treating patients who had myxedema and cretinism with raw or lightly cooked sheep thyroid gland or with glycerin extract of thyroid (Murray 1891; Howitz 1893). Ireland (1898) wrote

> The results of this treatment upon children affected with pachydermic idiocy are so rapid and striking that they rather resemble the transformation in a fairy tale than the slow gains of the healing art against chronic disease. (p. 243)

> It has been a disappointment to our warm hopes that under thyroid treatment the mental improvement has not kept pace with the bodily growth though almost all patients have shown a quickening of intelligence. Naturally the improvement has been greater the earlier the age at which they were treated. (p. 245)

In 1895, Bauman reported that high concentrations of iodine occurred in the thyroid gland. In 1915, Kendall derived crystalline tetraiodothryronine (thyroxine) from thyroid tissue. Harington (1925b) and Harington and Barger (1927) elucidated the chemical structures of the different forms of thyroxine (T3 and T4). Mott (1917) reported on the changes in the central nervous system in hypothyroidism.

It is important to note that endemic cretinism still occurs. As recently as 1980, in communities in Nepal and Central Africa (most notably the Democratic Republic of the Congo), 5%–10% of the population displayed cretinism, characterized by varying degrees of growth retardation, mental retardation, neurological symptoms, and deaf mutism (Stanbury and Hetzel, 1980).

In some communities, cretinism appeared when rock salt was no longer available and was replaced with low-iodine industrial salt. In other communities, for example, in Bangladesh, cretinism occurred following a decision by village elders to stop purchasing iodized salt because it was more costly than noniodized salt (*The Rain Plague*, BBC London, 1991). In 2002, the

World Health Organization (WHO) reported that in countries such as Colombia and Guatemala, where there was initially success in combating iodine deficiency and its consequences, political and social upheavals have led to the reemergence of the problem. The WHO also reported recurrence of iodine-deficiency diseases in a number of countries of the former Soviet Union. (http://www.who.int/nat/idd.htm) Iodine deficiency during pregnancy leads to deficiency of thyroxine in the fetus because there is a reduction in thyroid hormone transferred from the mother and because the fetus produces less hormone (Morreale de Escobar et al. 2004).

Sporadic hypothyroidism occurs today in approximately 1 in 4000 newborn infants in the United States. Fortunately, through newborn screening programs, this condition is detected early and can be vigorously treated (Dussault and Laberge 1973). Most commonly it is due to abnormal development of the thyroid gland. In some cases, congenital hypothyroidism is an inborn error of metabolism (Madeiros and Stanbury, 1994).

Education of the Mentally Retarded

As the study of neurology advanced in France in the nineteenth century, there was increased interest in the causes of mental retardation. Between 1839 and 1842, Edouard Seguin began to treat and educate retarded children at the Hospice des Incurables and at the Bicêtre in Paris. In 1848, when a revolution began in Paris, he moved to the United States and continued working as a consultant with a special interest in mentally retarded children in New York (Seguin 1866; Scheerenberger, 1983).

In the second half of the nineteenth century, along with increased social sensitivity to the plight of the disadvantaged came an increase in efforts to educate the mentally retarded. Between 1841 and 1865, Charles Dickens, in novels such as *David Copperfield, Nicholas Nickleby*, and *Our Mutual Friend*, realistically and sympathetically portrayed the plight of the poor and the handicapped.

In 1849, Samuel Gridley Howe, a physician, successfully lobbied the state of Massachusetts to establish a 3-year experimental school for "idiot" children. Howe reported gratifying improvements in the status and behavior of the children. Howe and Horace Mann worked together to promote the well-being of the mentally retarded population.

During the 1880s, William Ireland established a school for the mentally retarded in Scotland. He stressed that to produce improvement it was important to act upon the whole being, the body and the mind. He emphasized the importance of cultivating the senses of hearing, smell, taste, and touch and of open-air exercise. Ireland proposed assessing intelligence through comparison of the patient's skills with performance skills of children at different ages. He placed great importance on the teaching of language to retarded children. He also promoted the teaching of vocational skills.

In Rome, Maria Montessori, who in 1896 was the first Italian woman to graduate as a physician, came into contact with mentally retarded children housed along with adults in an "insane asylum." She began an active campaign for the education of mentally retarded children (Montessori 1896).

In the early years of the twentieth century, Alfred Binet in Paris analyzed intelligence and education. In response to legislation that required schools to design programs to educate mentally retarded children, Binet and Théodore Simon designed the intelligence test that bears their name. A paper describing this test was published in 1905. Binet believed that intelligence could be improved through learning.

Intolerance Reemerges

In the early decades of the twentieth century, attitudes toward the mentally retarded changed and intolerance reemerged, perhaps fueled by the emerging pseudoscience of eugenics. In Britain, the Mental Deficiency Act of 1913 resulted in a greater role for public authorities in the ascertainment and institutionalization of persons judged to be mentally defective. Kevles (1985) noted that the Eugenics Education Society took the Mental Deficiency Act as a victory for the eugenics movement. Penrose wrote later of the new attitude that became prevalent in the twentieth century: "the defective was no longer an innocent sufferer deserving only of pity. He was gradually becoming recognized as a menace."

In the United States, the concept that heredity was the prime cause of mental retardation provided part of the impetus to impose sterilization. Scheerenberger (1983) noted that by 1912 sterilization laws were imposed by eight U.S. states. Sterilization laws were applied to "idiots, imbeciles, feeble minded, epileptics, drunkards and prostitutes" (Van Wagenen 1914). In 1912, the American Breeders' Association had produced a report on the best practical means to cut off defective germ plasm in the human population.

Clarence Darrow, as a lawyer and humanist, in 1925 and 1926 attacked genealogical studies designed to demonstrate inferiority in particular families: He noted that eugenists ignored facts such as inadequacy of education, lack of opportunity and poverty.

Studies on Behavior and Mental Conditions That Predispose to Mental Retardation

During the 1930s, more emphasis was placed on the study of behavior. At the Vineland School in New Jersey, Edgar Doll studied adaptive behavior (Doll 1936); and in 1936, he introduced his Vineland Social Maturity Scale. Medical conditions that predisposed to mental retardation received more attention in the 1930s. Following a survey of 3548 retarded children in the Detroit public schools, Jackson (1935) reported that 281 were hypothyroid. Biochemical disorders and dysmorphology syndromes associated with mental illness were described with greater frequency throughout the 1930s. Most notable was the discovery of phenylketonuria (PKU) by Folling in 1934. This was the first described disease that led to mental retardation and conformed to the postulates proposed by Garrod in 1908 and published in 1909 for a disorder due to an inborn error of metabolism.

Physicians realized soon after the discovery of PKU that treatment was possible. In 1946, Penrose stated

> There may be ways of alleviating the condition, even though it is inborn, in a manner analogous to the way in which a child with clubfeet may be helped to walk or a child with congenital cataract enabled to see.

We will return to a discussion of PKU and inborn errors of metabolism in the section on the history of biochemistry (Penrose 1946, p. 197 in 1998 reprint).

Environmental Causes of Developmental Delay and Mental Retardation

Key to our understanding of an important nongenetic cause of mental retardation was the discovery in 1941 by Norman Gregg, an Australian ophthalmologist, that rubella virus infection during pregnancy could lead to deafness, blindness, and mental retardation.

Another key element of progress with respect to understanding the causes of mental handicap in children and its prevention was the realization that birth injury and profound jaundice in the newborn period leads to retardation, along with other neurological symptoms. An increasing interest in the birth process and in the care of newborn infants began in the latter part of the nineteenth century. Thomas Cone (1979) noted that intense investigation into the cause of fetal and infant mortality took place in France in the 1870s. The Franco-Prussian War caused the loss of many lives. During that period, the decline in birthrate and the incidence of early infant death further contributed to the fall in population numbers. This fall was much steeper in France than in Germany and England. The government of France therefore established the Commission on Depopulation. Following the report of this commission, France became a pioneer in organizing maternity and infant hygiene programs.

In 1916, La Fetra published a landmark paper in the American medical literature on the hospital care of premature infants.

In 1932, Diamond, et al. recognized that stillbirths due to universal edema of the fetus (fetal hydrops), severe jaundice, and anemia of the newborn are related. Landsteiner and Weiner (1940) described the Rhesus (Rh) blood group antigen. In 1941, Levine and coworkers published a key paper on the role of Rh blood group incompatibility in the etiology of hemolytic disease of the newborn. Edith Potter in 1947 described the consequences of profound jaundice due to hemolysis associated with Rh blood group incompatibility. Deposition of unconjugated bilirubin derived from hemolyzed blood cells led to brain damage, particularly to damage of specific nuclei in the brain. She noted that severe neonatal jaundice could lead to mental retardation associated with other neurological symptoms, including uncoordinated and uncontrolled movements and general muscle weakness. Wallerstein began treating severe jaundice of the newborn with exchange transfusions in 1946. In 1958, phototherapy was introduced to treat neonatal jaundice following the demonstration by Cremer and coworkers that bilirubin deposited in the tissues of newborns is highly photosensitive. After 1963, Rh screening of mothers and the use of RhoGAM shortly after delivery in Rh-negative women who carried an Rh-positive fetus reduced the frequency of the problem.

During the 1940s, as more data accumulated on the physiology of the newborn and premature infant, care of the low-birth weight infant improved dramatically. This coincided with a progressive decrease in the incidence of long-term central nervous system deficiencies (Lubchenco 1983).

An important environmental cause of retardation was delineated through the studies of Jones and Smith, who described fetal alcohol syndrome in 1973.

The Post–Second World War Period: Significant Breakthroughs in Science and Politics Relevant to Mental Retardation

There can be no doubt that the credibility and the power of the eugenics movement and of the Breeders' Association rapidly diminished as the Nazi atrocities became known. Particularly relevant to the history we are considering was the Nazi extermination of individuals considered "subhuman" because of physical or mental handicaps or "undesirable" racial or ethnic origins. As the world recovered from the ravages of war, scientists returned to the study of biochemistry and genetics with great vigor.

The discovery of the structure of deoxyribonucleic acid (DNA) in 1953 by Watson and Crick was key to the development of molecular genetics. It did not, however, have an impact on studies of the etiology of mental retardation for several decades. Of more immediate relevance was the report by Tjio and Levan in 1956 that the correct chromosome number for humans is 46. This was followed by reports from Lejeune et al. (1959a, b) that an extra small acrocentric chromosome was present in individuals with Down syndrome (previously called "mongolism"). In 1959, the first reports of an abnormal number of sex chromosomes were published by Ford et al. and Jacobs et al. By 1963 geneticists had discovered that structural chromosomal abnormalities such as translocations and deletions of segments of chromosomes could lead to malformation syndromes and mental retardation. The first structural chromosomal anomaly reported was deletion of part of the short arm of chromosome 5 (Lejeune et al. 1963).

In 1965, Senator Robert Kennedy visited institutions for the mentally retarded and publicized the scandalous conditions that existed there (Kennedy 1965). Late in 1965, Dr. Burton Blatt and professional photographer Fred Kaplan toured several of these institutions. Blatt wrote that he was in no way prepared for the degradation and despair he encountered. He stated that the experiences caused him a chronic sorrow that would remain with him until the American people became aware of and did something about the treatment of certain mentally retarded beings in state institutions (Blatt and Kaplan 1976).

One thousand copies of Blatt and Kaplan's photographic essay *Christmas in Purgatory* (reprinted in Blatt B 1976, pp. 345–60) were distributed to physicians, legislators, and commissioners. Through the work of the Kennedy family and the efforts of others who became interested in the cause of the mentally retarded, a period of great progress began (see Shorter 2000). Scheerenberger (1983) noted that No other 20 year period saw as many humanitarian changes as the 1960–1970's: These changes included rights, mainstreaming, advocacy, individual plans, interdisciplinary teams, normalization, developmental models and deinstitutionalization. . . . He emphasized that countless mentally retarded persons benefited from opportunities never before available.

In 1971, the United Nations General Assembly adopted the Declaration of General and Special Rights of the Mentally Retarded (see Scheerenberger 1983, pp. 250–1).

The period 1960–1980 was characterized by a rapid expansion in biochemical genetic, cytogenetic, and molecular genetic research that was relevant to understanding the etiology of mental retardation. Much of this research also has implications for genetic counseling and for prevention of some forms of mental retardation.

Aspects of the History of Developments in Biochemistry

Over the past 70 years, investigations into the causes of mental retardation have revealed the importance of inborn errors of metabolism due to deficiency of specific enzymes. We will therefore consider discoveries of the pathways of metabolism and biological oxidation and the development of concepts regarding enzyme action. We will also briefly review studies that culminated in the determination of protein and enzyme structure. In the latter half of the twentieth century, researchers discovered that deficiency of enzymes normally located in intracellular organelles gives rise to disorders associated with mental retardation and neurological symptoms. We will therefore briefly discuss aspects of the discovery and analysis of cellular organelles.

Metabolism, Energy, Biological Oxidation, and Enzymes

The biochemical definition of metabolism began with detailed studies of fermentation carried out by Justus Liebig, Louis Pasteur, and others between 1839 and 1900. Studies on the fermentation of glucose revealed that this process in yeast led primarily to the formation of alcohol. Under certain conditions, lactic acid was produced. Through the studies of the physiologist Claude Bernard (1853) it became clear that the metabolism of glucose in animal muscle produced lactic acid.

Studies on fermentation and metabolism also led to the growth of concepts regarding enzymes. Emil Fischer studied sugar substrates and the function of saccharase-containing solutions. In 1894 he proposed that the structure of the enzyme and its substrate are such that they fit together like a lock and key. Michaelis and Menten (1913) proposed the theory of enzyme action and guidelines for enzyme quantitation and kinetic analysis.

Between 1900 and 1940, biochemists intensely studied the processes involved in metabolism, the generation of energy, and the processes of biological oxidation. By 1940 the steps and enzymes involved in the conversion of glucose to pyruvate and lactic acid and the conversion of glucose to glycogen were established through the efforts of Emden and Lacuer (1921), Meyerhof (1930), Cori et al. (1939), and many others. In 1937, Krebs and Johnson elucidated the steps involved in the energy-yielding metabolism of carbon compounds, the tricarboxylic or citric acid cycle. Enzymes involved in the processes in intermediary metabolism were shown to frequently require cofactors.

Enzyme Cofactors and Vitamins

In 1912, Hopkins published his landmark paper "Feeding Experiments Illustrating the Importance of Accessory Factors in Normal Dietaries." Hopkins wrote of "the urgent call of the body for a number of organic substances. . . . Required in so small an amount that they contributed little or nothing to energy requirements." Casmir Funk (1912) proposed the name *vitamins* for these substances. Many of the cofactors required for the function of enzymes in metabolic pathways turned out to be derived from vitamins.

In the period 1915–1938, the efforts of hundreds of investigators led to isolation and characterization of vitamins A, B, C, D, E, and K. It rapidly became clear that some vitamins were fat-soluble while others were water-soluble. The water-soluble B vitamins constituted a class composed of seven different types. The first indication of the function of vitamins emerged in 1937 with the studies of Lohman and Schuster, who demonstrated that vitamin B_1 acts as a cofactor for the enzyme involved in the decarboxylation of pyruvic acid. Subsequently, it became clear that administration of specific vitamins in quantities higher than the minimum daily requirements was sometimes of value in the treatment of a number of different enzyme deficiencies.

Inborn Errors of Metabolism

In 1908, in the Croonian lectures (published in 1909) Archibald Garrod, a London physician, first presented his concept that certain diseases of lifelong duration are due to the absence or reduced activity of an enzyme that governs a single metabolic step. He published an account of a family where members in several generations passed urine that turned black on exposure to air. The condition was called "alcaptonuria." Patients with this disorder developed arthritis and bony changes. Bateson alerted Garrod to Mendel's work and to the concepts of dominant and recessive inheritance. In 1909, Garrod proposed the concept of inborn errors of metabolism transmitted as recessive characteristics. Garrod's work on alcaptonuria, which he published between 1908 and 1923, served as a foundation for biochemical genetics. In 1923, Garrod reported that when patients with this disorder were fed precursors of homogentisic acid, namely phenylalanine and tyrosine, the quantities of homogentisic acid that they excreted increased.

Later, Garrod defined additional inborn errors of metabolism including cystinuria and pentosuria. The concept of inborn errors of metabolism first described in 1909 was not incorporated into the armamentarium of physicians to the mentally retarded until much later in the twentieth century.

Amino Acids and Proteins

Between 1820 and 1920, chemists isolated a series of nitrogen-containing compounds from the albumin of egg white, from gelatin, and from casein present in milk and cheese. The nitrogen-containing substances derived by heating in the presence of acids or alkali came to be known as *amides* and later as *amino acids*. The first amino acid isolated from egg whites was leucine. By 1906, 12 amino acids were known: glycine, alanine, leucine, phenylalanine, tyrosine, serine, aspartic acid, glutamic acid, lysine, arginine, histidine, and cysteine. Later, valine, proline, hydroxyproline tryptophan, methionine, and threonine were isolated. Emile Fischer (1906) demonstrated that enzymatic cleavage of proteins with pepsin and trypsin generated peptones (peptides). Furthermore, it was known that amino acids were derived from protein. However, elucidation of the structure of proteins was not completed until 1952.

Isolation, Purification, and Characterization of Proteins

Methods of protein purification improved progressively throughout the first half of the twentieth century. Many of these methods built on earlier observations. Between 1856 and 1859, P. S. Denis reported methods for the precipitation of protein using salting-out procedures. Using these procedures, he accomplished the separation of a number of distinct serum proteins, including albumin, globulin, and fibrin. He also precipitated out a substance from red blood cells that he named *hematoglobulin*. Later, this became known as *hemoglobin*. Measurement of the size of different molecules and separation of molecules based on size were facilitated when Thomas Graham in 1861 developed an instrument that he referred to as a "dialyzer." This was a sealed bell jar with parchment covering the large end. The apparatus was immersed in water or other solutions. Substances added to the jar diffused across the membrane rapidly or very slowly depending on their size and solubility. In 1900, the biochemist G. Hardy published results of his studies on the movement of different proteins in an electric field and separation of proteins by charge. These methods that separated proteins by size and charge later facilitated the separation of the normal and variant or mutant forms of a specific protein.

Svedberg (1937) introduced size fractionation and isolation of proteins according to position in a gradient following ultracentrifugation. This technique enabled more precise estimations of the size of different proteins and high molecular weight compounds.

Sanger (1952) determined the linear structure of insulin and provided proof of the linear arrangement of amino acids in proteins.

Inborn Errors in the Metabolism of Amino Acids

Phenylketonuria due to defective metabolism of the amino acid phenylalanine constitutes one of the most important inborn errors of metabolism that plays a role in mental retardation. Also, PKU is important for heuristic reasons (Centerwall and Centerwall 2000). Asborn Folling discovered this condition in 1934.

Folling obtained a degree in biochemistry and then began his medical studies. During the course of his studies, he wrote a thesis on mechanisms of acidosis. In 1932, he was appointed as professor of nutritional research at the School of Medicine at Oslo University. In 1934, a young mother brought her two children to him for consultation. The children, a girl and a boy, appeared normal during the first few months of life; thereafter, their development was delayed. The children failed to develop language. The mother noted that the children had a peculiar musty odor. Their father, who was a dentist, thought that the odor was particularly strong in the children's urine. Folling ruled out urinary tract infection as a cause for the odor. He then carried out a ferrichloride test on the urine. A 10% solution of ferrichloride turns red–brown when ketones and acetone are present in the urine (e.g., in cases of ketoacidosis in diabetic patients). On addition of ferrichloride to the urine of the two retarded children, a green color appeared. The color was noted in several urine samples obtained from the children at different times. Folling set out to identify the abnormal compound, a process that required the mother to collect 20 l of urine from the children. Within 1 month he isolated a pure compound from the extracted urine, and within 6 weeks after purification he defined the chemical nature of the compound. He demonstrated that this compound was phenylpyruvic acid and hypothesized that it was derived from abnormal metabolism of the amino acid phenylalanine.

Folling then carried out analyses of urine from several hundred individuals; this survey included attendees of a school for the mentally retarded. He identified eight more cases of PKU, and these cases included another two sibling pairs. Within 5 months of examining the two children brought to him by a concerned mother, Folling published a report on a new metabolic disease, PKU. This was the first described disease that led to mental retardation and conformed to the postulates proposed by Garrod in 1908 for a disorder due to an inborn error of metabolism.

After the Second World War, scientists and clinicians returned to the study of PKU and its role in the causation of mental retardation. In 1953, Jervis discovered that PKU is due to deficiency of the phenylalanine oxidizing system. Subsequently, the deficient enzyme became known as phenylalanine hydroxylase. Between 1952 and 1954, Bickel and coworkers developed a low-phenylalanine diet that was adequate with respect to other amino acids. Their documentation of the improvement in behavior of a child affected with PKU on administration of the low-phenylalanine diet was dramatic and influential. Screening of infants to detect PKU before the onset of symptoms began a few years after development of the diet. Screening was initially accomplished by ferrichloride application to the diaper or urine. Later, in part through the work of Guthrie and Susi (1963), analysis of phenylalanine in blood samples from newborns was initiated.

The discovery of PKU stimulated research into the biochemical and metabolic bases of mental retardation. These studies served as a stimulus in part because they demonstrated that the brain damage that resulted from the underlying defect was preventable if the disorder was detected and treated soon after birth. Throughout the 1950s and 1960s, considerable progress was made in characterizing inborn errors of metabolism that resulted in the excretion of abnormally large quantities of amino acids in urine. This progress was initially due to the development of paper and thin layer chromatographic procedures to separate different urinary amino acids coupled with quantification of amino acids using ninhydrin reagent. Later, amino acid analyzers were developed.

Among the first identified aminoacidopathies were those caused by defects in enzymes involved in the urea cycle. Through this process (first described by Krebs and Henseleit in 1932), amino groups released through enzymatic cleavage of amino acids become transformed into ammonia and urea. Deficiency of enzymes in this cycle present with elevations of blood ammonia levels and urinary excretion of large quantities of amino acids that precede the metabolic block. In 1963, McMurray et al. described the occurrence of neurological damage and mental retardation in cases of citrullinemia, a disorder associated with high blood and urine levels of the amino acid citrulline (an intermediate in the urea cycle) and high levels of blood ammonia. Descriptions of patients with other urea cycle defects soon followed. In 1977, Cederbaum et al. reported that mental retardation and evidence of neurological damage occurred in patients with arginase deficiency. They documented that blood arginine and ammonia levels were normalized on a diet low in protein (Cederbaum et al. 1982).

In 1965, Gerritsen and colleagues identified hyperglycinemia (nonketotic), an aminoacidopathy not due to deficiency of an enzyme in the urea cycle. Hyperglycinemia was first described in an infant with intractable epileptic seizures and developmental delay.

Inborn Errors of Metabolism Leading to Organic Acidemias

The carbon skeletons that result from the deamination of amino acids and from the metabolism of fatty acids undergo further degradation before entering the tricarboxylic acid cycle (Krebs citric acid cycle). These degradative steps give rise to organic acids. In certain inborn errors of metabolism, excessive quantities of organic acids are produced. Analysis of organic acidemias was enabled by the development of gas chromatography and mass spectrometry. Tanaka et al. (1966) were the first to characterize a specific form of organic acidemia, isovaleric acidemia. This discovery was soon followed by characterization of methylmalonic acidemia (Oberholzer et al. 1967; Stokke et al. 1967) and propionic acidemia (Hommes et al. 1968; Hsia et al. 1969).

The organic acidemias often present in early infancy with acidosis, ketosis, and seizures. Survivors of these episodes of severe illness often develop mental and physical handicaps. An important aspect of the organic acidemias is that several forms of these disorders are responsive to specific treatments. A number of them are vitamin-responsive. Rosenberg and colleagues (1968) determined that the metabolic abnormalities in some cases of methylmalonic acidemia are normalized by vitamin B_{12} therapy. Certain forms of propionic acidemia are biotin-responsive (Barnes 1970). In 1977, Sweetman and coworkers reported that the health of children with multiple carboxylase enzyme deficiency often improves following administration of biotin.

Blass and colleagues (1970, 1971) first described inborn errors of pyruvate metabolism that lead to lactic acidosis and result in neurological symptoms. Progress in the elucidation of abnormalities of lactic acid and energy metabolism was facilitated by detailed analysis of mitochondria and peroxisomes.

Cellular Organelles and Inborn Errors of Metabolism

Between 1940 and 1960, electron microscopy facilitated the visualization and morphological description of subcellular organelles. Development of differential centrifugation techniques enabled the fractionation of subcellular components. Biochemists then analyzed the separated organelles to determine their specific functions.

Pallade published detailed studies of the structure of mitochondria in 1953. Chance and Williams (1956) defined mitochondria metabolism in particular steps in the respiratory chain and oxidative phosphorylation. Green and Tzagaloff described the mitochondrial electron transfer system in 1966. Between 1970 and 1990, scientists and clinicians achieved a more complete delineation of the role of deficiencies of mitochondrial proteins and enzymes in inborn errors of metabolism (Robinson et al. 1980; Robinson 1983).

Anderson and coworkers published the complete DNA sequence and organization of the mitochondrial genome in 1981. Through this sequence analysis it became clear that only a few of the enzymes that are present in mitochondria are encoded by mitochondrial DNA; the majority are nucleus-encoded and imported into the mitochondria.

Through analysis of pedigrees Giles and coworkers (1980) established that mitochondria are maternally inherited. At fertilization, a number of different mitochondria are passed on from the egg cytoplasm to the zygote. In subsequent cell division of the zygote, the mitochondria do not segregate equally, so the mitochondria in each cell are heterogeneous with respect to their DNA sequence. This cellular heterogeneity of mitochondria helps explain the clinical heterogeneity in disorders due to mitochondrial DNA mutations or structural changes.

Lysosomes

De Duve in 1963 published results of extensive studies on the isolation and physiological characterization of lysosomes. Within the interior of lysosomes, there are a series of hydrolytic enzymes, each involved in the degradation of different complex macromolecules. Within the lysosomes, pH is maintained between 3.0 and 6.0. Most lysosomal enzymes function at low pH optima. Hers in 1965 discovered that glycogen accumulates in the lysosomes in Pompe's disease. This is a genetic disorder characterized by profound muscle weakness, hepatomegaly, hypotonia, congenital heart disease, and developmental delay. Hers determined that the accumulation of glycogen was due to deficiency of the lysosomal enzyme α-1,4-glucosidase. He proposed that many other storage diseases might be due to deficiency of specific lysosomal hydrolases.

In 1969 Okada and O'Brien demonstrated deficiency of lysosomal hexosaminidase in classical Tay-Sachs disease (GM_2 gangliosidosis). Sandhoff and Harzer (2001) discovered that hexosaminidase B is deficient in the less common variant of Tay-Sachs disease known as GM_2 gangliosidosis. In Tay-Sachs disease, as in most lysosomal storage diseases, clinical signs are typically not present at birth. The severe psychomotor regression develops in early childhood, typically between 3 and 5 years of age. The high frequency of Tay-Sachs disease in the Ashkenazi Jewish population led Kaback and Zeiger in 1972 to promote development of carrier testing and prenatal screening programs and community-based Tay-Sachs disease education throughout the United States. Similar programs were also developed in Israel, Australia, and South Africa.

Throughout the 1970s and 1980s, a growing number of lysosomal enzyme deficiencies were documented among patients with the hallmark clinical signs and symptoms of storage disease. These included psychomotor regression after a period of normal development. Sometimes patients manifested hepatosplenomegaly and evidence of abnormal storage in bones and soft tissues. The specific signs and symptoms varied according to the tissue distribution of the defective enzyme.

Peroxisomes

De Duve and Baudhuin in 1966 developed density gradient methods to separate subcellular particles that contained catalase and D-amino acid oxidase. These bodies had the morphological characteristics of the organelles described by Rhodin (1954). Goldfischer et al. (1973) reported absence of peroxisomes in Zellweger syndrome. This syndrome is characterized by congenital craniofacial anomalies, neurological symptoms, and psychomotor retardation. Lazarow and De Duve (1976) demonstrated that enzymes present in peroxisomes carried out β-oxidation of fatty acids. Further insight into the functions of peroxisomes was obtained when Brown in 1982 discovered accumulation of very long chain fatty acids in patients with Zellweger. Clinical and laboratory research throughout the 1980–1990 period led to the development of key insights into the biogenesis of peroxisomes and into the range of metabolic functions performed in these organelles. These included synthesis of cholesterol and metabolism of bile acids, prostaglandins, ω-3 unsaturated fatty acids, dolichol and xenobiotics (Masters and Crane 1995).

Aspects of the History of Genetics

In tracing the history of genetics relevant to mental retardation, it is essential to consider the development of basic concepts relating to heredity, structures that carry genetic material, the chemistry and structure of the gene, and the nature of the gene product. Knowledge of basic concepts in genetics evolved through studies in plants, *Drosophila*, and microorganisms.

Heredity and Mendel's Laws

Genetics traces its origins to the work of Gregor Mendel. In 1854, in the garden of the monastery in Brunn, Austria, Mendel cultivated 34 strains of peas. He then studied the effects of crossing the different strains and carefully documented the characteristics of the parent plants and their first- and second-generation offspring. He followed characteristics such as flower color, seed coat color, texture, shape, and stem length. From the results of his experiments, he formulated two laws. Mendel's first law is known as the law of segregation: hereditary factors are transmitted from one generation to the next as discrete factors. Mendel's second law is the law of independent assortment: different traits (for example, flower color and seed shape) are inherited independently.

In 1865, Mendel presented the paper describing his results at a meeting of the Brunn Society of Natural History, and his paper was published in the proceedings of the society in 1866. The proceedings were regularly distributed to libraries in Europe. However, Mendel's work failed to gain attention until 1900.

Chromosomes as Units of Heredity

In 1879, Hermann Fol presented results of his studies on fertilization and drew attention to the role of the nucleus in this process. In 1883, W. Roux documented the linear nature of chromosomes contained in the nucleus and the fact that chromosomes spilt into two longitudinal halves during cell division.

In 1900, several papers that referred to Mendel's work appeared in the literature. De Vries authored one paper and Carl Correns, who replicated Mendel's studies with peas, authored another. Bateson (1902, 1909) described the work of Mendel and its confirmation by De Vries in a paper he presented to the Royal Horticultural Society in London in 1900. Bateson became very enthusiastic in promoting Mendelian concepts. He was responsible for introducing terms such as *zygote* for the fertilized egg and *heterozygote, homozygote*, and *allelomorphs* (later shortened to *alleles*) for the alternate forms of a specific hereditary factor.

The analysis of linkage began with the demonstration by Correns in 1900 that traits did not always segregate independently.

In 1902, Boveri published results of his studies on sea urchin egg fertilization and embryonic development. He demonstrated that in normal development the embryo required a haploid set of chromosomes from each parent. In 1902 W.S. Sutton described the somatic chromosomes of the grasshopper and documented that pairs of chromosomes occurred in somatic nuclei. He ended his paper with this statement, "I may finally call attention to the probability that the association of paternal and maternal chromosomes in pairs and their subsequent separation during reduction division may constitute the physical basis of the Mendelian law of heredity" (Sturtevant 1965, p. 37).

It is interesting to consider that during the period 1910–1913, when the eugenics movement in Britain and the Breeders' Association of America were directing legislation based on their concepts of heredity and mental retardation, scientists were developing the basic concepts related to genetics and transmission of characteristics.

The Function of Chromosomes

Thomas Hunt Morgan began his work on the function of chromosomes in 1910. In his research, Morgan brought together a number of different methodologies, including breeding and crossing of experimental organisms, phenotype analysis, microscopy, and statistical genetic analysis as described by Mendel. He chose *Drosophila* as an experimental organism because of its many advantages for research. These include the readiness with which it can be maintained in the laboratory, its short generation time, and the fact that it has only four chromosomes which can be readily distinguished from each other. Morgan and his group provided experimental observations and generated concepts regarding the linear arrangement of hereditary factors (genes) on chromosomes. They confirmed the observations of Janssens regarding the occurrence of chiasmata during meiosis. They provided experimental support for recombination by correlating recombination of traits and the exchange of parts of chromosomes. His group generated the first genetic maps of the elongated salivary gland chromosomes in *Drosophila* larvae (see Sturtevant 1965). Through staining and careful microscopy, Painter, Bridges, and others determined that each of the chromosomes has a definite constant morphology, made up of a series of dark bands interspersed between light areas. Painter noted "If the position of one or more segments is shifted by some form of dislocation (translocation, inversion, etc.), the exact morphological point or points of breakage can be determined and the segments identified in their new position" (Painter 1933, p. 585).

Defining the Nature of the Gene Product

In 1935 and 1936, Ephrussi and Beadle studied eye color development in *Drosophila*. They determined that eye color is dependent on a series of reactions, each of which is controlled by a gene.

Beadle and Tatum then went on to study the mold *Neurospora*. Through X-ray irradiation, they induced mutant forms of this organism with new specific nutritional requirements, for example, requirement of a specific amino acid in the growth medium. They postulated that the nutritional requirement in a particular mutant arose because of loss of a particular "function" which facilitated endogenous synthesis of that nutrient by the organism. In 1941, Beadle and Tatum published a landmark paper on the genetic control of biochemical reactions in *Neurospora*. They stated, "It is entirely tenable that these genes which themselves are part of a system, control or regulate specific reactions in the system either by acting directly as enzymes or determining the specificity of enzymes" (Beadle and Tatum 1941, p. 490).

Isolating the Gene and Defining Its Chemical Structure

In 1944, Avery et al. demonstrated that DNA is the primary genetic material. They isolated a DNA fraction from encapsulated Type III pneumococcus and introduced this into the R variant unencapsulated Type II pneumococcus. This resulted in conversion of the Type II cells to fully encapsulated Type III cells. Avery et al. wrote

> The data obtained by chemical, enzymatic and serological analysis together
> with the results of preliminary studies by electrophoresis, ultra-centrifugation,
> and ultraviolet spectroscopy indicate that, within the limits of the methods,
> the active fraction contains no demonstrable protein, unbound lipid or
> serologically reactive polysaccharide and consists principally, if not solely,
> of a highly polymerized, viscous form of desoxyribonucleic acid (p. 157)

In 1952, Norton Zinder and Joshua Lederberg reported results of their experiments on transformation of different strains of *Salmonella typhimurium* bacteria. They demonstrated that genetic information might be transmitted from one strain of bacteria to another by phage, a form of virus. This work provided the means for manipulation of genetic information and was one of the cornerstones of recombinant DNA technology.

When James Watson and Francis Crick undertook experiments to determine the molecular structure of DNA, it was known that DNA is composed of nitrogen-containing purine and pyrimidine bases and that it contained a sugar, deoxyribose, and phosphate. Chargaff (1950) and Magasanik and Chargaff (1951) reported that the ratios of adenine to thymine and of guanine to cytosine were close to 1. Rosalind Franklin's X-ray crystallographic images of DNA crystals provided evidence for the helical structure of DNA (Franklin and Gosling 1953). In 1953, Watson and Crick published their landmark paper in which they proposed that DNA consists of two helical chains composed of phosphate and sugar residues and that the chains are held together by paired purine and pyrimidine bases. They noted that the purine and pyrimidine bases were present in their keto form and that hydrogen bonding occurred between specific bases. The purine base adenine paired with the pyrimidine thymine and the purine guanine paired with the pyrimidine cytosine. Watson and Crick (1953) wrote, "It has not escaped our notice that the specific pairing we have postulated immediately suggests a possible copying mechanism for the genetic material."

Deciphering the Code

In the decade following the discovery of the DNA double helix, a number of molecular biologists carried out experiments to determine the steps by which this genetic material determined the structure and function of proteins. Brenner et al. (1961) discovered a new form of ribonucleic acid (RNA). This form, known as messenger RNA (mRNA), synthesized from DNA strand templates through the activity of RNA polymerase, interacted with polyribosomes and transfer RNA. Brenner (1961) and Crick et al. (1961) calculated that a triplet nucleotide code most likely constituted the genetic code. In that same year, Nirenberg and Matthaei determined that the mRNA code UUU specified the amino acid phenylalanine. Ghobind Khorana and others set about synthesizing RNA nucleotide triplets, which they then tested in cell-free protein synthesis experiments. These experiments resulted in establishment of the genetic code by 1966.

Recombinant DNA Technology

By 1973 recombinant DNA technology was established. It became possible to isolate segments of DNA from any organisms, including humans, through the use of restriction endonucleases that cleaved DNA. These DNA segments could then be inserted into the DNA of other organisms through the action of ligase enzymes. By ligating DNA segments into the DNA of virus-like organisms, such as plasmids and bacteriophages, and then using these to infect organisms such as Escherichia coli, it became possible for scientists to produce large quantities of specific cloned DNA segments. Analysis of relatively unstable mRNA was facilitated by isolation of reverse transcriptase by Temin and Baltimore in 1970. Reverse transcriptase permits the transcription of mRNA sequence into cDNA fragments that may be readily ligated into plasmids or phage.

Advances in DNA Sequencing and Amplification

In the latter half of the 1970s, techniques were developed to determine the nucleotide sequence of DNA. In 1977, Maxam and Gilbert developed a method based on chemical degradation of DNA. Sanger et al. (1977) developed a method based on the use of DNA polymerase, an enzyme that copied DNA and addition of modified nucleotides, dideoxynucleotides. Incorporation of a dideoxynucleotide into a growing DNA chain leads to termination of chain synthesis. Through electrophoresis DNA chains of different lengths are separated and the sequence of DNA is read (Sanger et al. 1977, Sanger and Coulson 1978).

In analyzing DNA of genes in eukaryotic organisms, molecular biologists soon realized that in these organisms the protein-coding regions of DNA, exons, are interrupted by noncoding sequences, introns (Leder 1978).

DNA sequencing and analysis were greatly facilitated by the development of polymerase chain reaction (PCR) technology by Mullis in 1986. In PCR, a DNA fragment that lies between known sequences can be readily amplified in the presence of nucleotides and heat-stable DNA polymerase. Known sequences used to design primers to initiate the DNA synthesis reaction may, for example, be the cloning sites present in a bacteriophage used to ligate in segments of DNA from another organism.

Use of PCR technology greatly facilitated the extensive DNA sequencing required to determine the sequence of humans in the Human Genome Project.

Human Gene Mapping

Development of linkage maps of human chromosomes depended initially upon the development of polymorphic markers (e.g., proteins that differ in size and/or electrophoretic mobility) or of variant antigens that may be distinguished with the use of specific antibodies (Harris 1972; Harris et al. 1973). Polymorphic markers were analyzed in families to determine if any cosegregated during meiosis in a high proportion of cases, indicating that they were closely aligned on a particular chromosome. Linkage mapping is also used to determine if a phenotypic trait segregates with one or more polymorphic markers. Lawler and

Sandler published the first report of linkage of a polymorphic marker and a human autosomal trait, the Rh antigen system and elliptocytosis, in 1954. In 1955, Renwick and Lawler reported linkage between the ABO blood group locus and a locus that determined nail-patella syndrome.

Development of methodologies for restriction endonuclease digestion of DNA, PCR, and methods to separate DNA fragments of different length greatly expanded the number of polymorphic markers available for linkage analysis. Analysis of DNA sequence has yielded further polymorphisms for analysis in families. These include polymorphisms due to differences in the number of dinucleotide repeats and single nucleotide polymorphisms. Through linkage mapping, the relative positions of pairs or strings of markers (haplotypes) on chromosomes may be determined.

Mapping of genes to chromosomes was greatly facilitated by somatic cell genetics and analysis of somatic cell hybrids. In 1967, Mary Weiss and Howard Green published results of their studies on rodent–human somatic cell hybrids grown in tissue culture. They noted that during the first few cell divisions after fusion, such hybrid cells rapidly lose human chromosomes. Thereafter, chromosome numbers stabilize. If individual hybrid cells are cloned at that stage, their progeny have a full complement of rodent chromosomes and a few human chromosomes. Correlations may then be established between the presence of human chromosomes and the presence of specific human proteins and human genes.

Advances in Cytogenetic Analysis: Molecular Cytogenetics

More precise identification of each of the human chromosomes was achieved in 1970 when Caspersson et al. developed techniques of banding of human chromosomes by staining with fluorescent dyes such as quinacrine or acridine orange. Seabright (1972) demonstrated that chromosome banding is achieved through trypsin digestion of chromatin followed by Giemsa staining.

Molecular cytogenetics began in 1977 with the in situ hybridization of DNA probes to human chromosomes. This technique was greatly facilitated by the introduction of methods for labeling DNA probes with nucleotides that are tagged with fluorescent dyes.

In 1991, Oberle and coworkers made a key molecular genetic discovery in cases of syndromic mental retardation characterized by fragility at a specific site on the X chromosome. Fragile X syndrome is a common form of inherited mental retardation. Oberle and coworkers discovered that X-chromosome fragility in these patients is due to an abnormally large and unstable DNA repeat element. Their discovery opened the way for a specific form of DNA testing and genetic counseling in families with mental retardation.

Human gene mapping and sequencing progressed rapidly in the last decade of the twentieth century. The availability of gene mapping and sequence information has and will continue to impact studies designed to determine the etiology of developmental disabilities and mental retardation. This information is readily accessed through different databases (e.g., http://www.ncbi.nlm.nih/gov). Human genome mapping and sequencing and implications of these endeavors for studies in individuals with mental retardation are reviewed in Chapter 8 of this book.

Improved Methods to Analyze Gene Function and Consequences of Mutation: Gene Targeting and Development of Transgenic Mice

An important recent breakthrough, which has facilitated analysis of the effects of gene changes on the phenotype of the organism, was the development of methods to generate mice in which a specific gene is disrupted and/or replaced by a mutated gene. The laboratory mouse is primarily used in these experiments to develop models of specific human diseases. Development of such mouse models was enabled by methods to introduce and target genes to specific sites in the mouse genome through injection of fertilized mouse oocytes or embryonic cells.

Gene targeting refers to the process through which a DNA fragment that is introduced into the nucleus (e.g., the nucleus of a mammalian cell) locates and recombines with closely similar (homologous) sequences in the nucleus. Among the earliest studies in this field were those of Folger et al. (1982), who described the pattern of integration of DNA microinjected into mammalian cells. They noted that a subset of the microinjected DNA fragments corresponding to a specific gene recombined with the homologous gene present in the host nucleus.

Lau et al. (1984) introduced a globin gene, carried in a plasmid vector, into fibroblasts. They demonstrated that the introduced gene was present at the globin locus in the fibroblast nuclei. They reported that in addition to specific targeting to the homologous loci, introduced sequences were randomly targeted. Identification of cells that had incorporated the introduced gene at the target locus was facilitated by the development of selectable markers. Genes to be introduced are often linked to specific regulatory elements that control their expression.

Minimal gene targeting vectors are composed of a plasmid or viral backbone and sequences that are homologous to the host gene to be replaced.

Mouse Embryonic Stem Cells and Transgenic Mice

Evans and Kaufman (1981) and Martin (1981) developed embryonic stem cell lines from mouse blastocysts. Genetic changes may be introduced into embryonic stem cells or into blastocysts. Blastocysts are implanted into hormonally treated mice, which then carry the blastocysts as a pregnancy.

Transgenic mice may be created by injection of gene-carrying vectors into fertilized oocytes. If these mice are viable, the phenotypic consequences of the heterozygous form of a mutation may be studied. Gene-carrying vectors may also be injected into blastocysts or embryonic stem cells, resulting in animals in which a proportion of cells contain the transgene. Through subsequent matings of these mice, it may be possible to generate mice that are homozygous for the mutant gene in all of their cells.

Targeting of genes through homologous recombination to study the effects of mutation is costly to perform. Alternate methods to analyze the effects of gene silencing have been developed.

RNA Interference

Fire et al. (1998) first described the introduction of double-stranded RNA into cells to silence genes. Through this technique, designated *RNA interference*, the expression of a gene that is homologous to the introduced double-stranded RNA is blocked. Short interference RNAs (siRNAs) may silence gene expression at the transcriptional level or at the translational level (Hannon 2002).

Most frequently, siRNAs are designed to target coding sequences in the 5'gene regions. However, siRNAs corresponding to sequences in the 3' noncoding regions have also successfully been used to inhibit gene expression (He and Hannon 2004). Initially, in experiments in mammalian cell systems, 21 nucleotide siRNAs were synthesized and injected into cells. Subsequently, vector-based strategies were developed to transfer siRNAs (McManus and Sharp 2002; Shi 2003). The potential medical applications of siRNA technology are founded on the high degree of specificity of a section of siRNA to inhibit gene expression. Shi (2003) noted that through this specificity it is possible to selectively alter the expression of genes with point mutations, insertions, deletions, or trinucleotide expansions.

Incorporation of Elements of Progress in Human Genetics into Evaluation of Mentally Retarded Individuals to Establish Etiology

Developments in human cytogenetics and human biochemical genetics during the past 50 years led to the formulation of guidelines for evaluation of patients with developmental delay and mental retardation in 1997. These guidelines include evaluation of pedigrees extending for at least three generations and of pre- and postnatal history, physical examination for evidence of congenital anomalies and dysmorphology and for evidence of neurological deficits and metabolic defects, and assessment of behavior. Laboratory tests recommended in 1997 included banded karyotype analyses, assessment for fragile X, and metabolic studies based to some degree on information obtained from history and physical examination (Curry et al.). More recently, these recommendations have been updated; they are discussed more fully in Chapter 9.

Increasingly, evaluation of patients with mental retardation includes computerized axial tomographic (CAT) scanning and magnetic resonance imaging (MRI) studies of the brain. In some cases, these studies demonstrate structural brain anomalies that likely play a role in the etiology of mental retardation. The combination of studies of brain structure by MRI or CAT scan, chromosomal analysis, and genetic linkage studies in families where more than one member has a brain malformation has led to the identification of genes that, when mutated, may lead to defects in brain development. A number of noninvasive methods have been developed to facilitate investigation of dynamic brain responses. These include functional MRI; positron emission tomographic scans, which measure metabolism in brain regions coincident with a specific activity; and magnetoencephalography.

During the past 50 years, most progress has been made in understanding the etiology of syndromic forms of mental retardation (i.e., mental retardation that occurs in a child who has dysmorphology or other congenital malformations or clinical metabolic abnormalities). Increasingly, clinicians and geneticists are seeking to understand the etiology of nonsyndromic forms of mental retardation. These analyses are facilitated by the development of a comprehensive gene map and availability of an almost complete sequence of the human genome.

Nonsyndromic mental retardation may represent a complex genetic disorder where the phenotype is due to the interaction of a number of different genes. However, many monogenic causes of mental retardation have been identified in recent years. A pattern that has emerged is that genes that are important in the etiology of mental retardation initially come to light through analysis of the genes that map in the region of structural chromosomal abnormalities. Precise delineation of deletions, duplications, translocations, and abnormal fragile sites through molecular genetic studies and availability of DNA sequence information enable scientists to determine which genes map in the affected regions. In this way, candidate genes for mental retardation may be identified. Sequencing of these candidate genes in DNA from patients with nonsyndromic mental retardation has, in some instances, led to identification of genes specifically involved in the etiology of mental retardation. Through use of these approaches, there has been substantial progress over the past 5 years in identification of genes on the X chromosome that play a role in the etiology of mental retardation.

2

Neurogenesis, Neuronal Migration, Maturation, and Function: Insights into Learning and Memory

Neurons transmit signals and are in turn modified through this transmission. Activity-dependent changes in synapses and neurons underlie information storage in the brain. Problems at any step in the formation or function of neural circuits may lead to mental retardation.

In this chapter, we will explore steps in the development of the nervous system: the generation of neurons, migration from place of origin, and maturation, including development of axons and dendrites and establishment of synaptic contacts. While synaptogenesis occurs primarily in prenatal life, it continues throughout childhood into puberty. There is evidence that neurogenesis continues at some level during adult life. Neurons are generated from stem cells that occur at a number of different locations in the adult brain. These neurons then become integrated into neuronal circuits.

We will discuss aspects of neuronal function, including neuronal activation, signal transduction, learning and memory, as well as synaptic plasticity. We will then consider specific gene defects that impact one or more of these processes and result in developmental delay or mental retardation.

Understanding of processes involved in neurogenesis and neuronal migration has evolved through morphological, cytological, and immunohistochemical studies of the brain of humans, and other animals at different stages of development. Knowledge of the molecular bases of these processes has grown rapidly during the past decade through studies on patients with mental retardation and the application of brain imaging, molecular cytogenetics, analysis of deoxyribonucleic acid (DNA) markers, gene mapping, and DNA sequencing. The oligophrenin gene, e.g., was initially isolated through analysis of genes that were interrupted as a result of an X;12 chromosome translocation that occurred in a patient with mental retardation. This gene has recently been shown to determine the growth and morphology of neuronal dendrites (Govek et al. 2004).

Pedigree analysis and gene mapping studies on families where a number of affected individuals had mental retardation and microcephaly led to identification of mutations in a gene, designated *ASPM* (abnormal spindle-like microcephaly-associated), that plays a role in cell cycle control (Pattison et al.

26

2000). Mutation in the *ASPM* gene leads to abnormalities in neurogenesis and neuronal proliferation. This finding will be discussed in more detail later in this chapter.

Increasingly, the role of a specific gene or genes in brain development is analyzed in "knockout" mice, i.e., mice where recombinant DNA technology is used to eliminate or interrupt a gene. The pathological and neurophysiological consequences of this change may be analyzed, provided the knockout mice survive at least through embryonic life. The exact function of a specific gene identified on the basis of molecular genetic and mapping studies as playing a role in mental retardation may be analyzed through studies in cell culture. This is true, e.g., of genes in signal transduction pathways. Increasingly, small inhibitory ribonucleic acids (siRNAs) are being used to inhibit translation of a specific messenger RNA (mRNA) transcript and to analyze consequences of absence of a specific protein. Through use of genomic approaches, there has been significant progress in the identification and characterization of genes that play a role in mental retardation. Progress in identifying X-linked genes has been particularly striking. A number of the genes thus identified are involved in intracellular signal transduction pathways, cytoskeletal organization, synaptic vesicle functions, and anchoring neurotransmitter receptors. These developments have led to new concepts of mental retardation.

Table 2–1 includes a partial list of genes that function in neurogenesis, neuronal migration, signal transduction, or synaptic function and in which specific mutations occur that lead to mental retardation.

Neurogenesis

Early in embryogenesis, cells in the ectoderm of the luminar or ventricular surface of the neural tube evolve as progenitor or stem cells capable of differentiating into neurons or glia. Glial cells constitute the support system for neurons. This process, referred to as *induction*, is dependent upon expression of a number of specific growth factors. Bally-Cuif and Hammerschmidt (2003) reported that neural induction and neurogenesis appear to be dependent upon cell cycle control systems. It is these systems that determine whether a cell remains as a stem cell or whether it undergoes proliferation, specification, and differentiation. In humans, neurogenesis takes place primarily between the fifth and the twentieth weeks of prenatal life. Brain-derived neurotrophic factor (BDNF) plays an important role in brain development (Binder and Scharfman 2004).

Studies on the *ASPM* gene, described above, revealed that it regulates mitotic spindle orientation during neurogenesis. Neuronal progenitor cells have a specific pattern of mitotic activity. Symmetric cell divisions result when the mitotic spindle is in the same plane as the neuroepithelium, the primitive neuron-generating cell layer. Symmetric cell divisions yield two neuronal cells. Asymmetric cell divisions result when spindles are perpendicular to the

Table 2–1

Genes That Play a Role in Neurogenesis, Neuronal Migration, and Signaling and When Mutated, May Lead to Mental Retardation

Gene Symbol	Gene Name	Function	Disorder
ASPM	Abnormal spindle-like microcephaly	Cell cycle control Neurogenesis	Microcephaly type 5
MCPH1	Microcephalin	DNA repair	Microcephaly type 1
FLNA	Filamin A	Neuronal migration	Heterotopia; MR
TM4SF2	Tetraspanin 4	Interacts with extracellular matrix and cytoskeleton	MR
14-4-3e	14-4-3	Modulates actin cytoskeleton influences migration	Miller-Dieker syndrome
DCX	Doublecortin	Ca signaling, neuronal migration	Lissencephaly, band heterotopia
PAK3	p21 GTPase-activated kinase	Dendritic spine formation, synaptic plasticity	X-linked MR
LIS1	Lissencephaly 1	Nucleokinesis, neuronal migration	Lissencephaly
L1CAM	L1 adhesion molecule	Cytoskeletal interactions	X-linked hydrocephalus
RLN	Reelin	Cortical layering	Lissencephaly
OPHN1	Oligophrenin	Rho GAP, dendritic growth	X-linked MR
SYNJ1	Synaptojanin	Phosphoinositide phosphatase, synaptic vesicle recycling	Overexpressed in Down syndrome
GDI1/RABGDIA	RAB GDP dissociation inhibitor	Synaptic vesicle budding and transport	X-linked MR

Gene	Protein	Function	Disorder
SAP102	Synapse-associated protein	Anchors neurotransmitters	MR
SNP1	Synapsin 1	Controls neurotransmitter release	X-linked behavioral and learning difficulties
ARHGEF	RHO GEF	Guanine nucleotide exchange factor	X-linked MR
TSC1	Tuberous sclerosis	Hamartin and tuberin interact and inactivate Rheb GTP and PI3K	Tuberous sclerosis, neuronal migration defects; associated with MR, autism.
TSC2	Tuberous sclerosis		
5GD1	Rho GEF	Binds Rho GTPase	Nonsyndromic MR, syndromic MR
NF1	Neurofibromin 1	Inactivates Ras GTP	Neurofibromatosis, may be associated with cognitive deficits
BDNF	Brain-derived neurotrophic factor	Synaptic plasticity	Polymorphism impacts learning
RSK2	Ribosomal S6 kinase 2	Links ERK–MAPK signal cascade and gene expression	Coffin Lowry syndrome
CREB	cAMP responsive element binding protein	Influences gene transcription	Rubinstein–Taybi syndrome
ATRX	Alpha thalassemia X-linked MR	Impacts gene expression	Alpha thalassemia X-linked MR
MECP2	Controls gene expression, impacts synapse refinement and pruning	Rett syndrome	

MR, mental retardation; GTPase, guanosine triphosphatase; GAP, GTPase activating protein; GDP, guanosine diphosphate; PI3K, phosphatidylinositol-3-kinase; GEF guanine nucleotide exchange factor; ERK, extracellular signal-regulated kinase; MAPK, mitogen activated protein kinase.

plane of the neuroepithelium. These cell divisions give rise to one neuronal cell and one progenitor cell.

Evans and coworkers (2004) analyzed the degree of amino acid divergence between apes and humans. They found evidence of advantageous amino acid changes in the *ASPM* gene, indicating that the *ASPM* gene underwent strong adaptive evolution in *Homo sapiens*. These findings indicate that *ASPM* gene mutations played an important role in the evolutionary enlargement of the human brain.

Following completion of rounds of proliferation, postmitotic neurons evolve. It is these neurons that migrate from their place of origin, in the ventricular zone that surrounds the cerebral ventricles (cavities). Postmitotic neurons migrate to the surface of the cerebral vesicles, where they form the preplate or neocortex. In humans, this migration takes place primarily between the fifth and twenty-second weeks of gestation (Meyer et al. 2001). Neurons that reach the neocortex may survive, differentiate, and become integrated into the neural circuitry. However, a number of neurons die before differentiation. As the preplate is invaded by additional postmitotic neurons, it becomes split into a superficial marginal zone and a deeper subplate. With the exception of layer 1 of the cortex, the subpial layer (where the Cajal-Retzius cells, the pioneer or earliest migrating neurons reside), the layers of the cortex have an inside-out sequence. Thus, the neurons that originate earliest are located deep in the cortex and the later derived neurons are located in the superficial layer. The Cajal-Retzius cells play a key role in the lamination of the neocortex that leads to the development of a six-layered cortex.

Formation of Cortical Layers

A single progenitor cell type gives rise to neuroblastic and glioblastic lineages. The glioblastic lineage gives rise to three branches of oligodendrocytes, astrocyte precursors, and radial glial cell precursors. Radial glial cells form a structural connection between the ventricular zone in the inner brain and the outer cortex. Neuroblasts generated in the ventricular zone migrate along the radial glial structures to the cortex. Later, the radial glial cells are transformed to astrocytes and ependymal cells. Astrocytes, through their expanded end feet, play a role in metabolism and nutrient support of neurons. The spatial and temporal expression of different integrin protein subunits plays a critical role in cortical layer formation. Integrins transduce signals from the extracellular matrix to the cytoskeletal compartment. This will be discussed in further detail below.

Mountcastle (1997) determined that the basic unit of the mature neocortex is the minicolumn. This is a vertical chain of neurons that extends from cortical layer 2 to layer 6. Cells in the minicolumn are connected vertically. The cells within each minicolumn represent all of the cortical neural cell types. Short horizontal connections bind individual minicolumns. Mountcastle proposed that the iterative division of a cluster of progenitor cells produces minicolumns. He proposed further that neurons that are generated in the same location migrate from the periventricular region along the same or adjacent radial glial fibers.

Postnatal and Adult Neurogenesis

During the postnatal period, there is a wave of secondary neurogenesis that produces the interneurons (connecting neurons) of the cerebellar cortex, the hippocampal formation, and the olfactory bulb (Hatten 1999).

The first evidence of neurogenesis in adult vertebrates came from the studies of Nottebohm in 1981, who demonstrated that new neurons were generated in the vocal nucleus and hippocampus when songbirds learned new songs. There is now evidence that in higher vertebrates, including humans, new neurons may be generated in two discrete areas of the brain. One such area is the dentate gyrus of the hippocampal formation. Another is the sub-ventricular zone (adjacent to the lateral ventricles) and its projection through the rostral migratory system. In addition, neural stem cells exist in most structures of the adult brain (Gage 2002). van Praag et al. (1999) and Kemperman (2002) demonstrated a link between hippocampal neurogenesis and the learning of new skills and physical activity.

Howell and coworkers (2003) reported that neuropeptide (NPY) has a proliferative effect on hippocampal neuroblasts. Through studies in NPY receptor knockout mice and by in vitro studies in the presence of selective NPY receptor agonists and antagonists, Howell et al. (2003) demonstrated that the neuroproliferative effect of NPY in the hippocampus is mediated through its receptor, R1 (NPYR1). They postulated that the effect of NPY on learning and memory may be mediated through NPY-induced neurogenesis.

Neuronal Migration

Progress in brain imaging techniques and their application to the evaluation of patients with mental retardation and/or seizures has furthered our understanding of processes involved in neuronal migration. Molecular genetic studies in patients with neuronal migration disorders, e.g., neuronal heterotopias, have led to elucidation of specific genes and molecular pathways involved in migration. Neuronal heterotopias are collections of neurons that failed to reach their final destination during migration. They may be found at different positions along the path of neuronal migration. Gene defects that lead to heterotopias will be discussed later in this chapter and in Chapter 3.

Neurons generated in the periventricular zone migrate primarily along the radial glial fiber network to reach their final destination. The growth factor neuregulin plays a critical role in the interactions between migrating neurons and radial glial cells (Rio et al. 1997; Anton et al. 1997).

When neurons reach their final destination, they extend processes, establish synaptic connections with other neurons, and respond to signals. All of these processes are dependent upon interactions between the cell and extracellular matrix, signal transduction processes, and cytoskeletal structural changes. Integrins transduce signals from the extracellular matrix to the cytoskeletal compartment. Integrin receptors interact with the tetraspanin family of proteins and with G protein–coupled receptors. One member of the tetraspanin family of proteins, TM4SF2, is disrupted in a subgroup of patients with mental retardation (Zemni et al. 2000).

Cytoskeletal Proteins Associated with Migration

To set the stage for the examination of genetic defects that impact the cytoskeleton and lead to neuronal migration disorders, we will briefly review cytoskeletal structure and dynamics. Within the cytoplasm of the cell are networks of distinct protein polymers that together constitute the cytoskeleton. There are three broad classes of polymers in the cytoskeleton: actin filaments, intermediate filaments (neurofilaments), and microtubules. Actin filaments are assembled from actin monomers. Actin plays a key role in neuronal membranes, where it serves to anchor protein complexes including neurotransmitter receptors. Neurofilaments are ropelike strands that extend through neuronal cell bodies and their processes. They are polymers of cytokeratin proteins and the products of at least three different genes. Microtubules assemble from dimeric tubulin subunits. Their assembly occurs in an energy-dependent process that utilizes nucleotide triphosphates, in particular guanosine triphosphate (GTP). Microtubules radiate out from a central point near the nucleus, centriole, or centrosome, which acts as a microtubule organizing center. In addition to the function of maintaining cellular structure, the cytoskeleton, particularly the microtubules, serve to transport vesicular material between different cellular compartments. The cytoskeleton also plays a role in the transduction of signals from the cell surface to the nucleus (Bielas and Gleeson 2004).

At the periphery of migrating neurons, actin filaments are concentrated and closely associated with the cell membrane. Microtubules form a cage around the nucleus, and within the leading process of the migratory neuronal cell, microtubules are ordered in a parallel array. This arrangement may be in part determined by the microtubule organizing center. Leading edge extension of neuronal cells during migration is directed by microfilament polymerization.

During migration, movement of the neuron nucleus occurs in a process known as *nucleokinesis* and in neuronal migration. Specific microtubule-associated genes and genes that affect the cytoskeleton were first identified because there are deleted or mutated in specific forms of neuronal disorder in humans (Bielas and Gleeson 2004). The 14-3-3 proteins, which modulate the actin cytoskeleton, are deficient in Miller-Dieker syndrome, a disorder that is associated with abnormalities of cortical organization and mental retardation. The 14-3-3 proteins interact with the phosphorylated amino acid residues phosphoserine and phosphotyrosine in actin cytoskeletal proteins (Toyo-oka et al. 2003).

Neuronal Maturation and Development of Neuronal Processes

After neuronal cells take up their final position, they extend processes, the dendrites and axons. Development of neuronal circuits is dependent on dendritic branching and outgrowth from the growth cone localized at the tip of the axon (Gupta et al. 2002).

Axon Development

The axonal process extended by a differentiating neuron terminates in a structure known as a growth cone. In addition to growth at the primary growth cone, secondary growth cones form along the axon shaft and give rise to collateral branches of the axon. Growth cone path finding appears to be determined by cell surface contact and factors within the extracellular matrix (Tessier-Lavigne 1994). Molecules that modulate axon growth include receptor protein tyrosine kinases and protein tyrosine phosphatases. Axon guidance molecules include netrins, semaphorins, laminins, and cadherins, the adherence molecules. These axon guidance molecules modulate axonal growth through their repellent or attractant properties (Goodman and Shatz 1993; Goodman et al. 1993).

The patterns of neuronal connection that are established during development fall into two categories. The first category includes connections that are independent of electrical activity. This category includes growth cone guidance and target recognition. In the second category, connectivity is established after electrical activity is established.

Cytoskeletal reorganization underlies growth cone motility. Reorganization includes polymerization and depolymerization of actin filaments and microtubules. Changes in the configuration of actin fibers of the cytoskeleton in the early stages of neurite outgrowth are likely mediated through Rho and Rac GTPases.

Dendrite Development

Dendrites develop from the opposite pole of the neuron than the axon. Development of neuronal circuits is dependent on dendritic branching. Microtubules and neurofilaments constitute the skeleton of the dendritic tree. In addition to branching, dendrites produce small extensions on their surface; these form dendritic spines that are usually found at the site of synaptic contact.

The most active stage of dendritic spine formation occurs in the first 6 months after birth. Dendritic spine formation continues into adult life (Yuste and Bonhoeffer 2004).

Among the most consistent histological abnormalities associated with mental retardation are reductions in the number of dendritic spines and abnormalities in spine morphology. Huttenlocher (1974) reported that in the brains of individuals with nonspecific mental retardation, Golgi staining revealed a reduction of dendritic branching. Purpura (1979) introduced the term *spine dysgenesis* to describe the abnormalities found in nonspecific mental retardation. These abnormalities included a predominance of long, thin spines that resembled immature dendritic spines and an absence of mushroom-like spines.

Abnormalities of dendritic spine morphology also occur in syndromic forms of mental retardation including Down syndrome, fragile X mental retardation, and phenylketonuria Kaufman and Moser 2000 (Ramakers 2002). Reduced and immature dendritic spines also occur in hypothyroidism and severe malnutrition (Berbel et al. 1985; Ramakers 2002) (Fig. 2–1).

Synaptogenesis

When an axon reaches its destination or target, it forms a presynaptic terminal. The target neuron undergoes change to produce postsynaptic elements,

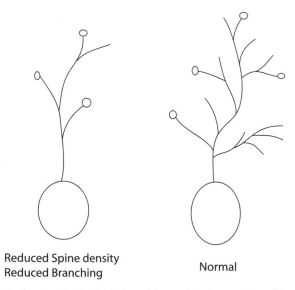

Reduced Spine density
Reduced Branching

Normal

Figure 2–1. Reductions in dendritic branching and in the number of dendritic spines occur in several forms of syndromic mental retardation (Huttenlocher 1974) and in hypothyroidism and severe malnutrition (Berbel et al. 1985; Ramakers 2002).

including neurotransmitter receptors and second messenger–generating systems. The concept of synaptic plasticity that has evolved over the past decade implies that for synapses to become stabilized, the postsynaptic cell must respond to the signal transmitted from the presynaptic neuron. In addition, it must generate a retrograde signal back to the presynaptic cell. Dendritic spines constitute the most common sites of synaptic contact. Key to the process of dendritic spine formation is neurotransmission through glutamatergic neurotransmitter receptors. The actin cytoskeleton plays an important role in establishing neuronal connections and synaptic function (Chechlacz and Gleeson 2003).

Synaptic Vesicles

In the presynaptic element, a collection of vesicles that contain neurotransmitters are formed by budding from the Golgi apparatus. Synaptic vesicle membranes are composed of a lipid bilayer that is spanned by protein molecules such as synaptophysin and synaptobrevin. The vesicle membranes also contain transporter proteins that are specific for particular types of neurotransmitter. Synaptic vesicles are transported from the Golgi on the cytoskeleton to the presynaptic terminal, where they aggregate within active zones of the presynaptic membrane. Mitochondria aggregate close to the pre- and postsynaptic membranes to supply energy for neurotransmission.

When an electric action potential passes into the presynaptic terminal, there is an influx of calcium through voltage-modulated channels. This causes synaptic vesicles to dock at specific sites in the presynaptic membrane. Following fusion of the synaptic vesicle membrane with the presynaptic membrane, the vesicles release their contents into the synaptic cleft. Neurotransmitter molecules then traverse the synaptic cleft to bind to receptors on the post-synaptic membrane.

Two types of synaptic vesicle occur, small vesicles and large dense core vesicles. Small vesicles contain small molecule neurotransmitters such as γ-aminobutyric acid (GABA), glutamate, glycine, and acetylcholine. Large dense core synaptic vesicles contain primarily the neuropeptide neurotransmitters. In the hypothalamus and pituitary, large dense core synaptic vesicles contain neurohormones. In these locations, the vesicles are sometimes referred to as "neurosecretory vesicles."

Synaptic vesicles undergo a trafficking cycle that is comprised of alternating rounds of exocytosis and endocytosis. Exocytosis of synaptic vesicles is triggered by a rise in intracellular Ca^{2+} concentration. During exocytosis, synaptic vesicle membranes fuse with cell membranes in the active zone of nerve terminal. This results in release of neurotransmitters. During endocytosis, synaptic vesicle membranes are recycled and the vesicles are primed with neurotransmitters (Sudhof 2004).

G proteins, especially RAB GTPases, play an important role in vesicle budding, vesicular transport, and vesicle membrane fusion. An important part of this process is recycling of RAB guanosine diphosphate (GDP) mediated through GDP dissociation inhibitor (GDI) proteins. RAB GDI forms a complex with RAB GDP and retrieves it from membranes. In 1998, D'Adamo and colleagues reported that mutations in the gene encoding GDIα occur in a subgroup of patients with X-linked mental retardation (Fig. 2–2).

Synapses and Neurotrophins

Once synapses form, they may stabilize and mature, or they may be eliminated. Stabilization is dependent upon synaptic activity, i.e., communication between pre- and post-synaptic neurons. Neurotrophins play key roles in neuronal connectivity through modulation of axonal and dendritic branching and through synaptic remodeling.

Neurotrophins include nerve growth factor (NGF), BDNF, and neurotrophins 3–5 (NT3, NT4, NT5). Biological activity of neurotrophins is dependent upon their binding to a neurotrophin receptor. The neurotrophin receptor p75NR binds to all neurotrophins; in addition, neurotrophins bind to tyrosine kinase (TRK) receptors TRKA, TRKB, and TRKC. Upon binding of neurotrophins to the TRK receptors, the receptor subunits dimerize and undergo autophosphorylation, which leads to activation. Activated TRK receptors then initiate signal transduction in cascades such as the mitogen-activated protein kinase (MAPK) kinase pathway, the phosphatidylinositol-3-kinase (PI3K) pathway, or the phospholipase C pathway.

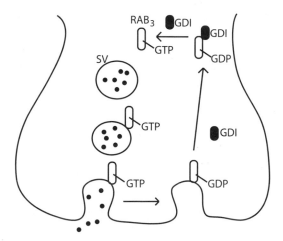

Figure 2–2. The signal transduction factor RAB guanosine triphosphate (GTP) plays an important role in synaptic vesicle (SV) budding, transport, and fusion with synaptic membranes. RAB guanine dissociation inhibitor (GDI) retrieves RAB from the membrane. RAB GDI deficiency leads to one form of X-linked mental retardation (D'Adamo et al. 1998). GDP, guanosine diphosphate.

Neurotrophins also modulate the expression of synaptic vesicle–associated proteins. One of the most important neurotrophic factors is BDNF (Cohen-Cory and Lom 2004). In the developing nervous system, BDNF regulates cell survival, proliferation, and synaptic growth (Tyler et al. 2002). Through modulation of synapses in the hippocampus, it plays a role in the long-term potentiation that is associated with memory and learning. This will be discussed further below. Mccp2 influences BDNF expression (Chen et al. 2003).

Deficiency in activity of the neurotrophin neurofibromin leads to neurofibromatosis; some patients with this disorder manifest learning problems. Neurofibromatosis is discussed later in this chapter.

Neuronal Function and Signal Transduction

Signal transduction may be defined as the process whereby an extracellular signal is turned into an intracellular signal. The extracellular signal may be a change in action potential generated through activity of ion channels; it may be mediated by the interaction of ligand and receptor, for example, binding of neurotransmitters to receptors or binding of growth factors to receptors.

Binding of ligand to receptor leads to conformational changes in the receptor protein and to exposure of tyrosine groups. The receptor tyrosine residues become phosphorylated. This may then lead to activation of several signaling cascades. These include G proteins and second messenger systems based on cyclic nucleotides, calcium, membrane lipids, and phosphatidylinositol. Nitric oxide may also act as a second messenger.

G Proteins

G proteins are membrane-associated proteins that act as signal transducers. They have a high affinity for the nucleotides GTP and GDP. The interaction of a ligand (first messenger) with its receptor in the cell membrane stimulates an exchange reaction on G proteins. In this reaction, the G protein–GDP complex is converted to a G protein–GTP complex. This activation reaction involves a conformational change in the G protein. Guanine nucleotide exchange factors (GEFs) catalyze the exchange of GTP for GDP on G proteins.

G proteins are trimeric, composed of α, β, and γ subunits. Different forms of each subunit occur. The diversity of forms of G protein subunits and the fact that different subunits can combine to form different types of G protein are key factors in the roles played by these proteins in many different forms of signal transduction.

The Ras superfamily of small G proteins includes five primary families: Ras, Rho, Rab, Ran, and Arf. Rho GTPase signal transduction factors serve to integrate extracellular cues and intracellular processes (Ramakers 2002). Genes encoding Rho GTPase signal transduction factors have been shown to be defective in at least four different forms of X linked mental retardation (Fig. 2–3).

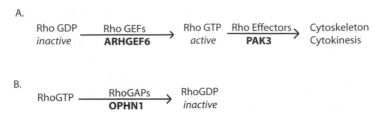

Figure 2–3. Rho guanosine triphosphate (GTPase) signal transduction factors (shown in bold) are deficient in several forms of nonspecific mental retardation. GDP, guanosine diphosphate; GEF, guanine nucleotide exchange factor; GAP, GTPase-activating protein.

Second Messenger Systems

Cyclic Nucleotides

The most common second messenger system is cyclic adenosine monophosphate (cAMP). This compound is formed from adenosine triphosphate (ATP) upon activation of the membrane-bound enzyme adenyl cyclase. When activated, adenyl cyclase converts the nucleotide ATP to cAMP. Cyclic AMP activates protein kinases that are in turn responsible for activation of specific intracellular target proteins. Target proteins may alter cytoskeletal elements to produce changes in structure, shape, or motility. They may enter the nucleus and promote gene expression. In some cases, the target protein of protein kinase may be another enzyme whose activity may be either stimulated or inhibited, thus affecting intracellular metabolic activity. Cyclic GMP (guanine monophosphate) may also act as a second messenger system. Nitric oxide acts as a messenger through its effects on GMP (von Bohlen und Halbach and Dermietzel 2002).

Calcium Ions

Calcium ions are considered second messengers since the cellular response to specific stimuli involves alteration in cellular calcium concentrations. Calcium acts as a messenger directly or through the protein calmodulin. In many nerve cells, activation of cAMP leads to activation of calcium channels and influx of calcium ions. The interaction of neurotransmitter ligand with ionotropic neurotransmitter receptor leads to influx of calcium. Control of calcium storage and release is mediated in part by the phosphoinositide system (Augustine et al. 2003).

The release of calcium from intracellular stores serves to activate intracellular proteases such as calpains. This activation plays an important part in the cytoskeletal reorganization that occurs as part of the cellular response

(Bozoky et al. 2004). The catalytic subunit of calpain cleaves proteins at the microfilament–actin interface. Calpain also cleaves other cellular proteins such as calmodulin, a major intracellular calcium-sequestering protein.

Phosphatidylinositol System

In the phosphatidylinositol system, the binding of ligand to receptor activates a G protein that functions as a phospholipase C activator. Phospholipase C cleaves a membrane-associated molecule, phosphatidylinositol-4,5-biphosphate (PIP2), resulting in generation of a molecule of 1,2-diacylglycerol and a molecule of inositol-1,4,5-triphosphate. These two molecules constitute second messengers (effectors). Other phosphatidylinositol second messengers result from activation by G proteins of specific kinases, such as PI3K. The kinase PI3K leads to the generation of inositol phosphate compounds including phosphatidylinositol-3,4-biphosphate and phosphatidylinositol-3,4,5-triphosphate. The phosphoinositides stimulate release of calcium from intracellular stores (Fruman et al. 1998).

Inositol triphosphate is hydrolyzed to yield inositol and phosphate, and this reaction ensures generation of cellular inositol. This reaction is inhibited by lithium, a chemical that is sometimes used to treat manic-depressive psychosis.

Synaptojanin is a polyphosphoinositide phosphatase that plays a role in the metabolism of phosphatidylinositol-4,5-biphosphate, which in turn is involved in synaptic vesicle recycling. Synaptojanin1 is encoded on chromosome 21 and overexpressed in Down syndrome. Arai et al. (2002) noted that the expression pattern of synaptojanin in fetal brain indicates that it is involved in neuronal migration and synaptogenesis. Phosphoinositol phosphorylation and the function of synaptojanin are shown in Figure 2–4.

The phosphoinositide system is affected by the gene mutations that cause tuberous sclerosis, a condition that may be associated with cognitive impairment. This is discussed further below in the section on signal transduction mutations that may lead to cognitive deficits

Modulation of the Phosphorylation of Targets by Kinases and Phosphatases

Signals at the cell surface frequently lead to activation of intracellular kinases by phosphorylated compounds (cAMP, cGTP) that are present in the inner cell membrane. Active phosphate groups are then passed on from one kinase to another, initiating a cascade of activity. The transfer of phosphate groups also involves the activity of phosphatases.

Phosphatases catalyze phosphate removal from proteins, including kinases. In some instances, removal of phosphate from a kinase results in inactivation of the kinase. In other instances, where inhibitory phosphate bound

Phospho-inositol Phosphorylation

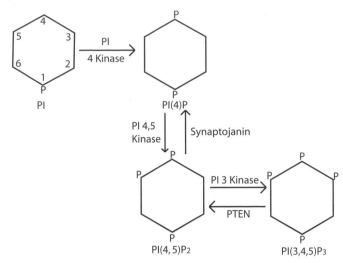

Figure 2–4. Synaptojanin is a polyphosphoinositide phosphatase that is involved in synaptic vesicle recycling. It is encoded on chromosome 21 and overexpressed in Down syndrome (Arai et al. 2002). P, phosphate; PI, phosphatidylinositol.

to a kinase is removed by the phosphatase, kinase activation results. Phosphatases may be associated with receptors or they may be intracellular, e.g., nonreceptor tyrosine phosphatases.

One signal transduction pathway that plays an important role in learning and memory is the extracellular signal–regulated kinase (ERK)–MAPK pathway. The components of the ERK–MAPK pathway are abundantly expressed in neurons (Sweatt et al. 2003a,b). This pathway will be discussed in further detail below.

Neurotransmitters and Receptors

Neurotransmitters are most often small molecules, such as the amino acids glutamate, GABA, and glycine or the amines serotonin (5-hydroxytryptamine) and dopamine. We will concentrate on the neurotransmitters and their receptors that play important roles in communication and brain development.

Glutamate Receptors

Glutamatergic neurons are particularly abundant in the cerebral cortex, hippocampus, caudate nucleus, and cerebellum. Glutamate is an excitatory amino acid that plays a role in fast synaptic transmission and in postsynaptic depolarization. Glutamate receptors are important in learning and memory. Molecular cloning studies have revealed that at least 24 different genes encode glutamate receptor subunits. Of these, 16 are ionotropic receptor subunits and eight are metabotropic receptor subunits. Ionotropic neurotransmitter receptors form ion channels; these channels open when ligand binds to receptor. In metabotropic neurotransmitter receptors, ligand binding is linked to activation of different intracellular signal transduction pathways, including G protein–coupled and second messenger pathways (von Bohlen und Halbach and Dermietzel 2002). Many of the genes that encode glutamate receptor subunits are expressed primarily in fetal life (Lujan et al. 2005).

There are several classes of ionotropic glutamate receptors. They are named for the pharmacological agonists that activate them.

α-Amino-3-hydroxy-5-methyl-4-isoxazole Propionate Glutamate Receptors

These receptors are responsive to glutamate and to α-amino-3-hydroxy-5-methyl-4-isoxazole propionate (AMPA). An AMPA glutamate receptor forms an ion channel, and binding of the ligand to the receptor is followed by an influx of ions—sodium, potassium, or sometimes calcium—into the neuronal synapse. The AMPA glutamate receptors are composed of four subunit types— GluR1, GluR2, GluR3, and GluR4—each encoded by a separate gene. Receptors may be composed of identical subunits or different subunits.

The AMPA glutamate receptors achieve high density in the cerebral cortex, hippocampus, amygdala, caudate, putamen, nucleus accumbens, and olfactory bulb. They occur in the pyramidal layer of the hippocampus and in layers 2 and 3 of the cerebellar cortex. Neurotransmission mediated by AMPA receptors plays a key role in several aspects of developmental and adult synaptic plasticity (Bear and Abraham 1996).

N-Methyl-D-aspartate Glutamate Receptors

These receptors are activated by glutamate, aspartate, and the pharmacological substance N-methyl-D-aspartate (NMDA). They play an important role in the response to excitatory amino acids. Each receptor is composed of five subunits, which together form an ion channel that is permeable to calcium, sodium, and potassium. Two genes, NR1 and NR2, encode NMDA receptor subunits. Alternate splice variants of each gene transcript occur. The NMDA receptors are abundant in the cerebral cortex, hippocampus, basal ganglia, hypothalamus, and olfactory bulb. Each NMDA receptor is composed of four subunits; usually, two are NR1 subunits and two are NR2 subunits, either NR2A or NR2B.

Kainate Glutamate Receptors

These ion channel receptors respond to glutamate and to the pharmacological substance kainate. They are formed from two classes of subunits. The first subclass includes GluR5, GluR6, and Glu R7, which are 80% homologous to AMPA glutamate receptor subunits. The second subclass includes KA1 and KA2, which are only 40% homologous to AMPA glutamate subunits. KA1 mRNA expression is restricted to the hippocampus. KA2 is expressed in the cerebral and cerebellar cortices and in the hippocampus. GluR6 mRNA is found in the hippocampus, caudate, putamen, and cerebellum. GluR5 occurs in the cingulate cortex and in the medial nucleus of the amygdala.

Metabotropic Glutamate Receptors

The metabotropic glutamate receptor genes give rise to eight different subunits, mGluR1–mGluR8. There are eight different receptor subtypes. Each receptor is dimeric and composed of only one type of subunit. Metabotropic glutamate receptors are widely distributed in the brain.

Early embryonic neurons express glutamate receptors. Lujan et al. (2005) reviewed glutamate receptor expression during development and concluded that expression of these receptors plays a role in neuronal proliferation and differentiation.

γ-Aminobutyric Acid Neurotransmitter Receptors

The most abundant inhibitory neurotransmitter in the brain is GABA. It is expressed at 30% of synapses. It is synthesized from glutamate through the activity of the enzyme glutamate decarboxylase. This synthesis requires the coenzyme pyridoxal phosphate (vitamin B_6). Two genes encode glutamate decarboxylase (GAD), and these two genes differ in their site of expression. GAD67 is expressed primarily in cell bodies and dendrites, while GAD65 is expressed primarily in axons. The GABA transporters serve to remove GABA from the synaptic cleft. The GABAergic neurons are particularly abundant in the striatum and in the interneurons of the globus pallidus, substantia nigra, thalamus, hippocampus and cerebral cortex. The GABA receptors occur on neurons and glial cells in the central nervous system. They also occur in the ganglia of the autonomic nervous system (von Bohlen und Halbach and Dermietzel 2002).

Twenty-one different genes encode ionotropic GABA receptor subunits. There are eight different families of GABA receptors. These receptors form ligand-gated chloride ion channels. Assembly of α, β, γ, and δ subunits forms the most common functional receptor, $GABA_A$. Two different genes encode subunits that form the metabotropic $GABA_B$ receptor. Alternate splice forms of these subunits occur. $GABA_B$ receptors utilize G protein signal transduction pathways. GABA$_B$ receptors occur primarily in the cerebral cortex, thalamus, and cerebellum.

Lujan et al. (2005) reviewed the role of GABA receptors in the developing brain. They reported that these receptors play a role in neuronal migration.

Dopamine Receptors

Five different genes encode receptors for the neurotransmitter dopamine. Dopaminergic neurons are particularly abundant in the substantia nigra and the striatum. They are also abundant in areas of the hypothalamus, in the limbic cortex, and in structures of the limbic system. Song et al. (2002) reported that dopamine receptors play an important role during development in the regulation of dendritic growth in cortical neurons.

Serotonin Receptors

At least 18 different genes encode receptors for the neurotransmitter serotonin. Beique et al. (2004) examined serotonin receptors in the developing brain. They determined that serotonin plays a key role in prefrontal cortex development, particularly during the period of synaptic outgrowth.

Glycine Receptors

Glycine and GABA are the main inhibitory transmitters in the central nervous system. Glycine acts through ionotropic receptors. In addition, it modulates NMDA glutamate receptors. The glycine receptor is a glycoprotein composed of five subunits. Together the subunits form glycine-gated chloride channels. Glycine receptors occur in the spinal cord, brain stem, hippocampus, amygdala, striatum, and cortex. Okabe et al. (2004) demonstrated that glycinergic membrane responses occur early in embryonic neocortical development in the cortical plate neurons and Cajal-Retzius cells.

Synapse-Associated Proteins

The *DLG3* gene, a human homolog of the *Drosophila* gene Disc Large, encodes the synapse-associated protein SAP102. The SAP102 protein serves to anchor NMDA glutamate receptors in the plasma membrane (Lau et al. 1996). The NMDA and AMPA glutamate receptors play a role, particularly in the hippocampus, in long-term potentiation and long-term depression of synaptic activity, respectively, functions that are involved in learning and memory.

Synapsins are neuronal phosphoproteins that are encoded by a family of genes. They are located on the cytoplasmic surface of synaptic vesicles. These proteins play a role in modulating the release of neurotransmitters. Different synapsin proteins encoded by different members of the gene family have common domains and, in addition, each synapsin protein has a unique domain. The gene that encodes synapsin 3 is located on chromosome 22q12.3.

Learning, Memory, and Synaptic Plasticity

Changes in synaptic plasticity are thought to play key roles in learning and memory. *Synaptic plasticity* may be defined as experience-dependent alterations in the strength of transmission at excitatory synapses (Malenka 2003). Specific changes in synaptic activity include long-term depression (LTD) and long-term potentiation (LTP). The latter involves an increase in synaptic response to a given signal, and the former involves a decreased response.

Milner et al. (1998) demonstrated that recall of experiences, or episodic memory, is dependent on the hippocampus and related mesial temporal lobe and on modification in synaptic activity. The hippocampus plays an essential role in learning and memory, particularly in spatial memory, Maguire et al. (2000) reported that the posterior hippocampi of London taxi drivers are significantly larger than those in control subjects. In 2000, Maguire et al. demonstrated that enlargement of the hippocampus is specifically associated with spatial learning. They noted that in the London taxi drivers hippocampal volume increase correlated with the amount of time spent driving. Maguire et al. concluded that these findings are consistent with the hypothesis that spatial representation of the environment is stored in the posterior hippocampus. Furthermore, the posterior hippocampus may increase in size to accommodate additional information.

Long-term potentiation occurs in different stages (Egan et al. 2003). Several components are involved: neurotransmitter receptor formation and activity, activity of neurotrophins, increases in intracellular calcium, activation of protein kinases and intracellular signaling pathways, changes in gene transcription and protein synthesis.

Neurotransmitter Receptor Changes in Long-Term Potentiation

Glutamate is the most abundant excitatory amino acid neurotransmitter. Glutamate receptors are particularly important in postnatal learning. Hippocampal glutamate receptors play a key role in establishing new memories. Synapses that are silent at resting potentials contain NMDA glutamate receptors but few AMPA glutamate receptors. Glutamate that is released by the presynaptic neuron may bind to an NMDA receptor. This interaction increases Ca^{2+} concentration in the postsynaptic neuron. The AMPA receptors move from the neuron cytosol to the plasma membrane of the dendrite and then to the synapse.

Synaptic plasticity is particularly dependent on regulation of the number of receptors at the synapse. Regulation of the formation of glutamate receptors occurs at the level of transcription and translation of receptor subunits and at the level of subunit assembly. Receptor numbers at the synapse can be increased through exocytosis or decreased through endocytosis.

Long-term depression involves a decrease in the number of AMPA receptors in the membrane. This decrease occurs through removal of AMPA receptors during endocytosis. The AMPA receptors move from the synaptic membrane back into the cell cytosol.

Both NMDA and AMPA receptors are associated with SAP102 in the endoplasmic reticulum and in the Golgi apparatus of the neurons. This interaction appears to play an important role in the trafficking of receptors to the surface of the synaptic membrane. SAP102 may be the first example of a neuronal synapse-associated protein that is mutated in mental retardation (Tarpey et al. 2004). This is discussed later in the chapter.

Activity of Neurotrophins in Long-Term Potentiation

The entry of Ca^{2+} into the postsynaptic neuron also promotes the release of neurotrophic factors such as NGF and BDNF. It also enhances NMDA receptor activity and Ca ion channel activity (Tyler et al. 2002).

The gene that encodes BDNF has multiple promoter elements, which are used to generate a series of mRNA transcripts that differ in their spatial and temporal expression. Martinowich et al. (2003) reported that increased synthesis of BDNF occurred in neurons after depolarization. Furthermore, this increase in synthesis correlated with a decrease in methylation of CG dinucleotides within a regulatory region of BDNF. They demonstrated that increased BDNF transcription resulted when the Mecp2 Sin3A–histone deacetylase complex dissociated from the BDNF promoter.

Brain-Derived Neurotrophic Factor Polymorphism and Memory Performance

The BDNF gene transcripts give rise to a precursor peptide, pro-BDNF. This is then cleaved by proteases to produce a mature peptide. A polymorphism in the BDNF gene results in an amino acid substitution, valine 66 to methionine (Val66Met), (val 66met, V66M) that affects intracellular processing and secretion of BDNF. Egan et al. (2003) investigated the effects of mutant BDNF on neurons in vitro. They demonstrated that the mutant protein differed from the normal form in that it did not localize to the secretory granules of synapses. Egan et al. studied groups of human subjects who were heterozygous for the val66met mutation. They used functional magnetic resonance imaging to examine hippocampal activity during a memory task that involved decoding and then retrieving a complex scene. They determined that in individuals with the Val/Met polymorphism there was a 25% decrease in memory performance.

Increases in Intracellular Calcium, Activation of Intracellular Signaling in Long-Term Potentiation

The earliest stage in the LTP process is dependent upon an increase in intracellular calcium and activation of protein kinases. Binding of ligand to receptor leads to conformation changes in the receptor protein and to exposure of tyrosine groups. The receptor tyrosine residues become phosphorylated. This in turns leads to the binding of intracellular proteins and to activation of small G proteins (guanine nucleotide–binding proteins). Activation of small G proteins, such as members of the Ras and Rho family, leads to activation of the MAPK–ERK cascade.

The MAPK pathway plays a role in the phosphorylation of cytoskeletal proteins. This in turn leads to structural changes in neuronal processes. Such changes constitute one form of adaptation of neurons to synaptic activity. The activation of intracellular proteins by phosphorylation facilitates the fusion of synaptic vesicles to cell membranes, thereby regulating neurotransmitter release. Activation of signaling pathways in postsynaptic neurons increases the synthesis of AMPA receptors.

The later stage of LTP involves the cAMP responsive element binding protein (CREB) signaling pathway, activation of gene transcription, and protein synthesis. Proteins in the ERK cascade, ERK1 and ERK2, are translocated to the nucleus of the neuron. Through phosphorylation they activate ribosomal S6 kinase and the cAMP response element (CRE) transcription factor. This factor activates gene transcription directly; in addition, it activates expression of other transcription factors. The proteins ERK1 and ERK2 also activate protein synthesis from mRNA bound to ribosomal complexes in the cytoplasm (Weeber and Sweatt 2002). The ERK–CREB signal transduction pathway is shown in Figure 2.5.

Impairment of Learning and Memory

Mutations leading to disruptions in cell surface receptors, receptor-linked proteins, signaling pathways, or transcription factors may lead to deficits in synaptic plasticity and to impairment of learning and memory.

Signals transmitted through the intracellular signal transduction pathway pass to the nucleus of the neuronal body, where they influence gene transcription. Over the past decade, several genetic disorders that lead to mental retardation have been found to be due to dysregulation of gene transcription. Several of these disorders involve DNA methylation and chromatin structure, e.g., Rett syndrome, X-linked mental retardation with α-thalassemia syndrome (ATRX), and RSK3 deficiency.

Johnston (2004) noted that disorders that disrupt the synthesis of new transcripts produce more profound intellectual impairment. Such disorders

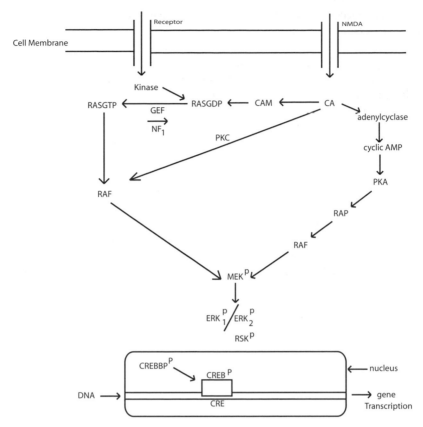

Figure 2–5. Protein kinases in the mitogen-activated protein kinase kinase (MEK)–extracellular signal–regulated kinase (ERK) pathway play an important role in long-term potentiation and in facilitation of signal transduction from receptors in the cell membrane to the nucleus, where they influence gene transcription (Sweatt et al. 2003a,b). NMDA, N-methyl-D-aspartate; CAM, cell adhesion molecule; GTP, guanosine triphosphate; GDP, guanosine diphosphate; GEF, guanine nucleotide exchange factor; PKC/PKA, protein kinase C/A; NF, neurofibromatosis; AMP, adenosine monophosphate; RSK, ribosomal S6 kinase; CRE, cAMP responsive element; CREBBP, CRE binding protein.

include cretinism, Rett syndrome, Coffin-Lowry syndrome, and Rubinstein-Taybi syndrome. In cretinism, thyroid hormone is deficient; in the absence of thyroid hormone, the thyroid hormone receptor acts as a transcriptional repressor. In Rett syndrome, the protein MECP2 is defective or deficient. This leads to altered control of gene expression. This altered gene expression disrupts the refinement of synapses that occurs during maturation. Rett syndrome, Coffin-Lowry syndrome, and Rubinstein-Taybi syndrome are discussed below. They are also discussed in further detail in Chapter 4.

Genetic Defects Associated with Mental Retardation and Due to Defects in Neurogenesis

Microcephaly is defined as a condition where the head circumference is more than 3 standard deviations below the mean. The reduction in head size results from severe reduction of brain size. In *primary microcephaly*, the brain is most often structurally normal and there are no other malformations or metabolic defects. Primary microcephaly is usually inherited as an autosomal recessive trait. Through gene mapping studies in families, at least six different gene loci have been shown to determine this condition. The clinical phenotype is indistinguishable in the defects determined by the different loci. A number of microcephaly-determining loci have been mapped through the use of homozygosity mapping.

Homozygosity mapping is used particularly to identify chromosomal regions that contain genes involved in the pathogenesis of recessively inherited diseases. In this form of mapping, DNA from affected and unaffected members in a pedigree is used to determine which alleles are present at specific polymorphic loci. The loci may be scattered throughout the genome. If there is some evidence that a disease gene maps to a specific chromosome or chromosomal region, polymorphic loci in that chromosomal region will be selected for analysis. The purpose of these studies is to identify segments of chromosomes where all affected members have the same alleles at specific marker loci.

Primary Microcephaly Type 1

The primary microcephaly type 1 locus (*MCPH1*) was mapped when all affected members of a consanguineous family were found to carry identical alleles for a series of markers on chromosome 8. Jackson et al. (2002) examined the gene map in the region on chromosome 8 where all affected members with primary microcephaly shared the identical ancestral haplotype. They noted that there were two protein-encoding genes in that region. DNA sequence analysis revealed that in affected family members a DNA mutation was present in exon 2 of one of these genes. They designated the product of this gene locus *microcephalin*. The gene mutation they detected at the MCPH1 locus generated a premature stop codon that resulted in premature termination of gene transcription. In carriers of the microcephaly trait, the microcephalin mutation was present in heterozygous form; that is, carriers had one normal *MCPH1* gene and one mutated *MCPH1* gene. Microcephalin contains specific domains referred to as BRCAT domains (BRCA1 C-terminal domains). These domains are characteristic of genes that are involved in the repair of double-stranded DNA breaks. In cases where the *MCPH1* gene product is deficient, repair of DNA breaks is less efficient.

Interestingly, previous studies on syndromes characterized by defective repair of DNA breaks, e.g., Nijmegen DNA breakage syndrome, revealed that microcephaly occurred consequent to excessive cell death during neurogenesis. It is likely then that in *MCPH1* inefficient repair of DNA breaks leads to abnormal rates of cell death during neurogenesis and to microcephaly.

Primary Microcephaly Type 5

Pattison et al. (2000) mapped microcephaly type 5 (MCPH5) to chromosome 1q31, based on their finding of a region of homozygosity in consanguineous families in northern Pakistan. In this geographic region, MCPH5 accounts for 43% of cases of primary microcephaly. Different families within this geographic region did not share a specific founder haplotype. However, within a particular family, affected members shared the same alleles in the 1q31 region.

Analysis of expressed genes encoded by loci in the 1q31 region led to identification of defects in a specific gene known to control the function of the mitotic spindle during cell division. The gene was named "abnormal spindle-like microcephaly associated" (*ASPM*). In different families with microcephaly, different mutations occurred within the *ASPM* gene. Studies in model organisms confirmed that the *ASPM* gene plays a key role in embryonic neuroblasts in determining the generation of neuronal progenitor cells. As noted earlier in this chapter, *ASPM* affects the orientation of the mitotic spindle.

In the process of evolution, the *ASPM1* coding gene underwent enlargement in humans. The *ASPM1* gene in humans differs from that in mice in that a large calmodulin binding domain is inserted. Furthermore, advantageous mutations in human *ASPM* have occurred at a much higher rate than in higher primates. These studies indicate that *ASPM* is a key factor in the evolution of human intelligence.

Genetic Defects in Neuronal Migration Leading to Mental Retardation

Neuronal migration defects may lead to cortical malformation syndromes. Cognitive impairment and epilepsy usually occur in these syndromes.

Lissencephaly Type 1 and Miller-Dieker Syndrome

The brain in lissencephaly shows varying degrees of absence of convolutions (*agyria*), or abnormally wide convolutions (*pachygyria*). Frequently, the ventricles are distorted and there is hypoplasia of the corpus callosum. Histological examination of the cortex reveals that it is disorganized and that the normal six-layered cortex is replaced by a cortex with four layers. Lissencephaly is caused by aberrations in neuronal migrations between the ninth and thirteenth weeks of gestation.

Miller-Dieker syndrome is characterized by lissencephaly and variable degrees of facial dysmorphology, including prominent forehead, bitemporal hollowing, upturned nose, flat face, prominent upper lip, and small jaw. Almost all children with Miller-Dieker syndrome have deletions of chromosome 17p13.3 (Cardoso et al. 2003).

In a subgroup of patients with lissencephaly and no facial dysmorphology, chromosome 17p13.3 deletions were shown to be much smaller than in Miller-Dieker patients. Molecular genetic studies in these patients and in patients where chromosome 17p13.3 was interrupted by translocation led to identification of a gene that was deleted or interrupted, the *LIS1* gene. It is important to note that defects in one copy of the *LIS1* gene are sufficient to cause the isolated lissencephaly phenotype (ILS).

The *LIS1* gene is comprised of 11 exons, and the coding sequence is 1,233 bp in length. The protein encoded by this gene is part of an evolutionarily conserved pathway that plays a role in cell motility through its effects on the cytoplasmic motor protein dynein. The LIS1 protein influences neuronal migration through its effects on nucleokinesis. The LIS1 protein binds to the product of the NUDEL gene *NDE1*; the product of this gene is essential for mitotic spindle assembly. It also interacts with tubulin in microtubules (Feng et al. 2000; Feng and Walsh 2004).

Analysis of the region of chromosome 17p13.3 deleted in patients with Miller-Dieker syndrome led to identification of a second gene that plays a role in neuronal migration. This gene is designated *14-4-3e* (Toyo-oka et al. 2003). The protein encoded by this gene is a member of a family of homologous proteins that bind to phosphoproteins and protect them from dephosphorylation. The 14-4-3 proteins are ubiquitously expressed in the body, with high levels of expression in the brain. Other members of the 14-4-3 protein family play a role in neuronal migration.

Subcortical Band Heterotopias and the Doublecortin Gene DCX

A gene locus that causes lissencephaly or subcortical band heterotopias was mapped to Xq22.3-q24 through linkage studies and analysis of an X;2 chromosome translocation in a patient with lissencephaly by Matsumoto et al. (1998). In male individuals, mutations in the *DCX* gene lead to lissencephaly. Female individuals heterozygous for *DCX* mutations develop varying degrees of subcortical band heterotopia. *Heterotopias* are collections of neuronal cells that form gray matter within white matter. The variability in extent of heterotopia in female individuals with *DCX* mutations is most likely due to random inactivation of the X chromosome. In some cells, the normal X chromosome may be inactivated and the amount of doublecortin produced in that cell is dependent on whether or not the mutant *DCX* gene produced functional protein. In other neurons where the *DCX* mutant–bearing X chromosome is inactivated and X chromosome carrying the normal doublecortin gene is expressed, doublecortin levels are normal. Expression of the *DCX* gene is most abundant in the frontal cortex (Guerrini et al. 2003).

The product of the *DCX* gene, doublecortin, has calmodulin and kinase domains. It plays a role in neuronal migration through its effects on calcium signaling. Studies in mice where siRNA was used to block *DCX* expression revealed that doublecortin plays a role in radial glial migration.

Periventricular Heterotopia

In periventricular heterotopia, neuronal migration arrest leads to the formation of neuron-containing nodules in the ventricles or subventricular zones. Mutations in the X-linked gene filamin A (*FLNA*) lead to periventricular heterotopia (Fox et al. 1998). The *FLNA* gene encodes a protein with multiple domains, including an actin binding domain and domains that bind membrane receptors. Periventricular heterotopias due to filamin A mutations occur most frequently in female individuals. It is thought that filamin A mutations may be lethal in male individuals. Occasionally, filamin A mutations occur in male individuals with periventricular heterotopia. In these cases, it is possible that the highly homologous gene product, filamin B, compensates for loss of filamin A. These proteins overlap partially in their patterns of expression. Filamin A is widely expressed, whereas filamin B is expressed primarily in periventricular regions. Both are expressed in neuronal precursors and in migratory neurons.

Lissencephaly Due to Reelin Defects

A form of lissencephaly that is inherited as an autosomal recessive trait and associated with abnormalities of the cerebellum, hippocampus, and brain stem maps to chromosome 7q22. Affected children are cognitively impaired, and they cannot sit or stand unaided. They may have visual problems and seizures. Hypotonia and lymph edema are frequently present. Hong et al. (2000) noted that the brain abnormalities in this form of lissencephaly are similar to those found in mice with reelin deficiency. In humans, the *reelin* gene (*RLN*) maps to chromosome 7q22. Studies in families with this autosomal recessive form of lissencephaly revealed mutations in the *reelin* gene. Reelin protein is secreted by Cajal-Retzius cells in the embryonic cortex and by cells in the hippocampus. It is also secreted by granule cells in the cerebellum and by ganglion cells in the retina and spinal cord (Bar et al. 2003). Reelin expression occurs within selected populations of neurons throughout life (Deguchi et al. 2003). Cell surface receptors for *reelin* include lipoprotein receptors, the very low-density lipoprotein receptor (VLDLR), and the apolipoprotein E receptor (ApoE). Studies in mice revealed that *reelin* binding to lipoprotein receptors leads to activation of the intracellular adaptor molecule Dab1 by the Src family of kinases. Activated Dab1 together with Lis1 and the Nudel–dynein complex lead to development of the layers of the cerebral cortex

Assade et al. 2003. Reelin is present in serum and detectable on electrophoresis as three bands. The presence of abnormal forms of reelin in serum may be related to the lymph edema found in association with lissencephaly in patients with *RLN* gene mutations.

Defects in Extracellular Matrix Interactions and Cortical Layering

The spatial and temporal expression of different integrin protein subunits plays a critical role in cortical layer formation. Integrins transduce signals from the extracellular matrix to the cytoskeletal compartment. Integrin receptors interact with the tetraspanin family of proteins and with G protein–coupled receptors. One member of the tetraspanin family of proteins, TM4SF2, is disrupted in a subgroup of patients with mental retardation (Zemni et al. 2000).

Mutations in Genes in Signal Transduction Pathways That May Lead to Cognitive Deficits

Tuberous Sclerosis

Tuberous sclerosis (TSC) is a dominantly inherited condition due to mutations in the *TSC1* gene on chromosome 9q34.3 or in the *TSC2* gene on chromosome 16p13.3. There is, however, a high frequency of new mutations in this disorder so that in at least 50% of cases there is no family history of the disorder. Discrete areas of abnormal neuronal migration and abnormal cortical maturation are characteristic of TSC. Within the cortical tubers, the characteristic lesions of TSC, cortical architecture is abnormal and neuronal cells have abnormal morphology (O'Connor et al. 2003). Brain abnormalities are not present in all cases of TSC. However, when present, they may lead to intellectual impairment, seizures, autism, and other behavioral problems. A number of the hamartomas that occur in other regions of the body in TSC, e.g., angiomyolipomas of the kidneyand lymphangiomyomatosis of the lung, show evidence of deletion or mutation of the normal allele in addition to the germline mutation or deletion (Green et al. 1994). There is, however, no evidence that a second hit is involved in the generation of the cortical tubers and regions of abnormal migration. Rarely, a brain tumor, giant cell astrocytoma, may develop in TSC; and in these lesions, there is evidence of loss or mutation of the normal allele.

The *TSC1* gene encodes hamartin; *TSC2* encodes tuberin. These proteins interact with each other to form a complex. The tuberin–hamartin interaction serves to stabilize both proteins and tuberin increases the solubility of hamartin in the cytosol (Nellist et al. 1999). Mutations that lead to a reduction in the quantity of tuberin in the cytosol also lead to a reduction in the quantity of hamartin.

Within the catalytic domain of tuberin, in the C-terminal region of the gene, there is a region that has sequence homology to the catalytic domains of GTPase-activating proteins. These proteins convert active forms of small G proteins to inactive forms. Recent studies reveal that tuberin acts as a GTPase-activating protein for the small G protein Rheb (Marygold and Leevers 2002).

A more complete picture of the role of the tuberin–hamartin complex is now emerging (Manning and Cantley 2003a,b). This is illustrated in Figure 2–6. In quiescent cells, in the absence of growth and mitogenic stimuli or in the absence of adequate nutrients, levels of phosphatidylinositol-3,4,5-triphosphate (PIP3) are kept low through the activity of the *PTEN* gene. The product of this gene converts PIP3 to PIP2. Under quiescent conditions, the tuberin–hamartin complex acts as a Rheb GTPase-activating protein and Rheb is maintained primarily in its inactive form, Rheb GDP.

In the presence of growth factors or mitogenic stimuli, quantities of PIP3 increase, and this leads to phosphorylation and activation of the kinase AKT. Phosphorylation of AKT (a serine threonine protein kinase) has several effects, including subsequent transfer of phosphate groups to tuberin, binding of 14-4-3 to the tuberin–hamartin complex, and formation of increased quantities of Rheb GTP. Rheb GTP activates mammalian target of rapamyein (mTOR), and this in turns activates ribosomal S6 kinase and 4EBP1 protein (Pende et al. 2004).

Overexpression of tuberin and hamartin inhibits mTOR signaling. Deficiency of tuberin or hamartin likely leads to increased quantities of active Rheb and increased mTOR signaling, i.e., effects similar to those that occur in the presence of mitogenic stimuli.

It is of interest to note that tuberin and hamartin operate in the same pathway as the *PTEN* gene product, (Cantley and Neel 1999) (Fig. 2–6). All three of these proteins serve to limit cell proliferation (Li et al. 2002). The *PTEN* gene is deleted in several disorders that are associated with hamartomas, e.g., Cowden syndrome and Bannayan-Riley-Ruvalcaba syndrome (Eng 2003). As noted above, hamartomas occur as a complication of TSC.

Neurofibromatosis

Neurofibromatosis is characterized by the propensity to develop neurocutaneous tumors (e.g., neurofibromas) and nervous system tumors (e.g., meningiomas). Darkly pigmented skin lesions, known as *café-au-lait spots*, are characteristic manifestations of this disorder. The rate of mental retardation in neurofibromatosis NF1 patients is twice that in the normal population. In the nonretarded NF1 patient population, the mean intelligence quotient (IQ) range is lower than that in the general population (North et al. 2002). Costa et al. (2002) studied a mouse model of NF1. They demonstrated that mutations of the GTPase-activating protein (GAP) domain of the *NF1* gene resulted in learning problems but not the characteristic neurofibromas.

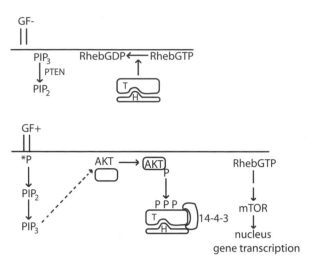

Figure 2–6. In quiescent cells, tuberin (T) and hamartin (H), the products of the tuberous sclerosis genes, cause Rheb to be present in an inactive form. In growth-stimulated cells, T and H are phosphorylated and bound to AKT. Rheb is then present in active form, and it acts in the mammalian target of rapamyein (mTOR) pathway to enhance gene transcription (Manning and Cantley 2003a,b). GDP, guanosine diphosphate; GTP, guanosine triphosphate; PIP_2, phosphatidylinositol-4,5-biphosphate; PIP_3, phosphatidylinositol-3,4,5-triphosphate. GEF, guanine nucleotide exchange factor AKT, alpha Thymine related kinase.

The GAP domain of NF1 influences its reaction with the GTP binding protein RAS (Fig. 2–7). RAS in turn activates the ERK MAPK kinase. There is thus evidence that the GTPase-activating domain of NF1, through its interaction with signaling pathway cascades, plays a key role in learning and synaptic plasticity.

Defects in RAB GDP Dissociation Protein

G proteins, especially RAB GTPases, play an important role in vesicle budding, vesicular transport, and vesicle membrane fusion. An important part of this process is recycling of RAB GDP mediated through GDI proteins. RAB GDI forms a complex with RAB GDP and retrieves it from membranes. In 1998, Thierry Bienvenu and coworkers as well as D'Adamo et al. (1998, 2002) reported that mutations in the gene encoding GDIα occur in a subgroup of patients with X-linked mental retardation.

Defects in Rho Signal Transduction Factors

Genes encoding Rho GTPase signal transduction factors have recently been shown to be defective in at least four different forms of X-linked mental re-

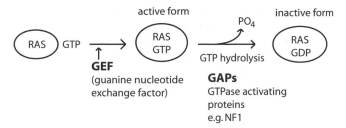

Figure 2–7. The guanosine triphosphate (GTPase) activating domain of the neurofibromatosis protein NF1 promotes transition of Ras protein from its active form, RASGTP, to its inactive form, RASGDP (Costa et al. 2002). GDP, guanosine diphosphate.

tardation (Bienvenu et al. 2000). These genes include *FGD1*, *ARHGEF*, *PAK3*, and *OPHN1*. They are listed in Table 2–1.

Defects in Genes in Nuclear Signaling Pathways

Activation of small G proteins, such as members of the Ras and Rho families, leads to activation of the ERK–MAPK cascade. Proteins in the ERK cascade, ERK1 and ERK2, are translocated to the nucleus of the neuron. Through phosphorylation they activate ribosomal S6 kinase (RSK) and the CRE transcription factor. Defects in RSK lead to a mental retardation syndrome known as Coffin-Lowry syndrome. Defects in CREB lead to a mental retardation syndrome known as Rubinstein-Taybi syndrome (Johnston 2004).

Overexpression of Phosphoinositide Phosphatase in Down Syndrome

Synaptojanin is a polyphosphoinositide phosphatase that plays a role in the metabolism of PIP2, which in turn is involved in synaptic vesicle recycling. Synaptojanin1 is encoded on chromosome 21 and overexpressed in Down syndrome. Arai et al. (2002) noted that the expression pattern of synaptojanin in fetal brain indicates that it is involved in neuronal migration and synaptogenesis.

Defects in Synapse-Associated Proteins That Lead to Mental Retardation or Behavioral Problems

SAP102

The *DLG3* gene, a human homolog of the *Drosophila* gene Disc Large, encodes the synapse associated protein SAP102. The SAP102 protein serves to anchor NMDA glutamate receptors in the plasma membrane (Lau et al. 1996). It may be the first example of a neuronal synapse-associated protein that is mutated in mental retardation. Tarpey et al. (2004) carried out mutation analysis in genes that map in the chromosome Xp13 region. In a number of families with X-linked mental retardation, there is evidence that affected individuals share haplotypes for markers in the Xp13 region. Sequence analysis revealed that in four families where nonsyndromic mental retardation mapped to chromosome Xp13, mutations were present in the *DLG3* gene.

Synapsins

Synapsins are neuronal phosphoproteins that are encoded by a family of genes. They are located on the cytoplasmic surface of synaptic vesicles and play a role in modulating the release of neurotransmitters. Synaptic vesicles that contain neurotransmitters are distributed in two pools, one that is ready for release and one that serves as a reserve pool (Pieribone et al. 1995). Synaptic vesicles in the reserve pool are linked to the actin cytoskeleton via synapsin (Ceccaldi et al. 1995).

Mutation in *Synapsin 1* (SYN) gene was recently shown to be associated with learning difficulties. Garcia et al. (2004) described a four-generation family where men had neurological and behavioral problems. The proband presented with learning difficulties and outbursts of aggressive behavior. He had two male relatives with similar problems as well as male relatives with normal intelligence and epileptic seizures. In all, there were nine affected individuals. Macrocephaly occurred in two of the nine affected individuals. All of the affected men were related through women who were unaffected. In individuals with seizures, nocturnal or tonic-clonic seizures occurred. Individuals with learning disabilities were also noted to have autistic behaviors that included impairments in reciprocal social interactions and restricted, repetitive behaviors, interests, and activities. Linkage analysis placed the gene on the X chromosome within a region of 25 megabases between two polymorphic markers, DXS1275 and MAOB (monoamine oxidase B). Garcia et al. (2004) noted that the gene encoding SNP1 maps in this interval. They determined that a mutation in exon 9 that generated a nonsense codon was present in all affected males and in transmitting females in this family.

Garcia et al. (2004) proposed that the episodic outbursts of rage that occurred without precipitating environmental incidents in some affected men in this family represent a form of epilepsy. This is consistent with the observation reported by Li et al. (1995) that synapsin 1-deficient mice have a lower seizure threshold than normal mice. In deficient mice, the axons of hippocampal neurons are shorter than those in normal mice and synapse formation is delayed.

3

Structural Brain Anomalies and Neural Tube Defects

This chapter focuses on neural tube defects and structural brain defects associated with mental retardation where, in each case, an underlying gene defect in a specific biochemical pathway occurs. The brain malformations discussed include defects due to homeotic gene mutations, structural defects due to mutations in genes involved in protein glycosylation, and X-linked hydrocephalus associated with spastic paraplegia due to defects in the adhesion molecule L1 CAM. Also described are structural brain defects due to mutations in genes in a signaling pathway known as the sonic-hedgehog pathway. Joubert's syndrome serves as an interesting example of a specific brain malformation associated with other variable malformations and genetic heterogeneity. This disorder maps to three different chromosomal regions; the disease gene at one of these loci was defined in 2004 and will be discussed here.

These disorders and their underlying gene defects account for a small percentage of cases with structural brain anomalies. However, the progress made in delineating underlying gene defects, defining the pathways in which these genes operate, and elucidating the pathogenesis of a subset of structural defects will facilitate elucidation of genetic defects that lead to other structural brain anomalies.

Neural Tube Defects

During neurulation, the neural plate folds to form the neural tube. The spinal cord is derived from the caudal neural tube, and the brain is derived from the rostral neural tube. The process of neurulation takes place during days 21–28 of gestation, i.e., in the first week after a missed menstrual period (Eskes 2002). Neural tube defects are relatively common human malformations. They occur in approximately 1 per 1000 pregnancies; however, the prevalence varies in different countries, ranging from 1 in 2500 in Finland to 1 in 80 in South Wales (Eskes 2002; Copp et al. 2003). Infants with the severest neural tube defect, anencephaly, do not usually survive for more than a few days or weeks. In anencephaly, the bony vault of the skull fails to form and underlying brain tissue is exposed. This tissue degenerates during pregnancy, resulting in absence of cerebral hemispheres. Infants with anencephaly do not usually survive for more than a few days or weeks after birth. Defects in the bony vault of the skull may lead to herniation of underlying tissue. In cephalomeningoceles, meninges herniate through the bone defect. In encephaloceles, both brain tissue and meninges herniate through the defect. These lesions are often incompatible with life; however, the prognosis is in part dependent on the position and size of the herniation.

Meningocele and myelomeningocele (spina bifida) are compatible with life, particularly when treated by surgical closure. Individuals with meningocele or myelomeningocele are at risk for hydrocephalus. Hydrocephalus is more likely to occur as a consequence of lesions in the cervical or thoracic vertebrae. It may also occur as a complication of lumbar–sacral myelomeningocele. Mental retardation may occur as a complication of hydrocephalus (Hunt 1973; Tolmie 2000; Norrlin et al. 2003).

In patients with meningocele, there is a defect in the vertebral bone and the meninges are fused with the overlying skin. In myelomeningocele, the meninges and the spinal cord tissue are fused with the skin. In some cases, a layer of skin tissue covers the meninges and spinal cord tissue so that the defect is closed. In open defects, the spinal cord tissue is exposed. Open lesions are usually associated with neurological deficit. However, closed lesions may or may not be associated with neurological deficit. Lifelong complications usually occur in patients where myelomeningocele leads to sensory loss above the level of T11 (eleventh thoracic vertebra) and in patients where hydrocephalus occurs. If hydrocephalus is complicated by episodes of increased intracranial pressure—e.g., due to blockage or failure of the surgical shunt designed to drain excess fluid from the ventricles of the brain—the incidence of complications, including mental retardation, is much higher (Hunt 1999). Renal damage and hypertension are also common complications of neural tube defects in patients who have no neurological enervation of the bladder (Muller et al. 2002).

Posterior encephalocele is considered part of the spectrum of neural tube defects, and they account for about 10% of these defects (Tolmie 2002). Anterior encephalocele including sphenoidal and frontoethmoidal encephaloceles are considered separate anatomical defects.

Prenatal Screening for Neural Tube Defects

Open neural tube defects (those not covered with a layer of skin) result in a flux of proteins from the fetus into the amniotic fluid. In 1972, Brock and Sutcliffe reported that open neural tube defects lead to elevated levels of alpha-fetoprotein in amniotic fluid. Subsequent studies in a large series of pregnancies revealed that screening of maternal serum alpha-fetoprotein levels between 16 and 18 weeks of gestation detected 88% of anencephalic fetuses and 79% of open spinal neural tube defects (UK Collaborative Study, Wald et al. 1977).

Follow-up procedures in cases with higher than normal serum levels of maternal alpha-fetoprotein include high-level ultrasound screening of the fetus and amniocentesis to determine levels of alpha-fetoprotein and other fetal proteins. The birth prevalence of anencephaly and open spina bifida has dropped dramatically in countries and cities where prenatal screening is offered and where termination of affected pregnancies is an option.

Neural Tube Defects and Folate

Smithells et al. (1976) analyzed serum and red cell folate levels as well as vitamin C levels in 900 women during the first trimester of pregnancy. Six of these women subsequently gave birth to infants with neural tube defects. In these six women, levels of folate were significantly lower than in women whose infants did not have neural tube defects. In 1981, Smithells et al. reported results of a study on women who had previously had a pregnancy complicated by fetal neural tube defects. They noted that 40 of 821 had a history of neural tube defects in more than one pregnancy. Women in this study were given a multivitamin containing folate prior to and during a subsequent pregnancy. They noted that administration of this folate multivitamin greatly reduced the occurrence of neural tube defects.

Results of a large multicenter study of more than 18,000 pregnancies (MRC Vitamin Study Research Group, 1991) demonstrated that periconceptual folate administration at a dose of 0.8 mg in a multivitamin reduced the incidence of neural tube defects by 70%.

McDonnell et al. (1999) reported results of an epidemiological study of neural tube defects in eastern Ireland. They noted that the birth prevalence decreased fourfold, from 46.9 per 10,000 in 1980 to 11.6 per 10,000 in 1994. They attributed this change primarily to dietary factors, including vitamin intake since termination of pregnancy is not permitted in Ireland.

Murphy et al. (2000) described results of an ecological study that measured dietary folate intake and annual neural tube rate prevalence in Britain and Ireland between 1980 and 1996, a period during which folate fortification of cereals was implemented. During this period, dietary folate intake increased between 1.4% and 1.6% and the annual rate of decline in neural tube defects was 5.2% in England, 8.2% in Glasgow, and 10.4% in Ireland.

Neural tube defects occur throughout the world. In many developing countries, the incidence is higher in rural communities than in the urban populations. Venter et al. (1995) reported that the incidence of neural tube defects in the northern Transvaal province of South Africa is 3.55 per 1000 in a rural black population and 0.69 per 1000 in an urban black population.

Genetic Variation and Folate Metabolism

There is evidence that genetic factors play a role in neural tube defects. Multiple cases of these defects may occur in one pedigree. However, within one pedigree, the severity of the neural tube defects may vary. This variation suggests that both environmental and genetic factors play a role and/or that genetic factors are likely to be polygenic (Relton et al. 2004a,b). It is likely that genetic factors influence the extent to which nutritional supplementation can decrease the frequency of neural tube defects.

Steegers-Theunissen et al. (1991) determined that women who did not have a vitamin shortage but had a defect in homocysteine metabolism had offspring with neural tube defects. van der Put et al. (1995) and Jacques et al. (1996) confirmed that high homocysteine levels occurred in association with reduced levels of methylene tetrahydrofolate reductase (MTHFR) activity (see Fig. 3–1). They reported that a DNA sequence variant in the MTHFR gene, C677T, results in lower levels of red cell folate and higher levels of homocysteine. In Dutch, Irish, and American populations, this mutation increases the risk for neural tube defects three- to fourfold.

Gaughan et al. (2001) reported on analysis of polymorphisms in the gene encoding methionine synthase reductase (MTRR). A common nucleotide polymorphism occurs in this gene: at position 66, there may be an A-to-G

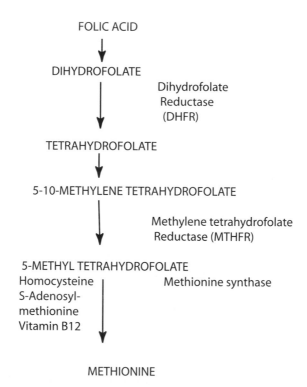

Figure 3–1. Folate metabolism and its relationship to homocysteine metabolism; a specific mutation in methylene tetrahydrofolate reductase leads to high levels of plasma homocysteine, low levels of folate, and an increased risk of neural tube defects.

substitution. This leads to an isoleucine-to-methionine substitution, I22M, in the protein. They determined that the *AA* genotype at position 66 was associated with elevated homocysteine levels: lower homocysteine levels occurred in *AG* heterozygotes and in *GG* homozygotes. Relton et al. (2004a,b) noted that the MTRR *66A-G* genotype acts as a protective factor against neural tube defects in a population from the northern region of the United Kingdom.

Polymorphic DNA sequence variations have been identified in genes encoding other enzymes involved in folate metabolism. No single polymorphism is implicated as a risk factor in all populations. Relton et al. (2004a,b) proposed that specific combinations of variant alleles at different loci most likely influence folate metabolism.

Christensen et al. (1999) reported that the maternal and fetal genotypes together influence the risk for neural tube defects. They noted an elevation in risk when both the mother and the fetus had the MTHFR *T677T* genotype.

The metabolism of folate and the relationship of folate to homocysteine metabolism are illustrated in Figure 3–1.

Vitamin B$_{12}$, Homocysteine Metabolism, and Neural Tube Defects

Vitamin B$_{12}$ (cobalamin) is also required for homocysteine metabolism. It is likely that availability and variation in metabolism of this compound may also play a role in neural tube defects.

Zetterberg (2004) reported evidence that increased concentrations of homocysteine may lead not only to neural tube defects but also to other developmental defects and to a higher frequency of spontaneous abortion. He proposed that fetal toxicity from high levels of homocysteine may be related to accompanying elevation of *S*-adenosylhomocysteine levels, which in turn leads to inhibition of methylation. This may lead to altered gene expression. The serum homocysteine concentration is dependent upon dietary intake of folic acid and vitamin B$_{12}$ (Mattson and Shea 2003). In addition, it is influenced by sequence variation in genes encoding enzymes involved in the metabolism of folic acid and vitamin B$_{12}$ and sequence variation in genes encoding vitamin B$_{12}$ and folate transport proteins. Vitamin B$_{12}$ bound to methionine synthase tends to oxidize. A reducing system is required to regenerate active methionine synthase. This is methionine synthase reductase.

Structural Brain Anomalies

As an introduction to the discussion of structural brain abnormalities and cognitive defects due to gene mutations, we will briefly review the development of specific brain structures.

Development of the Forebrain

The neural plate is converted to a neural tube, which then differentiates into the central nervous system, brain, and spinal cord. During the fourth week of gestation, before the rostral and caudal neuropores of the neural tube close, bulges appear along the rostral end of the neural tube. These are the primordia of the major brain regions: forebrain (prosencephalon), midbrain (mesencephalon), and hindbrain (rhomboencephalon). By the fifth week of gestation, further subdivision occurs and secondary vesicles develop. The prosencephalon divides and forms paired vesicles. This process gives rise to the telencephalon and the diencephalon. The telencephalic vesicles constitute the primitive cerebral hemispheres. Cavities within these vesicles form the lateral ventricles. The diencephalon differentiates to form the thalamus, the hypothalamus, and the neural part of the eyes. The mesencephalon does not subdivide. The rhombencephalon gives rise to the metencephalon and the myelencephalon (Nolte, 2001) (see Figs. 3–2 and 3–3).

Of all the primordial structures of the brain, it is the telencephalon that undergoes the most remarkable growth. A thin membrane, the lamina terminalis, connects the telencephalic vesicles in the midline. The portion of the telencephalon adjacent to the diencephalon thickens to form the basal ganglia. The diencephalon forms the hypothalamus and the thalamus. With

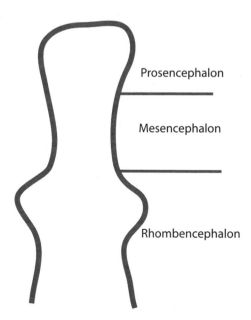

Figure 3–2. The primordia of the major brain regions, forebrain (prosencephalon), midbrain (mesencephalon), and hindbrain (rhombencephalon), develop from the neural tube during the fourth week of gestation.

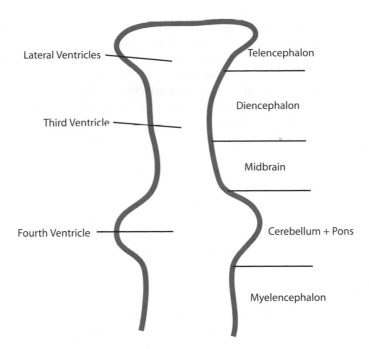

Lateral Ventricles

Telencephalon

Diencephalon

Third Ventricle

Midbrain

Fourth Ventricle

Cerebellum + Pons

Myelencephalon

Figure 3–3. Further subdivisions of the primordia give rise to the telencephalon, diencephalon, midbrain, and myelencephalon and to the cerebral ventricles.

further growth, the telencephalon folds down along the diencephalon, and the two then fuse. The portion of the telencephalon directly adjacent to the area of fusion is the insula.

The mesencephalon gives rise to the midbrain, the most rostral portion of the brain stem. The third and fourth cranial nerves, the oculomotor nerve and the trochlear nerve, arise in the midbrain; and in this structure nuclei develop that are essential for motor function. The midbrain also conducts ascending and descending tracts. The metencephalon gives rise to the pons and cerebellum. The myelencephalon forms the medulla, which is contiguous with the spinal cord.

Genes in Brain Development

Insight into the role of specific genes in brain development is continuously being expanded through studies on humans with brain malformations and cognitive deficits and through studies on organisms such as mouse and *Drosophila*. Homeotic genes were first isolated in *Drosophila*, where they play a key role in early embryogenesis in determining body plan and the development of body segments. Homologous genes occur in vertebrates, including humans, and there is a high degree of homology in homeobox structure and function in different organisms. In all organisms, these genes tend to occur in clusters. In humans, there are four clusters of homeotic genes. Homeotic genes encode proteins that contain a recurring amino acid sequence domain, comprised of 60 amino acids, referred to as the *homeodomain* (Gehring 1985a,b). The homeotic gene products act as specific transcription factors. Homeodomains bind to the regulator elements of target genes. There are at least 30 different classes of homeotic genes, each distinguished by a specific homeodomain consensus sequence. Homeotic genes that play an important role in brain development include *Hes1*, *Otx1*, *Otx 2*, *Pax6*, *Emx1*, *Emx2*, and *Six3*. (Note that mouse gene abbreviations begin with a capital and are followed by lower-case letters, whereas human gene abbreviations are all capitalized.)

Genes that encode proteins that function in specific signaling pathways also play an important role in brain development. These include the sonic-hedgehog signaling pathway and the transforming growth factor beta (TGF-β) and SMAD (homolog of Drosophila sma) transcription factor pathway (Lazaro et al. 2004).

Holoprosencephaly

Holoprosencephaly (HPE) is due to impaired cleavage of the embryonic forebrain. The prosencephalon may fail to undergo sagittal cleavage, resulting in absence of the cerebral hemispheres. Transverse cleavage of the prosencephalon may not occur, and this leads to malformation of the telencephalon and the diencephalon. Malformation of the olfactory and optic bulbs may arise due to defects in horizontal cleavage processes (Muenke and Cohen 2000).

In different patients, various degrees of HPE occur and are associated with varying degrees of facial dysmorphism. Patients at the mild end of the HPE syndrome spectrum may have mild to moderate mental retardation and mild facial dysmorphism, including hypotelorism, absence of nasal septum, and a central single incisor tooth. Brain malformations in mild forms of HPE include absence of the corpus callosum and malformation of the olfactory bulbs and tracts.

In severe HPE, cerebral hemispheres may be absent and in their place there is a monoventricular cerebrum. The most extreme variant of facial dysmorphology is *cyclops*, a single malformed eye, and the presence of a *proboscis*, a malformed nose. In families with HPE, phenotypic expression may be variable; in some individuals, the only clinical abnormalities may be mild hypotelorism and *anosmia* (inability to smell) (Wallis and Muenke 1999; Cohen 2003a–c).

Gene Mutations in Holoprosencephaly

Sonic Hedgehog (SHH)

Seventeen percent of HPE cases have mutations in the human homolog of a gene first identified in *Drosophila* and designated Sonic hedgehog (*SHH*).

In humans, *SHH* is expressed in the ventral neural tube and in the forebrain. A chromosome microdeletion associated with HPE was mapped to chromosome 7q36. Linkage studies in families with HPE confirmed the presence of a candidate gene in the 7q36 region. Since the *SHH* gene maps to chromosome 7q36, DNA from HPE patients was analyzed for *SHH* mutations. Ming et al. (2002) reported that heterozygous *SHH* mutations are present in 30% of cases of familial HPE but in only 3.7% of sporadic cases.

SHH is secreted as a proprotein, and it undergoes autocatalytic cleavage to yield a 19 kDa N-terminal protein and a 19 kDa C-terminal protein. Cholesterol binds to the C-terminal end of the SHH protein. It is interesting to note that HPE-like manifestations may occur following exposure to inhibitors of cholesterol biosynthesis and in humans with genetic defects involving cholesterol biosynthesis, e.g., Smith-Lemli-Opitz syndrome (Smith et al. 1964) (this syndrome is discussed in Chapter 4). The SHH signaling network interactions require addition not only of cholesterol to the C-terminal end of SHH but also of fatty acids, usually palmitic acid, to the N-terminal end (Tian et al. 2005). The lipid form of the SHH protein is further modified by the gene product DISP1, and it is then available as a signaling molecule.

Sonic-Hedgehog Receptors, Regulators, and Effectors

The transmembrane proteins Patched (PTC) and Smoothened (SMO) apparently function as SHH receptors. The PTC protein is a negative regulator of SHH signaling, while SMO is a positive regulator. The PTC protein inhibits signaling by blocking the action of SMO. The transcriptional effector of SHH signaling is a microtubule-associated zinc finger protein. The human homologs of this gene are known as glioma oncogene (*GLI*) genes. Zinc finger proteins have a characteristic repeating amino acid motif that forms a fingerlike structure that interacts with DNA. The protein folding that leads to formation of this structure may be elicited by zinc. Zinc finger proteins often act as transcription factors.

The *GLI3* gene is mutated in the human malformation syndromes acrocallosal syndrome and Greig syndrome. These disorders are characterized by absence of the corpus callosum, macrocephaly, hypertelorism (widely spaced eyes), cognitive deficits, and skeletal abnormalities including polydactyly (Wallis and Muenke 1999; Dahmane et al. 2001).

Other proteins that play a role in the transcriptional effector function of SHH include serine threonine kinases and a transcriptional coactivator that contains histone acetyltransferase. The end result of SHH signaling is modulation of gene expression. Gene targets of SHH signaling include the human homologs of the *Drosophila* Wingless (*WNT*) and Engrailed EN (*ENT*) genes (Wallis and Muenke 1999).

It is likely that mutations in other proteins in the SHH signaling pathway play a role in HPE. Stone et al. (1996) described HPE associated with a mutation in the *PTC* gene.

Chromosome Rearrangements in Holoprosencephaly and Associated Genes

Based on the presence of recurrent chromosome rearrangements in association with HPE, it is likely that genes in a least nine different chromosome regions play a role in HPE. These loci are listed in Table 3–1.

The ZIC2 Gene

The *ZIC2* gene maps on chromosome 13q32. Mutations in *ZIC2* associated with HPE include heterozygous insertions, deletions, frameshift and nonsense mutations, and expansions of an alanine repeat. Brown et al. (1998) reported that patients with *ZIC2* mutations often have mild facial dysmorphology, including hypotelorism, flat nasal bridge, and microcephaly. The *ZIC2* gene is expressed in the neuroepithelium and in the ventral midline of the neural tube. It apparently interacts with the gene targets of SHH signaling.

Homeotic Gene SIX3

The homeotic gene *SIX3* maps to chromosome 2p21. Heterozygous deletions or missense mutations in the homeodomain of *SIX3* lead to HPE. Mutations in *SIX3* occur in both familial and sporadic cases of HPE (Wallis et al. 1999). The clinical phenotype even within a single family is variable and may range from alobar HPE to microphthalmia associated with mi-

Table 3–1
Gene Loci and Chromosome Regions Associated with Holoprosencephaly (HPE)

Locus	Chromosome Region
HPE1	21q22.3
HPE2	2p21
HPE3	7q36
HPE4	18p
HPE5	13q32
HPE6	3p24-pter
HPE7	9q22.3
HPE8	14q13
HPE9	20p13

It is possible that deletions or translocations in these regions delete, interrupt, or alter the expression of HPE genes. Specific HPE-determining genes were identified in the 13q32 and in the 2p21 regions.

crocephaly and mental retardation. The phenotype may include bilateral cleft lip and cleft palate. The *SIX3* gene is expressed in the rostral neural plate, ventral forebrain, and developing eye. Genes in the *SIX* family apparently participate in transcriptional activation. Dubourg et al. (2004), in a study of 200 patients with HPE, identified eight patients with mutations in the *SIX3* gene.

Transforming Growth Factor Interacting Factor

The gene encoding human transforming growth factor–interacting factor (TGIF) maps to chromosome 18p11.3. TGIF is an atypical homeodomain protein. Heterozygous deletions and missense mutations in TGIF lead to HPE. TGIF is present in the cell nucleus, and it modulates the TGF-β signaling pathway by forming a complex with two members of that pathway, SMAD2 and SMAD4 (Melhuish and Wotton 2000). It also forms complexes with retinol binding protein II and plays a role in gene transcription mediated by retinoic acid. This is of interest given the observation that prenatal retinoic acid exposure leads to HPE (Cohen and Shiota 2002).

Schizencephaly

In schizencephaly there are full-thickness clefts in the cerebral hemisphere. The clefts may be unilateral or bilateral. The walls of the clefts are lined with gray matter. Clinical manifestations of schizencephaly include mental retardation, seizures, altered muscle tone (hypotonia or spasticity), speech defects, and blindness. At least 17 patients have been reported in the literature where mutations in the homeobox gene *EMX2* lead to sporadic schizencephaly (Granata et al. 1997; Faiella et al. 1997).

Septo-Optic Dysplasia

The cardinal features of septo-optic dysplasia are hypoplasia of the optic nerve and dysgenesis of the septum pellucidum that divides the two lateral ventricles. Functional defects in the pituitary and hypothalamus occur in more than 60% of patients.

Based on the observation that septo-optic dysplasia occurs in mice with defects in the *Hesx1* gene (homeobox-containing, embryonic stem cell transcription factor), Dattani et al. (1998) examined the human homolog of this gene in two consanguineous families with several members affected and in 18 sporadic cases. They identified a *HESX1* mutation in one consanguineous family. Carvalho et al. (2003) identified a *HESX1* mutation in a female child with septo-optic dysplasia. She was the offspring of consanguineous parents. This finding suggests that septo-optic dysplasia due to *HESX1* mutations represents a recessively inherited conditions (see Table 3–2).

Table 3-2
Homeotic Gene Mutations Associated with Brain Malformations

Homeobox Gene	Brain Malformation
SIX3	Holoprosencephaly
EMX2	Schizencephaly
HEXS1	Septo-optic dysplasia
PAX6	Polymicrogyria and aniridia
ARX	Lissencephaly, mid-brain malformations

Polymicrogyria

Polymicrogyria is a malformation of cortical development in which normal gyri are replaced by multiple small gyri, separated by shallow sulci, in specific regions of the brain. Histological analysis reveals that in the small gyri a four-layered cortex or an unlayered cortex replaces the normal six-layered cortex. The most common form of polymicrogyria occurs bilaterally in the perisylvian region. The sylvian sulcus is the posterior, inferior boundary of the frontal lobe. It lies on the undersurface of the brain and marks the boundary of the frontal and temporal lobes. Frontal and occipital polymicrogyria occur but are rare.

Villard et al. (2002) reported that, on the basis of brain magnetic resonance imaging (MRI) analyses, polymicrogyria occurs with a frequency of 1 per 2500 live births. Clinical manifestations of this disorder include mental retardation, epilepsy, and neurological deficits. Bilateral perisylvian polymicrogyria is associated with a typical clinical picture first described by Kuzniecky and colleagues in 1993. Features of this syndrome include mild mental retardation, epilepsy, and pseudobulbar palsy leading to difficulties in feeding and in articulation of language.

Polymicrogyria may be due to environmental or genetic factors. Environmental factors include cytomegalovirus infection and vascular perfusion deficits, e.g., due to twinning. Genetic factors include biochemical deficits, e.g., peroxisomal disorders such as Zellweger syndrome. Temporal polymicrogyria was reported in patients with deleterious mutations in the *PAX6* homeotic gene (Mitchell et al. 2003). Familial forms of polymicrogyria occur.

Villard et al. (2002) reported results of linkage analysis in five families in whom perisylvian polymicrogyria segregated as an X-linked trait. Affected subjects were predominantly male. Females were less commonly affected and, if affected, their symptoms were milder. Results of genotyping revealed that perisylvian polymicrogyria mapped to Xq28 distal to the marker DXS8103.

Piao and coworkers (2002) studied two consanguineous families from Palestine where a number of children manifested bilateral frontoparietal polymicrogyria. In these families, the disorder segregated as an autosomal recessive trait since the parents of the affected children did not manifest symptoms. Clinical symptoms included developmental delay, mild to moderate mental retardation, tonic-clonic seizures, oculomotor abnormalities, increased muscle tone, and mild ataxia. Head growth was normal, and the children did not have dysmorphic features. Results of genotyping and linkage analyses suggested linkage to chromosome 16q. Extended analysis of markers on 16q revealed that affected individuals within each pedigree were homozygous for a series of markers between 16q12.2 and 16q21, indicating that the polymicrogyria in these two families was likely recessively inherited.

These mapping studies will facilitate identification of the causative genes for the X-linked form of perisylvian polymicrogyria that maps to Xq28 and the autosomal recessive form of bilateral frontoparietal polymicrogyria that maps to the 16q12.2–16q21 region.

Lissencephaly

In lissencephaly, the normal folds in the brain that lead to gyri and sulci are not present.

Mutations in ARX, the X-Linked Human Homolog of the Drosophila Homeobox Gene Aristaless

Gene mutations in *ARX* lead to a variety of different manifestations that vary in severity. The phenotypic consequences of *ARX* gene mutations differ depending upon the nature of the mutation and its position within the gene (Sherr 2003). Mutations associated with premature transcription termination and with loss of a functional product lead to a syndrome characterized by X-linked lissencephaly, seizures, mental retardation, and ambiguous genitalia. Life span in these patients is shortened. Brain abnormalities include not only lissencephaly but also malformations of the midbrain, particularly the thalamus and hypothalamus. Cavities may occur in the caudate and putamen. Female carriers of the *ARX* truncating mutation frequently have agenesis of the corpus callosum and cognitive levels that range from normal to severely impaired. They may also be prone to epileptic seizures.

ARX mutations that do not lead to premature transcription termination are associated with mental retardation only, with or without autistic features, or in some cases with a constellation of symptoms referred to as Partington syndrome: mental retardation, myoclonic epilepsy, and spasticity. Non-truncating *ARX* mutations associated with mental retardation only or with mental retardation and seizures include GCG triplet expansion leading to polyalanine expansion in the ARX protein. Mutations leading to amino acid substitutions both within and outside of the homeotic domain may be associated with mental retardation. Poirier et al. (2004) analyzed ARX expression in the central nervous system. They reported that in the early stages of development a large number of neurons in the cortex express ARX. Later in development, in postnatal life, and in the adult, ARX expression occurs predominantly in regions that are rich in γ-aminobutyric acid-ergic (GABAergic) neurons. Poirier et al. (2004) postulate that ARX mutations lead to aberrant location or dysfunction of GABAergic receptors and to seizures, which commonly occur in patients.

Lissencephaly Associated with Other Structural Brain Anomalies and Muscle Disease

In lissencephaly, the normal folds in the brain that lead to gyri and sulci are not present. Cobblestone lissencephaly occurs in Walker-Warburg syndrome (WWS) and in Fukuyama congenital muscular dystrophy (FMD). This form of lissencephaly results when migrating postmitotic neurons fail to respond to stop signals and migrate through the neocortex and the glial limiting membrane to the subarachnoid space. Lamination of the cortex is absent in these syndromes, and the brain surface is irregular. The term *lissencephaly* is applied because normal cortical folding is not present.

Cobblestone Lissencephalies: Walker-Warburg Syndrome, Fukuyama Muscular Dystrophy

The most severe of the cobblestone lissencephalies is WWS. Other structural brain anomalies in this syndrome include agenesis of the corpus callosum, fusion of the cerebral hemispheres, cerebellar hypoplasia, dilation of the fourth ventricle, and hydrocephalus. Congenital muscular dystrophy and eye abnormalities are also characteristic of WWS. A similar constellation of defects is found in FMD and in muscle-eye-brain disease (MEB). Patients with WWS are very severely developmentally delayed and usually die before the third year of life.

Beltran-Valero and coworkers (2002) carried out homozygosity mapping studies in 10 consanguineous families with WWS. They determined that candidate regions of homozygosity existed, but no unique locus emerged. Further progress in identifying the gene responsible for this syndrome occurred later, following progress in defining the genetic etiology of the closely related disorders FMD and MEB (see below).

In the Japanese population, FMD has a high prevalence; it is characterized by severe muscle weakness and contractures of the hip, ankle, and knee joints that appear before 1 year of age. Ophthalmological lesions include abnormal eye movements, myopia, and cataract. Patients exhibit severe mental retardation, with intelligence quotient (IQ) scores between 30 and 50. Brain malformations include lissencephaly, pachygyria, agyria, and polymicrogyria in the cerebral hemisphere and cerebellum. Histological studies reveal absence of the normal six-layered cortex. Interhemispheric fusion and ventricular dilation may occur. The corticospinal tracts often exhibit hypoplasia. Pons hypoplasia and cerebellar cysts may occur (Toda and Kobayashi 1999; Toda et al. 2000).

Based on the description of a patient who had FMD and a rare skin disorder, xeroderma pigmentosum, that mapped to chromosome 9q, Toda and coworkers (2000) undertook an analysis of chromosome 9q polymorphic markers in 35 families with FMD. This study revealed that the disorder maps to chromosome 9q31. Through examination of haplotypes in 17 consanguineous families, the authors determined that all affected individuals had the same allele at each marker within a 200 kb region of chromosome 9q31. These findings strongly supported their proposition that the disease arose in a single founder in the Japanese population. Toda and coworkers (2000) analyzed patient DNA with a series of genomic DNA probes from this region. One of these probes identified a 3 kb insertion that occurred in all affected individuals and only in only 1 of 88 unaffected individuals. This probe was used to isolate a cDNA probe. This cDNA probe hybridized to mRNA from brain and muscle. Northern blot analysis of mRNA from patient tissues revealed much weaker hybridization. Sequence analysis of the gene represented by this cDNA clone revealed mutations in patients with FMD. Two independent mutations were found. One was a nonsense mutation in exon 3, and the other was a 2 bp deletion in exon 4. The protein encoded by this gene was designated Fukutin. The precise function of this protein is as yet unknown; most likely it plays a role in glycosylation (Kobayashi et al. 2001).

Beltran-Valero et al. (2002) described two Turkish patients with WWS who had mutations in the Fukutin-encoding gene.

Muscle Eye Brain Disease

A developmental disorder, MEB is characterized by congenital muscular dystrophy, brain malformations, mental retardation, and eye abnormalities including glaucoma and myopia. The brain exhibits evidence of disordered neuronal migration, such as pachygyria, a condition in which gyri are larger than normal. Cerebellar hypoplasia is also often present. This disorder has a higher prevalence rate in Finland than in any other country. Taniguchi et al. (2003) reported that it also occurs in Japan and Korea.

Linkage analysis and homozygosity mapping in families with MEB revealed that the gene responsible for this disorder maps to chromosome 1p32–p34 (Cormand et al. 1999).

In MBED and WWS, no α-dystroglycan is detectable on immunohistochemical analysis of skeletal muscle with an antibody to the glycosylated form of α-dystroglycan. This observation led Yoshida et al. (2001) to examine gene loci in the chromosome 1p31.3-p34 region where MEB maps, to determine if there was a locus involved in glycosylation. They determined that the gene encoding the enzyme O-linked mannose β-1,2N-acetylglucosaminyltransferase 1 (POMTGnT1) maps in this region. Molecular genetic analysis of DNA from patients with MEB established that this disorder is due to loss-of-function mutations in the gene encoding POMTGnT1.

Taniguchi et al. (2003) reported that POMTGnT1 mutations occur not only in Finnish patients with MEB but also in patients of Italian, Belgian, Turkish, Korean, and Japanese descent. They noted that a broad range of clinical phenotypes occurs in this disorder. Mutations in the 5' region of the POMTGnT1-encoding gene are associated with severe brain defects. Failure of binding of mannose to laminins and to molecules in the extracellular matrix may be responsible for abnormalities in muscle function and for abnormal migration of neurons in the developing brain (Akasaka-Manya et al. 2004).

Disorders of Glycosylation

Jacken et al. (1997) and Jaeken and Matthijs (2001) described congenital disorders of glycosylation. Glycans (polysaccharide complexes) are synthesized in the Golgi apparatus of the cell, and they are then covalently attached to other molecules including proteins and lipids. The most common form of linkage of glycans to proteins is N linkage, where the glycan moiety is attached to the amide group of the amino acid via N-acetylglucosamine. Glycans may also link to proteins in O linkages, where the saccharide moiety, e.g. N-acetylglucosamine or mannose, links to the hydroxyl group of serine or threonine. Among the few proteins known to exhibit O-mannosyl glycan linkages are α-dystroglycan, neural cell adhesion molecule, and Tenascin J (Jaeken 2003, Jaeken 2004a,b).

Based on the observation that a glycosylation defect causes MEBD, Beltran-Valero and coworkers (2002) used a combined homozygosity mapping and candidate gene approach to isolate the gene responsible for WWS. They established that the polymorphic marker D9S64, which shows genetic linkage to this syndrome, is located in intron 2 of the glycosylation-determining gene *POMT*. They demonstrated mutations in *POMT* in 5 of 15 consanguineous families. Subsequent studies revealed mutations in this gene in 6 of 30 WWS patients in nonconsanguineous families. Figure 3–4 illustrates defects in O-mannosyl glycan synthesis in WWS and MEB.

L1CAM Mutations Leading to X-Linked Hydrocephalus

Mutations in the neural cell adhesion molecule L1CAM lead to a group of disorders with overlapping clinical phenotypes. Manifestations include congenital hydrocephalus, mental retardation, hypoplasia or agenesis of the corpus callosum and corticospinal tracts, spastic paraplegia, and adducted (flexed) thumb. L1CAM phenotypes are inherited as X-linked recessive traits (Finckh et al. 2000; Weller and Gartner 2001).

L1CAM is expressed in neurons and Schwann cells, and it plays an important role in the development and function of the nervous system. L1CAM molecules serve as guidance forces during axonal growth (Kamiguchi 2003). In the mature nervous system, L1CAM molecules contribute to neuronal cell

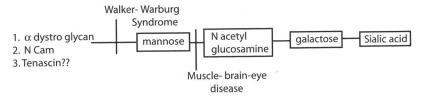

Figure 3–4. Glycans are attached to proteins through mannose and *N*-acetylglucosamine linkages. Defects in *O*-mannosyl glycan synthesis occur in Walker-Warburg syndrome and muscle eye brain disease (Beltran-Valero et al. 2002).

survival and function and particularly to long-term potentiation (Kenwrick et al. 2000).

Kutsche et al. (2002) summarized the results of comprehensive mutation analysis of the *L1CAM* gene in patients. They reported that 70%–75% of mutations are single nucleotide substitutions. The remaining mutations are predominantly short-length gene rearrangements leading to exon deletion. Kutsche et al. noted that the deletions in the *L1CAM* gene are located near the ends of L1 and Alu repetitive elements. They postulate that deletions result from non-homologous recombination between paired chromosomes during female meiosis. Mutations in the *L1CAM* gene region, which encodes the extracellular domain of the protein, are less deleterious than mutations in gene regions that encode the protein domains that are located within the cell.

Joubert Syndrome

Joubert syndrome is characterized clinically by neonatal breathing difficulties, hypotonia, oculomotor abnormalities, and mental retardation. The characteristic brain abnormality in Joubert syndrome is partial agenesis of the vermis, a structure located in the midline between the two cerebellar hemispheres. The malformed vermis takes on a typical appearance, the form of a molar tooth, which is readily distinguished on MRI. Clinical heterogeneity exists in Joubert syndrome. Some patients manifest other developmental defects, including ocular colobomas, retinal blindness, polydactyly, cystic changes, and fibrosis in the liver. Cortical polymicrogyria may also be present. Collectively, these different clinical forms are referred to as Joubert syndrome and related disorders.

Underlying the clinical heterogeneity there is locus heterogeneity. Defects at three different loci, JBTS1, -2, and -3, lead to clinical manifestations of Joubert syndrome. JBTS1 maps to 9q34.3, JBTS2 maps to 11p12-11p13.3, and JBTS3 maps to 6p23. In patients with JBTS3, cortical polymicrogyria is frequently present.

Dixon-Salazar et al. (2004) described studies in 18 consanguineous families. In each family, there were several affected individuals with Joubert syndrome. Prior linkage studies revealed that the disease locus in these families mapped to chromosome 6p23. They therefore concentrated their analyses on this chromosomal region. Using DNA markers, Dixon-Salazar et al. defined the smallest region of homozygosity that was common to all of the families. They then examined candidate genes in this region. This led to identification of frameshift mutations in a gene previously mapped to this region and designated *AHI1* (Abelson helper integration 1). The gene name was based on previous reports that the Abelson leukemia virus frequently integrated at this site.

In one family from Palestine, a frameshift mutation occurred in exon 8 of *AHI1*. In two families from Kuwait, a T1328A missense mutation leading to amino acid substitution V443D was present in exon 10. In a Turkish family, a dinucleotide deletion, 1188-1189delTG, occurred in the sequence that encodes exon 10. Dixon-Salazar et al. (2004) named the protein formed by the *AHI1* gene Jouberin. They studied expression of this protein in mouse brain and determined that it is predominantly expressed in the cerebellum and forebrain and that maximal expression occurs in late embryogenesis.

Ferland et al. (2004) reported that a V443D mutation occurred in the *AHI1* protein in a family from Saudi Arabia with several individuals with Joubert syndrome.

Elucidation of the precise function of this protein in the brain and of the pathogenesis of the malformation in Joubert syndrome await further research.

4

Mental Retardation Associated with Dysmorphology, Growth Retardation, or Overgrowth

Mental retardation associated with facial dysmorphology, congenital malformation, and growth retardation or overgrowth may be due to gene dosage imbalance. Extra copies of genes may result from the presence of an extra chromosome, e.g., trisomy 21. Dosage changes may also result from the presence of an extra chromosomal segment or from loss of a chromosomal segment. Contiguous gene syndromes are disorders where dosage changes in a number of genes that map within a chromosomal segment are thought to play a role in producing the characteristic clinical features of the syndrome. Syndromes characterized by mental retardation, growth retardation, and dysmorphology may also result from defects in specific single genes.

The discovery by Lejeune et al. (1959a,b) that Down syndrome resulted from trisomy 21 represented a landmark in our understanding of the role of chromosomes in mental retardation. Subsequently, abnormalities of sex chromosome number were reported to be associated with mild or severe mental retardation. During the past few decades, advances in cytogenetics and molecular genetic techniques have led to the recognition of a growing number of segmental chromosomal changes that lead to gene dosage changes and to specific syndromes. Gene dosage changes may involve deletion of a specific chromosomal segment or duplication of a segment. Molecular genetic techniques have facilitated identification of specific genes that are interrupted as a result of structural chromosomal changes such as breakage and rearrangement, inversion, or translocation of chromosomal segments. Many structural chromosomal changes lead to developmental delay, mental retardation, and varying degrees of dysmorphology.

Based on the use of standardized chromosomal banding techniques for karyotype analysis, Curry et al. (1997) reported that at least 12% of cases of mental retardation are due to chromosomal abnormalities. Standardized banding techniques will not detect abnormalities that are less than 2 Mb in size. Furthermore, conventional cytogenetic methods will not detect rearrangements that do not alter banding patterns. As more sophisticated methods of chromosome analysis developed, it became clear that the incidence of chromosomal abnormalities in mental retardation is in fact much higher.

Methodologies that provide a more comprehensive analysis of chromosomes include fluorescence in situ hybridization (FISH). In FISH analysis, deoxyribonucleic acid (DNA) probes for specific genes or chromosome segments, including subtelomeric regions of chromosomes, are directly hybridized to metaphase chromosomes of interphase nuclei on microscope slides. A number of different chromosome analysis methods make use of quantitative comparisons of chromosomal segments in DNA from controls and test subjects, e.g., comparative genomic hybridization. Loss or gain of specific chromosomal regions may also be indicated through DNA analysis of children and their parents using polymerase chain reaction to identify polymorphic DNA markers.

Chromosomal segments that are deleted or duplicated as a result of chromosomal rearrangements often contain a number of different genes. Dosage alteration in each specific gene may contribute to the phenotype. Examples of disorders where multiple contiguous genes each play a role in the generation of the final phenotype include Williams syndrome and Langer-Giedion syndrome. In these instances, the phenotype varies as the size and exact position of the deletion varies in different patients (Lupski 1998).

In several instances, detailed molecular analysis of the specific chromosomal changes in a group of patients with the phenotypic manifestations of a specific syndrome led to the conclusion that one gene in a particular chromosomal region is responsible for the predominant features of the phenotype. In Rubinstein-Taybi syndrome, e.g., the gene encoding the cyclic adenosine monophosphate (cAMP) responsive element binding protein (CREB) binding protein is disrupted as a result of deletion or chromosomal rearrangement (Coupry et al. 2004). This syndrome may also result from point mutations in the CREB binding protein gene (Bartsch et al. 2002).

It is important to consider that deletions or duplication may lead not only to loss of coding sequences or the presence of excess coding sequences but also to dosage changes of regulatory sequences.

A region-specific chromosomal deletion or duplication may also exhibit different effects depending on whether the change arose on a maternal or a paternal chromosome. This is the case, e.g., in chromosomal rearrangements in the 15q11–q13 region. In this region, a number of genes are imprinted so that they are expressed only from one member of the chromosome pair, i.e., the maternally derived chromosome or the paternally derived chromosome. If, for example, a deletion eliminates a maternally derived allele of the *UBE3A* gene on chromosome 15q12, Angelman syndrome results (Matsuura et al. 1997).

Chromosomes are composed of chromatin, and there is a growing body of evidence that chromatin remodeling plays an important role in gene expression. In recent years, several disorders of chromatin remodeling associated with mental retardation have been described. In the following section, I will review the more common aberrations of chromosomes and chromatin associated with mental retardation.

Chromosomal Aneuploidies Associated with Mental Retardation

Down Syndrome

John Langdon Down first described the clinical features of this syndrome in 1866. Characteristic features include upslanting palpebral fissures, small round head, small mouth, large tongue, flattened nasal bridge, incurving fifth finger (*clinodactyly*), single palmar crease, and spots on the iris (*Brushfield spots*). Many of these features of Down syndrome are present at birth. Congenital heart disease, particularly atrioventricular canal defects or septal defects, occurs in 45% of patients (Jones 1997).

Early developmental milestones may be achieved at appropriate times. Children experience special difficulties with language. Intelligence quotient (IQ) scores range from low normal to severely retarded, 85–20. Birth weight, length, and head circumference are usually between the tenth and fifteenth percentiles. By 3 years of age, most children are more than 3 standard deviations below average height and head circumference. Puberty usually occurs at the appropriate time, and final adult height is 56–60 inches. Down syndrome adults tend to be overweight.

Down syndrome patients may experience a number of other medical problems. These include gastrointestinal defects, duodenal atresia, celiac disease, enlarged colon, hypothyroidism; hearing loss frequently due to otitis media; ophthalmic disorders, including strabismus, nystagmus, congenital cataract, glaucoma; immune system deficiencies, particularly cell-mediated immune deficiencies; and higher frequency and earlier presentation of Alzheimer's disease than the normal population (Jones 1997; Holland et al. 2000). Trisomy 21 present in a G-banded karyotype is shown in Figure 4–1. Figure. 4–2 illustrates trisomy 21 resulting from a translocation between chromosomes 21 and 14.

A number of investigators have carried out studies on patients with partial trisomy 21, i.e., two intact copies of chromosome 21 plus an additional chromosome comprised of only part of chromosome 21. The purpose of these studies was to determine if specific segments of chromosome 21 contributed to specific aspects of the syndrome. Data collected by Olson et al. (2004) indicate that typical Down syndrome craniofacial features cannot be accounted for by duplication of any specific segment of the chromosome.

In 2000, Hattori et al. published the complete DNA sequence of chromosome 21. Availability of DNA sequence information has facilitated analysis of the structure and function of specific genes on chromosome 21 that may play a role in Down syndrome. Barlow et al. (2001a,b) studied patients with congenital heart disease and partial trisomy of chromosome 21. They defined a region on 21q22.3 that, when present in three copies, leads to congenital heart disease. They identified a candidate gene that likely plays a role in the pathogenesis of congenital heart defects. This gene encodes chromosome 21

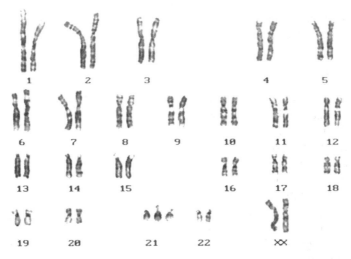

Figure 4–1. Trisomy 21 present in a G-banded karyotype. (Chromosome preparation and photography by K. W. Dumars and G. Dumars)

encoded cell adhesion molecule (DSCAM), which is expressed in the heart during development. It is also expressed in brain.

The phenotypic manifestations of Down syndrome are attributed to increased dosage of genes on chromosome 21. Several investigators have reported results of analyses on brain tissue from Down fetuses and control fetuses of the protein product levels of genes encoded by chromosome 21 genes. They determined that for a high proportion of chromosome 21 gene products the expression levels in Down fetuses do not differ from those in controls. Cheon et al. (2003) studied expression levels of six proteins in Down syndrome fetuses and controls. They determined that only one of the six proteins, Synaptojanin 1, exhibited increased levels of expression. Synaptojanin 1 is a polyphosphoinositide phosphatase that plays a role in synaptic vesicle trafficking, exocytosis, and endocytosis. It acts as a phosphatase that converts phosphatidylinositol-4,5-biphosphate (PIP2) to phosphatidylinositol monophosphate (PIP1). Synaptojanin also influences cytoskeletal organization through its effects on actin filaments (Sakisaka et al. 1997).

Arai et al. (2002) reviewed the neuropathology in Down syndrome. They noted that Down syndrome is characterized by congenital and developmental abnormalities as well as age-related neuropathology. Congenital and developmental neuropathology includes reduction in the number of granular cells in the cortex, reduction in the number of dendritic spines, and presence of aberrant spines. Age-related neuropathology includes the early formation of senile plaques and neurofibrillary tangles in the frontal cortex and hippocampus. Arai et al. (2002) reported that synaptojanin is expressed in cortical

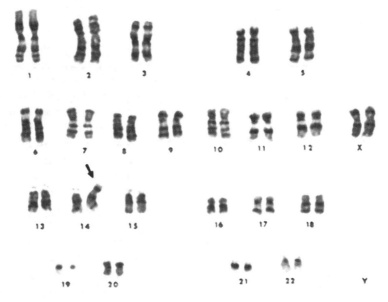

Figure 4–2. Trisomy 21 and translocation of chromosomes 21 and 14. (Chromosome preparation and photography by K. W. Dumars and G. Dumars)

plate neurons, intermediate neurons, germinal matrix cells, and the Cajal-Retzius cells in the fetal cerebrum. After birth, the highest levels detected by antibodies are in the neuronal cytoplasm.

Based on its widespread and early expression, Arai et al. (2002) proposed a broader physiological role for synaptojanin. They suggest that it is involved not only in synaptic recycling but also in the regulation of neuronal migration and synaptogenesis during fetal life.

Of particular interest to analysis of the neuronal manifestations in Down syndrome is the identification of the human gene corresponding to a gene first described in *Drosophila* and C. elegans and designated Minibrain, *Mnb* (Pang et al. 2004). In vertebrates, *MNB* expression is restricted to neurons. The timing and localization of *MNB* gene expression correlate with the final stage of neuronal differentiation and with dendritic tree development (Hammerle et al. 2003). In the dendritic tree, the MNB protein colocalizes with the protein DYN, a guanosine triphosphatase (GTPase) that plays a role in membrane trafficking. Neurons in Down syndrome undergo a dramatic cessation of dendritic growth late in fetal development. The final result of this is dendritic shortening and atrophy of neurons. Hammerle et al. (2003) emphasized the critical role that dendrites play in the development of the nervous system. Dendrites are essential for synaptogenesis and neuronal innervation.

Sex Chromosome Abnormalities

In considering the phenotype in sex chromosome anomalies, it is important to take the phenomenon of X-chromosome inactivation into account. Female mammals have two X chromosomes, and male mammals have one X and one Y chromosome. The Y chromosome in males is approximately half the size of the X chromosome. Furthermore, the Y chromosome is composed of many repetitive DNA elements and relatively few expressed genes. In nuclei of female mammals, one member of the pair of X chromosomes is inactivated over much of its length. Inactivation of one X chromosome in female mammals likely serves as a dosage compensation mechanism. The inactivated X chromosome is visible as a densely staining heterochromatic structure that adheres to the nuclear membrane. In each nucleus, all X chromosomes but one are inactivated in the nucleus. Thus, in individuals with three X chromosomes, there are two Barr bodies; in individuals with four X chromosomes three Barr bodies are present. In the case of structurally abnormal X chromosomes, for example, X chromosomes that are deleted, duplicated, or rearranged, the structurally abnormal chromosome is inactivated. In X-autosome translocations, the normal X chromosome is usually preferentially inactivated. In this way, the autosome that is translocated to the X chromosome is protected from inactivation.

On the inactive X chromosome, at least 40 genes escape inactivation. A large proportion of these genes are located on the distal part of the X short arm in a segment of DNA of approximately 15 Mb in length. Genes in this region are highly homologous to genes on the Y chromosome and are known as "pseudoautosomal" genes. Approximately one-third of the genes on Xp outside the pseudoautosomal region do not undergo inactivation; this includes a region encoding six genes that is located in Xp11.2. There are also genes at the end of the long arm of the X chromosome that do not undergo inactivation (Willard 2001). The fact that a significant number of genes on the X chromosome fail to undergo inactivation likely accounts for the abnormal phenotype observed in patients with an extra X chromosome. Furthermore, the phenotypic consequences of extra copies of segments of the X chromosome are likely to be more severe in cases where extra copies of Xp are present (Willard 2001).

The imprint control region, XIC, located on Xq13, determines the earliest steps in X-chromosome inactivation, (Brown 1991; Brown and Greally 2003). It is approximately 1 Mb in length and contains several elements that play a role in X inactivation (Clerc and Avner 2003). One of these elements, known as XIST, produces a 17 kb noncoding ribonucleic acid (RNA) that is essential for X-chromosome inactivation. The XIST RNA coats the X chromosome. Stabilization of inactivation is apparently achieved through recruitment of protein complexes to the inactivating chromosome. Thereafter, global hypoacetylation of histone occurs. A histone H2 variant, macroH2, replaces histone H2 in chromatin, and changes in the methylation pattern of histone occur. Hypermethylation of DNA then occurs at CpG dinucleotides (Avner and Heard 2001). Inactivation is in part regulated by TSIX, a reverse antisense transcript of XIST. It is one of the factors that regulate the function of XIST. It binds to XIST and blocks its expression.

There is evidence that the first function of XIC is a counting one, by which the ratio of the number of X chromosomes to autosomes is determined (Clere and Auner 2003). Counting ensures that only one X chromosome in each diploid cell is inactivated. Selection of the chromosome to be inactivated is influenced by another controlling element in the XIC region, known as XCE (Debrand et al. 1999).

XXY Klinefelter Syndrome and Variants

The IQ range in males with XXY Klinefelter syndrome is usually in the low normal range. In individual XXY patients, it is most often lower than that of sibling controls. Geschwind et al. (2000) reported that Klinefelter patients score below normal controls in language skills and verbal processing; their motor dexterity is frequently reduced compared with controls. Samango-Sprouse (2001) postulated that difficulties in language processing and expression in male Klinefelter patients led them to be at increased risk for social interaction difficulties. Speech delays and decreased verbal IQ are more pronounced in XXXY male patients.

Gonadal and hormonal dysfunction is an important feature of Klinefelter syndrome (Jacobs and Strong 1959). During infancy, testicular histology is normal; however, germ cell loss occurs throughout childhood, though some germ cells may persist beyond puberty. Testosterone levels are low in 50% of cases. Luteinizing hormone and follicle-stimulating hormone levels are elevated. These elevations may result in gonadotrophin stimulation and may partly normalize testosterone levels. Decrease in testosterone levels is more striking in XXXY male patients.

In children with Klinefelter syndrome, diagnosis is most commonly made when they present with behavioral problems; in adolescence, it may be made during the course of an evaluation of delayed puberty (Simpson et al. 2003). Adults are most commonly diagnosed during evaluation for infertility or gynecomastia (Allanson and Graham 2002).

Analysis of DNA polymorphisms revealed a parental origin of the extra X chromosome in 98% of cases (Hassold et al. 1985). In 50% of cases, the extra X chromosome arose in paternal meiosis. In 48% of cases, the extra X chromosome was maternal in origin. There is no evidence that paternal age is correlated with Klinefelter syndrome. The frequency of X chromosome nondisjunction in female patients is correlated with increasing maternal age.

XXYY male patients are often tall, and the degree of mental retardation is often severe.

In XYY male patients, the phenotype is normal, and most do not present for genetic evaluation (Iryns et al. 1995). Abramsky and Chapple (1997) reported that those who do present frequently have borderline mental retardation. Psychosocial integration problems occurred in 86% of XXY male subjects who presented with borderline mental retardation.

Effects of an Extra Sex Chromosome

Linden et al. (1995) and Rouet et al. (1995) reviewed the phenotype in subjects with sex chromosome anomalies. They concluded that there is a direct relationship between the number of extra sex chromosomes, X or Y, and the severity of the phenotype.

Warwick et al. (1999) studied 32 adult patients who were reported at birth to have sex chromosome aneuploidy (XXX, XXY, or XYY) and a matched control group. They analyzed IQ and brain volume as determined by MRI. They determined that in all subjects IQ was lower than in the control group. In XXX patients, the mean IQ was 82.5; in the matched XX control group, it was 100.2. The mean IQ in XXY patients was 87.2; in the matched XY control group, it was 101. In XYY patients, the mean IQ was 85; in the matched XY control group, it was 101.2.

Warwick et al. (1999) determined that brain volumes in the XXX and XXY patients were significantly reduced compared with age-matched controls. Brain volume was correlated with IQ. No reduction in brain volume was found in XYY patients. In XXY patients, there was a tendency to enlargement of the lateral ventricles.

XO Turner Syndrome and Variants

Turner syndrome due to the absence of one X chromosome (Jacobs et al. 1960), XO karyotype, is not associated with mental retardation. Verbal intelligence is usually normal; however, deficits in visual-spatial abilities may sometimes occur. Psychosocial adjustment deficits may be present.

Growth rate is reduced in childhood, and no prepubertal growth spurt occurs, resulting in reduced height in adults. Gonadal dysgenesis is present in the majority of patients with this syndrome, and hormone therapy is required at puberty. Dysmorphology is usually absent. Patients may have a broad and sometimes webbed neck and posterior rotation of the ears.

Ring X Turner Syndrome

Jacobs et al. (1997) reported that a significant proportion of patients who present with the Turner phenotype are mosaic: they have an XO cell line and a ring X, r[X], karyotype. A 46XX cell line may also frequently be present in these mosaic patients. Kuntsi et al. (2000) carried out a study on 89 XO Turner patients and on 33 patients with ring X cell lines. They concluded that the presence of a cell line with a ring X chromosome leads to a reduction in cognitive performance and poorer social adjustment: 63% of ring X patients and 38% of XO Turner patients had special education needs; 95% of XO Turner patients and 69% of ring X patients received education in mainstream schools. Most patients with ring X did not meet criteria for mental retardation. They determined that the parental origin of the ring X did not impact verbal or nonverbal IQ.

Kuntsi et al. (2000) analyzed the inactivation status of ring X and determined whether or not the XIST locus was deleted from the ring. Cases with smaller ring X chromosomes that were not inactivated had IQ scores in the 71–99 range. Individuals with extremely small ring X chromosomes that were not inactivated had IQ scores in the 88–102 range. Furthermore, the greater the proportion of cells with a ring X, the more severe the impact on cognitive performance.

In summary, the studies of Kuntsi et al. (2000) indicate that the degree of impairment in IQ is proportional to the size of the active ring and to the number of functional genes. Specific genes that impact brain development have not yet been identified.

The findings received further support from Kubota et al. (2002), who studied Turner syndrome patients who are mosaics for an XO cell line and a ring X cell line. They determined that the severity of mental retardation was directly related to the proportion of cells in which the ring X chromosome was not inactivated.

Segmental Chromosomal Defects

Molecular Mechanisms That Lead to Regional or Segmental Chromosomal Rearrangements and Dosage Changes

Terminal Deletions

Chromosomal breaks in the terminal region usually occur within repetitive DNA elements. Although some chromosomal deletions are described as terminal, they are not strictly speaking terminal since, following deletion, the chromosome breakpoint is healed by the addition of repetitive telomeric sequence elements, $(TTAGGG)_n$. Deletions of chromosome-specific, gene-rich subtelomeric regions play a role in the etiology of a number of syndromes associated with mental retardation.

Interstitial Deletions

Low copy repetitive DNA elements often flank genomic regions that are prone to rearrangement. The DNA sequences of these flanking repeat elements are often highly similar but not identical. Their sequences are sufficiently identical so that nonallelic repeats may align during meiosis.

Repetitive DNA elements may include genes, pseudogenes, and Alu-type repeats. Low copy repetitive elements that predispose to chromosomal rearrangements are particularly common in pericentromeric or in subtelomeric regions.

Aberrant recombination between blocks of closely similar repetitive sequence elements that are linearly ordered on a chromosome pair (nonhomologous recombination) may lead to deletions, duplications, or inversions. Low copy repeats often occur at translocation breakpoints and may play a role in translocation between chromosomes.

Chromosomal breakage leading to rearrangements does not always occur in repetitive DNA elements; it may also occur in unique-sequence DNA. There is some evidence that specific sequence motifs, e.g., TTTAAA, are frequently located at the breakpoints in unique-sequence DNA.

Role of Environmental Factors in Chromosomal Breaks and Rearrangements

There is some evidence that chromosomal breaks and recombination at repetitive elements are influenced by environmental factors. Prader-Willi syndrome is most commonly due to deletions that occur in duplicons comprised of repeats of the *HERC2* gene. Akefeldt et al. (1995) reported an association between paternal hydrocarbon exposure and Prader-Willi syndrome. Schiestl et al. (1994) reported increased genomic recombination at repetitive DNA following exposure to low-dose X-rays.

Terminal Deletions, Duplications, and Rearrangements of Chromosomes in Mental Retardation

Subtle abnormalities involving the telomeric ends of chromosomes are encountered more frequently in subjects with mental retardation than in the population with IQ in the normal range. Pooled data from studies carried out by a number of investigators in different countries indicate that telomeric chromosomal dosage changes occur in 5% of subjects with mental retardation (Flint and Knight 2003). Telomeric imbalances sometimes occur in individuals with normal IQ, and in these cases the imbalance seems to have no phenotypic effect. It is possible that the size and exact position of the chromosomal change play a role in determining long-term consequences. Martin et al. (2002) proposed that in cases where a telomeric imbalance is detected multiple probes within the subtelomeric region should be used to measure the size of dosage changes or telomeric rearrangement. These investigators stressed that in order to determine the relevance of telomeric dosage changes to the clinical phenotypic in a specific patient, it is important to carry out analysis of parental chromosomes and DNA and to assess parental phenotype. It is also important to examine unaffected family members before attributing mental retardation in a patient to a specific subtelomeric rearrangement.

Rossi et al. (2001) and Flint and Knight (2003) noted that in cases where dosage changes and rearrangements at chromosome ends lead to mental retardation, dysmorphic facial features and congenital anomalies are also present. Patients with may also exhibit prenatal or postnatal growth retardation and behavioral problems. Facial dysmorphology among patients with sub-telomeric deletions includes reduced head circumference, hypertelorism, nasal abnormalities, and ear abnormalities. In addition, patients may have hand abnormalities and undescended testes.

Flint and Knight (2003) summarized results of 22 studies of subtelomeric regions in patients with mental retardation. They reported that in approximately half of the mentally retarded probands studied, telomeric deletions occurred de novo, and there was no evidence of similar subtelomeric changes in parents. They reported that familial subtelomeric translocations that were balanced in unaffected family members and unbalanced in affected probands accounted for half of the cases

De Vries et al. (2003) reported that subtelomeric chromosomal changes occurred most frequently among patients who are severely mentally retarded. However, they do sometimes occur in mildly affected individuals. Subtelomeric deletions in specific chromosomal locations may lead to specific phenotypes, e.g., chromosomes 1pter, 4pter, 5pter, 22qter, and 2qter. However, in other subtelomeric regions, the phenotype is not specific (Riegel et al. 2001).

Structure of Telomeric and Subtelomeric Chromosomal Regions

Mefford and Trask (2002) presented a comprehensive review of DNA structures at the ends of chromosomes. They reported that chromosome ends are capped by arrays of short-sequence DNA repeats, $(TTAGGG)_n$. The telomere terminal transferase, a ribonucleoprotein enzyme, adds repeats of the TTAGGG to existing DNA sequences at telomeres.

Within subtelomeres, there are larger blocks of repeat sequence and duplications of these blocks. Genes and pseudogenes located in subtelomeric regions are also prone to duplication. Polymorphisms occur, and different individuals vary with respect to the size and number of blocks of subtelomeric repeats. Sequence within the subtelomeric repeats extends for distances of 10–500 kb, and it is common to most chromosomes.

Polymorphisms are common and different individuals vary in the number of repeats, and this polymorphism leads to variation in the intensity of staining of the telomeric regions. Centromeric of these blocks of repeats, chromosome-specific subtelomeric sequence occurs. DNA probes that are designed to examine subtelomeric regions of individual chromosomes are derived from a sequence located immediately proximal to the subtelomeric region, a sequence that is unique to each chromosome pair.

Contiguous Gene Syndromes Associated with Cognitive Deficits

In contiguous gene syndromes, the phenotype is due to deletion of a number of different genes that lie in close proximity and are usually functionally unrelated. Specific features of the phenotype may vary in different patients with the same syndrome depending on the extent of the deletion and on which specific genes are deleted. The discussion below does not include all known contiguous gene deletion syndromes. Rather, I chose to describe a few contiguous syndromes that play a role in mental retardation and that have been intensely studied to identify the genes involved in the pathogenesis of specific phenotypic features.

A number of disorders initially thought to represent contiguous gene syndromes were later shown to be due to deletions or mutations in one particular gene. One example of this is Smith-Magenis syndrome; Mowat-Wilson syndrome is another example.

Williams Syndrome

In patients with Williams syndrome, the 7q11.23 region is deleted from one member of the chromosome 7 pair. The syndrome is due to deficiency of 25–30 genes (Tassabehji et al. 1999). In most patients, the deletion is 1.5 Mb in length. In a few patients, smaller deletions occur.

Williams syndrome patients have distinct facial features; they are often described as "elfin-like," with wide mouth, full cheeks and lips, and stellate iris pattern. They have mild growth retardation. They often display poor visual motor integration. The IQ ranges 41–80. Williams syndrome patients are described as friendly and outgoing. About 15% of patients are reported to have behavioral problems, most commonly attention-deficit hyperactivity disorder.

Other features of the syndrome that may be present include hypercalcemia, vascular defects (particularly supravalvular aortic stenosis), pulmonary stenosis, and ventricular or atrial septal defects.

Williams syndrome is almost always sporadic; i.e., it is not passed on from parent to offspring. The deletion region is flanked by three low copy repeat elements that contribute to misalignment and unequal crossing over. Bayes et al. (2003) reported that in one-third of cases they found that a parent was heterozygous for inversion of the chromosome 7q11.2 segment between the centromeric and telomeric repeats. They stressed that a parent who is heterozygous for an inversion at 7q11.2 may be at increased risk for producing gametes with a 7q11.2 deletion. There are a few reports of familial cases of Williams syndrome. The most likely explanation for these cases was the presence of parental gonadal mosaicism. In one parent, somatic cells contained a normal chromosome complement. However, in the gonad, two cell lines were present: a normal cell line and a second cell line in which one chromosome 7q11.2 was deleted. A parent with this form of gonadal mosaicism is at risk for having a second child with Williams syndrome.

At least 20 genes map in the Williams syndrome critical region, and a number of investigators have carried out studies to determine whether or not deletion of specific genes contributes to a specific feature of the phenotype. There is evidence that deletion of the Elastin gene plays a role in the pathogenesis of supravalvular aortic stenosis (Morris and Mervis, 2000). This evidence comes both from studies in Williams syndrome and from studies in patients with isolated supravalvular aortic stenosis. The latter patients may have deletions or mutation in the Elastin gene.

Hoogenraad et al. (2004) reported results of studies in mice in which they induced targeted deletions in genes that corresponded to those that map in the Williams syndrome region. They concluded that deletions of two genes, *LIMK1* and *CYLN2* (also known as *CLIP115*), played a key role in generating the neurological features of Williams syndrome. In *Limk1* knockout mice, there are abnormalities of neuronal dendritic spine morphology and abnormalities of synaptic function. The mice exhibited behavioral abnormalities. *LIMK1* is a member of the *LIMK* family of serine threonine kinases. It plays a role in the cytoskeleton and in actin dynamics. *CYLN2* has a microtubular binding domain and appears to play a key role in regulating microtubule behavior. Hoogenraad et al. (2004) proposed that aberrant microtubule dynamics impacts outgrowth of axons and axonal transport.

Chromosome 22q11.2 Deletion Syndrome

Chromosome 22qll.2 deletion syndrome is sometimes referred to as velocardiol facial syndrome or DiGeorge syndrome if the full spectrum of phenotypic abnormalities is present. It is due to haploinsufficiency (deletion of one copy) of the 22q11.2 region. This deletion occurs with an incidence of 1 in 4000 live births, and it is therefore one of the most common segmental deletion syndromes. The phenotypic spectrum in patients with 22q11.2 deletion syndrome includes a variety of manifestations that differ in severity and that occur in different combinations. Characteristic facial features include ocular abnormalities (widely spaced, narrow eyes with heavy eyelids), nasal abnormalities (the nose appears to be divided into two parts), low-set ears and ear lobe abnormalities. Other typical features include cleft palate or submucosal cleft palate, absent or underdeveloped thymus, and parathyroid and congenital heart defects. Patients frequently have learning disabilities and behavioral problems. In children who do not have cardiac defects, learning disabilities and behavioral problems are often the reason for referral for genetic evaluation (Solot et al. 2001). The incidence of psychosis is reported to be higher in patients with 22q11.2 deletions than in the general population (Arnold et al. 2001).

McQuade et al. (1999) described a patient with a 22q11.2 deletion phenotype who had a small chromosomal deletion in the 22q11.2 region that encompassed only two genes, *TBX1* (T box transcription factor) and *COMT* (catechol-O-methyltransferase). Yagi et al. (2003) reviewed the literature and determined that in at least 250 cases with clinical features of the 22q11.2 deletion, investigators found no evidence of chromosome 22 deletions. Yagi et al. then undertook a study of 13 patients with clinical features of 22q11.2 deletion syndrome and no evidence of deletions. They carried out comprehensive FISH analysis to examine the appropriate chromosomal region. They also carried out mutation analysis. In 3 of the 13 patients, they identified mutations in the *TBX1* gene. In each case, the mutation occurred de novo in the patient and was not found in the parents. In two patients, the mutation led to replacement of a highly conserved amino acid. In the third patient, a frameshift mutation was present, and it generated a truncated protein. These three patients each exhibited several features within the spectrum of abnormalities common to the 22q11.2 deletion syndrome.

Yagi et al. (2003) proposed that part of the variability of the phenotype in patients with *TBX1* mutations was related to variability in genes that are regulated by *TBX1*. *TBX1* is a transcription factor. In mice, haploinsufficiency of this syndrome leads to defects in structures derived from the fourth branchial arch. In mice, a phenotype that includes many of the features of the 22q11.2 deletion results when both copies of the *Tbx1* gene are deleted.

Langer-Giedion Syndrome

Langer-Giedion syndrome is also known as trichorhinopharyngeal syndrome type II (TRPS II). It is caused by a microdeletion in the chromosome 8q24.1–8q24.3 region. The Langer-Giedion syndrome phenotype includes unusual facial features, bone changes such as cone-shaped epiphyses in metacarpals and phalanges, bony outgrowths on long bones (*exostoses*), and hypotonia. Mental retardation occurs in 70% of cases. The unusual facial features include heavy eyebrows, deep-set eyes, bulbous nose, thickened nasal septum, simple prominent philtrum, and large protruding ears. Hair is sparse, and skin is loose.

Molecular genetic studies revealed that this syndrome is due to a microdeletion that simultaneously deletes two genes, the Exostosis 1 gene (*EXT1*) and the *TRPS1* gene, which encodes a zinc finger transcription factor (Shin and Chang 2001).

In TRPS I, the *TRPS1* gene is mutated and the *EXT1* gene is not mutated or deleted. In a subgroup of patients with a specific class of mutations in *TRPS1*, the phenotype includes only short stature and short fingers, brachydactyly. This syndrome is sometimes referred to as TRPS III (Kobayashi et al. 2002).

Chromosome 17q11.2 Deletions Associated with Neurofibromatosis and Mental Retardation

Neurofibromatosis type 1 (NF1) is an autosomal dominant disorder due to deletion or mutation of the gene that encodes Neurofibromin. Clinical features of this disorder include benign and malignant tumors, such as neuro-fibromas, neurofibrosarcomas, optic gliomas, and peripheral nerve sheath tumors. Other characteristic features of NF1 are pigmented lesions, café-au-lait spots, freckling in the axilla or inguinal region, and nodules on the iris of the eye (Lisch nodules). Venturin et al. (2004) reviewed the literature on genotype–phenotype correlations in NF1. They determined that approximately 70% of NF1 patients reported have germline truncating mutations in the *NF1* gene and that in 5%–20% of patients NF1 was reported to be due to deletion of a 1.5 Mb segment of DNA in 17p11.2, leading to deletion of the *NF1* gene and flanking genes. These patients had additional symptoms including facial dysmorphism, developmental delay, and in some cases, mental retardation. Learning disabilities were present in 57% of the deletion patients and in 4%–8% of patients with *NF1* mutations.

Facial dysmorphism was present in 78% of patients with 1.5 Mb deletions on 17p11.2 and in 5%–15% of patients with *NF1* mutations. Specific facial dysmorphic features included hypertelorism (widely spaced eyes), epicanthic folds, downslanting eyes, prominent nose, and low posterior hairline. Cardiovascular malformations were present in 18% of deletion patients and in 2% of *NF1* mutation patients.

Venturin et al. (2004) noted that two genes in the *NF1* flanking regions might play a role in the etiology of mental retardation in patients with large deletions. These are *OMG* and *CDK5R1*; both of these genes are involved in the development of the central nervous system.

Mental Retardation Dysmorphology Syndromes That Are Each Due to Deletion, Disruption, or Mutation of a Specific Gene

Smith-Magenis Syndrome

In patients with Smith-Magenis syndrome, multiple congenital anomalies and mental retardation occur as a result of deletion of chromosome 17p11.2. Congenital anomalies include unusual head shape (*brachycephaly*), myopia, hearing loss, hoarse voice, and short fingers. Speech and motor development are delayed, and patients are moderately mentally retarded. Their sleep patterns are disturbed, and they may exhibit self-injurious behavior. The prevalence of this syndrome is 1 in 25,000.

Most cases of Smith-Magenis syndrome have a deletion of 4 kb in chromosome 17p11.2. In some affected individuals, smaller deletions occur. Specific phenotypic differences do not correlate with the size of the deletion. Three clusters of repeated sequence elements map within the 17p11.2 region. Vlangos et al. (2003) reported that the most common deletion occurs as a result of aberrant recombination between the proximal and distal repeat sequence elements. Twenty-five percent of the deletions are atypical and may result from aberrant recombination between the middle and proximal repeats or between the middle and distal repeats.

Slager et al. (2003) identified three individuals with clinical features consistent with this syndrome where no deletions could be detected. They undertook systematic sequencing of three genes located in the Smith-Magenis critical region. In one of the genes, retinoic acid–induced 1 (RAI1), they identified a 29 bp deletion. *RAI1* is expressed in neurons, and its protein has a nuclear localization signal. Slager et al. (2003) proposed that, in Smith-Magenis, deletions or defects in a single gene may be responsible for most of the clinical features and deficiencies in the products of other contiguous genes may influence the complete phenotype. They postulated further that defects in *RAI1* are likely responsible for the behavioral, neurological, craniofacial, and otolaryngological aspects of the syndrome; other genes may contribute to the etiology of the more variable features, including the cardiac and renal abnormalities.

Mowat-Wilson Syndrome

Mowat-Wilson syndrome, first described in 1998 by Mowat et al., is characterized by mental retardation and distinct facial features. Patients also frequently manifest symptoms of Hirschsprung's disease, in which segments of the colon are distended and immobile due to absence of nerve ganglia. The characteristic facial features include sunken eyes, broad flared eyebrows, pointed chin, and pointed nasal tip. The mouth has an *M* configuration and is often open and smiling; drooling may be a problem. The ears are posteriorly rotated, and the ear lobes are turned up. Microcephaly is usually not present at birth but may develop during infancy. Seizures are present in 90% of cases. Patients with this syndrome do not usually develop speech. Independent walking is achieved on average by 4 years of age. Children often walk with a wide-based gait and with arms raised and flexed at the elbows. Fingers are slender and tapered. Occasionally, patients with Mowat-Wilson syndrome may have cardiac malformation, including septal defect and tetralogy of Fallot.

Several of the features of this syndrome are suggestive of Angelman syndrome. Another consideration in the differential diagnosis of Mowat-Wilson syndrome is Goldberg-Shprintzen syndrome, in which mental retardation and Hirschsprung's disease also occur; however, facial features differ in the two syndromes. In Goldberg-Shprintzen syndrome, eyebrows are arched, eyelids tend to droop (*ptosis*), iris abnormalities occur, and patients may have a cleft palate.

Mowat et al. (1998) identified a deletion in chromosome 2q22-q23 in a patient with Mowat-Wilson syndrome. In 2004, Ishihara et al. reported that in nondeletion Mowat-Wilson syndrome loss-of-function mutations occurred in a specific gene located in 2q22-q23. This gene was initially named *SIP1* (Smad interacting protein 1). It is now designated *ZFHX1B*. It has three zinc finger domains and a homeobox domain. *ZFHX1B* intragenic mutations that lead to Mowat-Wilson syndrome are usually nonsense or frameshift mutations that result in absence of protein (Zweier et al. 2003). *ZFHX1B* is a transcription modulator in the transforming growth factor-beta SMAD signaling pathway (Bassez et al. 2004). It is expressed in many tissues throughout the body and in many brain regions. *ZFHX1B* interacts with SMAD proteins. Activated SMAD proteins then move from the cytoplasm to the nucleus, where they activate gene expression.

Mowat et al. (2003) reported that in a number of patients with clinical features of Mowat-Wilson syndrome no deletions or mutations occurred in *ZFHX1B*. This may be due to genetic heterogeneity. It is possible that other genes that act in the same developmental pathway may give rise to a similar clinical syndrome.

Cornelia de Lange Syndrome

Cornelia de Lange syndrome, which was first described by de Lange in 1933, is characterized by growth and cognitive retardation, facial dysmorphology, and hirsutism, with excessive hair growth particularly on the shoulders, upper arms, and upper back. Limb reduction abnormalities and malformations are often present. Malformations may be present in the urogenital tract, gastro-intestinal system, and heart. Autistic behaviors are present in some patients. Characteristic facial features include low anterior hairline, prominent arched eyebrows that often meet in the middle (*synophrys*), upturned nose with depressed nasal bridge, prominent upper jaw, thin lips, long philtrum, and carp mouth.

A number of different chromosomal translocations have been reported in cases with features that resemble Cornelia de Lange syndrome. In 2004, two independent groups of investigators mapped this syndrome to chromosome 5p13.1 and identified mutations in a specific gene in this region. Tonkin et al. (2004) defined the breakpoint in a 5p13.1-13q12.1 translocation in a patient with this syndrome. They concentrated their efforts in the breakpoint region on chromosome 5p13.1 because of a previous report of a Cornelia de Lange syndrome patient with deletion of 5p13.1-5p14.2. They determined that the 5p13.1 breakpoint mapped in the vicinity of a gene named Nipped B-like (*NIPBL*), the human homolog of a gene that is well characterized in *Drosophila*. They then screened DNA from other patients with Cornelia de Lange syndrome who did not have chromosomal translocations for *NIPBL* point mutations. They identified 10 patients with *NIPBL* point mutations. In all patients analyzed, the mutation was present on a single allele, i.e., in the *NIPBL* gene on one member of the chromosome 5 pair. The phenotype in these patients varied from mild to severe. They identified *NIPBL* mutations in approximately 50% of the patients they screened. This finding may indicate incomplete gene analysis or that there is allelic heterogeneity in Cornelia de Lange syndrome.

Tonkin et al. (2004) carried out expression analysis in human embryonic sections. They determined that *NIPBL* is expressed in cartilage of developing limbs and in skull bones of the head and face.

These investigators identified NIPBL homologs in a number of different organisms. The *NIPBL* homolog in *Drosophila* modulates the activity of a number of homeobox genes, including *DLX*. In yeast, the *NIPBL* homolog plays an important role in the metaphase of cell division in maintaining sister chromatid adhesion.

Krantz et al. (2004) carried out genomewide linkage analysis in nine families with more than one child with Cornelia de Lange syndrome. Evidence for linkage was obtained on five chromosomes, including 5p13.3-5p13.2. These investigators then concentrated on the chromosome 5 linkage region because of a previous report of a 5p13-p12 deletion in a patient with Cornelia de Lange syndrome. They analyzed 11 genes in this region for mutations and discovered *NIPBL* mutations in affected offspring in six of the nine families. All mutations found were of the type that would lead to truncation of the protein product of *NIPBL*. In all cases, the mutation found in the offspring was not present in the parents. The most likely explanation for this finding is that in each of these families gonadal mosaicism was present in one parent; i.e., in the gonad of one parent, there were two different cell lines, a cell line with two normal *NIPBL* genes and a second cell line with one normal and one mutant *NIPBL* gene.

Specific Syndromes Due to Deletions, Mutations, or Imprinting Defects

Chromosome 15q11-q13 is predisposed to deletions and duplications. The breakpoints of these structural changes lie within repeat sequence elements. Prader-Willi syndrome and Angelman syndrome are most commonly due to deletions in this region. A number of genes in 15q11-q13 are imprinted. Imprinting may be defined as differences in the expression of two alleles of the same gene depending on the parental origin of that gene (Ohlsson et al. 1998). Imprinting influences the clinical pictures that emerge in consequence of deletion or duplication; the phenotype varies depending on whether the deletion or duplication arose on a maternal or a paternal chromosome.

Buiting et al. (1992) first reported information on repeat sequence elements in 15q11-q13. They isolated a clone, D15S37 (MN7), and demonstrated that four copies of this clone sequence were interspersed along 15q11-q13. Amos-Landgraf et al. (1999) cloned large blocks of sequences in the 15q11-q13 breakpoint regions. They reported that these blocks of sequence contained the MN7 sequence and part of a novel unique gene, *HERC2*. They proposed that deletions and duplications in chromosome 15q11-q13 arise during meiosis as a result of misalignment of the repeat units during chromosome pairing, followed by unequal crossing over and recombination. There are three common and two rare breakpoints in 15q11-q13, BP1–BP5. The most common distal (telomeric) breakpoint in Prader-Willi syndrome is BP3. The proximal (centromeric) breakpoint may be located at BP1 or at BP2.

The functional *HERC2* gene maps to chromosome 15q13 and generates a 15.3 kb mRNA transcript. Numerous copies of partial *HERC2* genes occur in 15q11-q13, particularly at the breakpoint regions BP1–BP5. However, there are at least 12 regions on chromosome 15q11-q13 where sequences similar to HERC2 occur (Ji et al. 1999). Many of the *HERC2* duplicons and partial duplicons are transcribed; however, definitive data on the direction of transcription are not available for all of these duplicons (Amos Landgraf et al. 1999).

Pujana et al. (2001, 2002) postulated that other duplicated sequence elements in 15q11-q13 play a role in the generation of rearrangements. Low copy repeats include genes encoding a Golgin-like protein, an SH3 domain, an adenosine triphosphate (ATP) binding cassette protein, and a MYLE encoding gene. Smith et al. (2002) reported that duplicons similar to those in 15q11-13 also occur in 15q22-q23. Pujana et al. (2002) reported the presence of multiple copies of Golgin-like repeat sequence elements in 15q24-q26.

Imprinting on Chromosome 15q11-q13

Ohta et al. (1999a,b) identified two imprint control regions on chromosome 15 through molecular genetic analysis of microdeletions present in Prader-Willi syndrome patients and Angelman syndrome patients. The Prader-Willi imprint control region includes a 4.3 kb sequence that encompasses the SNRPN promoter and SNRPN exon 1. The Angelman syndrome imprint control region is an 880 bp DNA sequence located 35 kb upstream (centromeric) of the SNRPN transcription start site.

Genes expressed from the paternal chromosome include *MKRN*, *MAGEL2*, *NDN*, and *SNURF-SNRPN*. On the maternal chromosome, methylation occurs in the promoters of these genes, causing them to be silenced.

Two genes, *UBE3A* and *ATP10C*, are expressed from the maternal chromosome (Runte et al. 2004). Tissue-specific differences in *UBE3A* imprinting occur. Yamasaki et al. (2003) demonstrated that *UBE3A* is expressed only from the maternal allele in neuronal cells. In glial cells, *UBE3A* is expressed from maternal and paternal alleles. Promoter methylation does not apparently play a role in the silencing of *UBE3A* and *ATP10C*.

Runte et al. (2001) isolated a 460 kb transcript that starts at the imprint control region, and includes *SNURF-SRNPN* sense and *UBE3A* antisense sequences. A number of different splice products are derived from this transcript. It also gives rise to small nucleolar RNAs, termed SNOs. The SNOs are encoded in introns of the transcript. Exons 1–3 encode SNURF, a highly basic protein that occurs in the nucleus; exons 4–10 encode SNRPN, a protein that plays a role in RNA splicing. Toward the 3' end of the transcript, the *UBE3A* antisense sequence is present.

Runte et al. (2001) reported that the 435 kb transcript has important implications for understanding imprinting. Three of the four paternally expressed genes are located upstream and centromeric of the imprint control region. Expression of these genes and of the SNRPN gene is controlled by differential methylation of maternal and paternal alleles, determined by the imprint control region. They propose that imprinted expression of the *UBE3A* and *ATP10C* genes is likely controlled by means of an antisense transcript initiated at the imprint control region.

There is increasing evidence that antisense sequences may hybridize to the corresponding sense mRNA. This binding may be followed by degradation of the sense messenger. In some instances, the antisense sequences suppress translation of messenger RNA (mRNA) at the ribosome. In these cases, mRNA may remain intact. Later, in response to specific cellular signals, the sense RNA may be released from antisense RNA repression (Good 2003).

Angelman Syndrome

In 1965, Angelman described three children with a similar clinical phenotype, characterized by severe learning disability, ataxic jerky movements, easily provoked laughter, and failure to develop speech. They had mild dysmorphology that included wide mouth and pointed chin. These children were prone to seizures, and their electroencephalograms (EEGs) had similar distinctive features. This syndrome is sometimes referred to as "the happy puppet syndrome." In 1987, Magenis et al. described deletion of the 15q11-q13 region in two patients with this syndrome.

Since the original description, a number of investigators have described additional clinical features of Angelman syndrome. These include hyperactivity, sleep disorder, and evidence of frustration that may lead to aggressive behavior. Frustration is likely due to the severe communication difficulties these children experience. Children may manifest autistic behaviors. Motor milestones are usually severely delayed; children crawl by 18–24 months and walk by 4 years. Their muscle tone is increased, and they walk with stiff legs and raised arms. Later, they develop joint contractures. Seizure types vary and may include tonic-clonic, atonic, or absence seizures. Head circumference measurements do not increase with age so that children may be microcephalic by the age of 2 years (Williams and Frias 1982).

During the past two decades, studies have revealed that a number of different genetic mechanisms lead to Angelman syndrome. The genetic defect that is common to all patients is loss of expression of the maternal copy of the ubiquitin ligase E3 gene (*UBE3A*). Since features of this syndrome specifically involve loss of expression of a maternally derived gene, it is clear that imprinting plays an important role in the control of gene expression in this region.

Clayton-Smith and Laan (2003) reviewed the literature on Angelman syndrome. They determined that 70%–75% of cases have a deletion in 15q11-q13 detectable by FISH analysis. Deletion breakpoints are most commonly located within repetitive DNA elements composed of duplicons that are similar in sequence to the *HERC2* gene.

Angelman syndrome may be caused by uniparental disomy; i.e., both members of the chromosome 15 pair are paternally derived. One likely mechanism for this is that a sperm that contained two copies of chromosome 15 fertilized the egg so that the zygote was trisomic for chromosome 15. During early cell divisions of the zygote, one of the three chromosomes, specifically the maternal chromosome 15, was lost, leading the embryo to have two members of the chromosome 15 pair, both paternally derived. Uniparental disomy accounts for 2%–3% of cases.

Mutations in the *UBE3A* gene may lead to Angelman syndrome. *UBE3A* encodes a protein that modifies other proteins by transferring a ubiquitin group to that protein, thereby targeting it for degradation. Albrecht et al. (1997) demonstrated that in the brain *UBE3A* is expressed only from the maternal allele. It is most abundantly expressed in the hippocampus and the Purkinje cells in the cerebellum. Disease-causing mutations may arise at positions throughout the gene; however, they are most abundant in the HECT (homologous to E6-AP carboxyl terminus) domain of the gene. Approximately 20% of cases of Angelman syndrome are due to UBE3A mutations. In the majority of cases, these deletions arise de novo during formation of the egg. In rare cases, Angelman syndrome is familial. Mutations in *UBE3A* occur in 75% of cases with familial Angelman syndrome (Malzac et al. 1998; Fang et al. 1999). Familial *UBE3A* mutations manifest only when the affected chromosome is transmitted from the mother.

Prader-Willi Syndrome

Prader-Willi syndrome results from absence of products of genes located in the 15q11-q13 region of the paternally derived copy of the chromosome 15 pair. Infants with this syndrome are frequently hypotonic and have feeding problems. Later in childhood, they manifest developmental delay, mental retardation, and behavioral problems, including obsessive eating that leads to marked obesity.

In approximately 70% of cases, Prader-Willi syndrome results from deletions in the 15q11-q13 region. Approximately 25% of cases are due to maternal isodisomy of chromosome 15 (both members of the chromosome 15 pair are maternally derived). In 2.5% of cases, there are mutations in the Prader-Willi imprint control region, a 4.3 kb region that includes the *SNRPN* gene promoter and first exon (Ohta and Buiting 1999b).

Butler et al. (2004) examined the behavioral phenotype in Prader-Willi patients where the proximal breakpoint occurred in the most centromeric breakpoint (BP1) and in patients where the proximal break was at BP2. Prader-Willi patients with the longer deletions, i.e., deletions extending from BP1 to BP3, had significantly more compulsive behaviors and more visual perception difficulties. Chai et al. (2003) described four genes that are located in the DNA that lies between BP1 and BP2. These genes are *NIPA1*, *NIPA2*, *CYFIP1*, and *TUBGCP*. NIPA1 is particularly abundant in the brain.

NIPA1 and *NIPA2* are non-imprinted genes. NIPA1 is highly expressed in brain. The *CYFIP1* gene encodes a protein that interacts with the protein encoded by *FMRP1* (this is the gene that is underexpressed in fragile X mental retardation). *TUBGCP* encodes a γ-tubulin complex protein. This complex plays a role in the generation of microtubules. Studies of Butler (2003) suggest that one or more of these four genes influences behavior.

Clinical differences exist between patients where Prader-Willi syndrome is due to different mutational mechanisms. Prader-Willi patients with maternal uniparental isodisomy leading to absence of the paternal copy of chromosome 15 have higher verbal IQ and fewer behavioral problems than Prader-Willi patients with deletions (Dykens et al. 1999; Butler et al. 2004).

Segmental Duplication Syndromes

Duplication of Chromosomal Regions: 15q11-q13 Inverted Duplication and 15q11-q13 Interstitial Duplications in Mental Retardation and Autism

Instability in chromosome 15q11-q13 during meiosis may sometimes lead to duplication or triplication of segments of DNA. The extra segments may remain within the chromosome, giving rise to interstitial duplications or triplications. In some cases, duplications include the centromere of chromosome 15 as well as DNA between the centromere and a breakpoint; duplicated segments are then present as an extra small chromosome. The most common extra chromosome is a 15q inverted duplication chromosome; two centromeres are present (only one is active), the centromeres lie at opposite poles of the small chromosome, and in between them there are two segments of DNA representing DNA between the chromosome 15 centromere and repeat sequence elements in breakpoint region DNA. The two halves of the inverted duplication chromosome are not necessarily identical in size and gene content (Roberts et al. 2002). The frequency of 15q inverted duplication chromosomes is reported to be between 1 in 3500 and 1 in 9000 (Amos Landgraf et al. 1999).

Wandstrat and Schwartz (2000) demonstrated that 15q inverted duplication chromosomes that most commonly arise during meiosis may be derived from sister chromatids of a single chromosome or from two different members of the chromosome 15 pair. Inverted duplications derived from sister chromatids have identical alleles at polymorphic markers in the two portions of the duplication. Inverted duplications derived from two different members of the chromosome 15 pair will have different alleles at polymorphic markers in the two portions of the duplication.

Amos-Landgraf et al. (1999) proposed that in 15q inverted duplication and interstitial duplication, the duplication breakpoints occurred within HERC2 repetitive elements. Pujana (2002) postulated that other duplicated sequences on 15q11-q14 might play a role in the generation of the rearrangements. A number of these duplicons contain multiple copies of genes or pseudogenes.

Duplications of chromosome 15q11-q13 (including interstitial duplications and those that lead to the presence of an extra chromosome 15qinv dup) are considered by a number of investigators to be of clinical significance only if they are maternally derived and only if they include the Prader-Willi/Angelman region. Duplications are therefore significant only if the distal breakpoint occurs at BP3, as defined by Amos-Landgraf et al. (1999), or at a more telomeric site (Huang et al. 1997).

However, Chai et al. (2003) described four transcribed genes that map between BP1 and BP2: *NPA1*, *NPA2*, *CYFIP1*, and *TUBGCP5*. It is likely that duplication of these genes may in fact lead to a clinical phenotype. Of further interest is the fact that genes in this region do not carry a parent-specific imprint. Based on the fact that the two alleles of each of these genes seem to replicate asynchronously, it is likely that allelic exclusion occurs so that in some cells the maternal allele is expressed while in other cells the paternal allele is expressed. It is likely that phenotypic consequences of duplication of this region would therefore not be limited to cases where the duplication arose on a maternal chromosome.

Wolpert et al. (2000) reported that phenotypic features of chromosome 15q inverted duplication include hypotonia, tendency to seizures, delayed motor milestones, and severe speech delay. Autistic behaviors may be present; these include lack of social reciprocity and repetitive behaviors. Moderate to severe mental retardation may also occur.

Bolton et al. (2001) reported that maternally derived interstitial duplication of chromosome 15 that includes the Prader-Willi/Angelman region is associated with developmental delay and behavioral problems that do not necessarily fit the parameters of autism spectrum disorder. They noted too that within a sibship where one or more children carried the duplication, there was a wide range of clinical symptoms. Furthermore, even in subjects who met criteria for autism, the autism seemed "unusual." Thomas et al. (2003) reported that the phenotype of chromosome 15q interstitial duplications includes not only autistic behaviors but also attention-deficit hyperactivity disorders. Abnormal behavioral phenotype and developmental delay occur in a few cases of paternally derived 15q duplication (Mohandas et al. 1999; Roberts et al. 2002).

Kabuki Makeup Syndrome

The characteristic facial features of Kabuki makeup syndrome include long palpebral fissures, arched eyebrows, lateral eversion of the lower eyelids, and prominent ears. The facial features evoke the image of actors in Kabuki theater. Other features of the syndrome are persistence of fetal finger pads, skeletal anomalies including scoliosis, and short fingers (brachydactyly). Milunsky and

Huang (2003) carried out molecular cytogenetics studies on six patients with Kabuki makeup syndrome. They determined that in all patients duplication of the 8p22-23.2 region was present. Their studies in parents of these patients revealed that in two mothers an inversion occurred at 8p23.2 on one member of the chromosome 8 pair.

Mental Retardation Associated with Expansion of Triplet Repeats in DNA Aberrant Methylation and Changes in Chromatin Condensation: Fragile X Syndrome

Fragile X mental retardation is caused by loss of function of the *FMR1* gene, which maps to chromosome Xq27.3. This syndrome affects about 1 in 1000 male and 1 in 2000 female individuals; about 1 in 700 women is a carrier (Laxova 1994). Clinical features include a long narrow face, large protruding ears, and enlargement of the testes (*macrorchidism*). Height in childhood is frequently between the 50th and 97th percentiles. In adult life, it is frequently below the 50th percentile. Neurological symptoms include seizures in 10%–20% of patients; complex partial seizures are most common (Sutherland et al. 2002). The majority of male patients with this syndrome exhibit moderate mental retardation. Behavioral abnormalities include increased response to auditory stimuli, and touch avoidance. Patients may exhibit autistic behaviors or attention deficit (Laxova 1994; Stoll 2001).

Neuroimaging studies reveal a reduction in the size of the cerebellum, particularly of the vermis of the cerebellum. As fragile X syndrome patients grow older, there is often an increase in the size of the hypothalamus, the caudate nucleus, and the thalamus. The gray matter of the temporal lobe is reduced in volume relative to the white matter.

Histological analysis of postmortem brain tissue reveals striking changes in dendritic spines. Spines are long, thin, and tortuous; and there are increased numbers of spines per dendrite. Irwin et al. (2000, 2001) proposed that these findings suggest a failure of normal pruning.

The fragile X chromosome was first demonstrated in studies on metaphase chromosomes. Sutherland and Baker (1986a,b) reported that fragile sites on chromosomes are induced when cells are cultured in the presence of high concentrations of thymidine. Dewald et al. (1992) reported guidelines for fragile X studies on peripheral blood lymphocytes. They reported that culturing cells in the presence of excess thymidine or with 5-fluorodeoxyuridine induces fragile sites. There are two fragile sites on the X chromosome. The site that plays a role in the etiology of the most common form of fragile X mental retardation, FMR1, is located at Xq27.3 and is designated FRAXA1 (Webb 1991).

Oberle et al. (1991) and Yu et al. (1991) reported that a 550 bp segment of DNA in the region of the fragile site FRXA is subject to sizes changes in patients with fragile X mental retardation. They determined that this DNA segment is composed of repeats of the nucleotide CGG. They also reported that expansion in the size of the segment is associated with increased methylation of the CGG repeat. Verkerk et al. (1991) reported that the CGG repeat is located in the 5'-untranslated region of the gene *FMR1*.

In normal individuals, the CGG repeat is present in 6–55 copies. Male and female carriers are seen; these individuals have 55–230 copies of the repeat and do not express the fragile site. In female carriers, repeats at the FRAX site may undergo expansion during meiosis. If repeat size in their male offspring varies between 230 and 1000, the offspring will express fragile X mental retardation. The clinical picture in female offspring with repeat expansion of comparable size is variable and depends upon whether or not the normal X chromosome is primarily the active chromosome and whether or not the repeat-containing chromosome is silenced (Fryns et al. 2000).

Repeat expansion and associated hypermethylation lead to reduced or absent expression of the FMR protein. Methylation of the expanded CGG repeat is associated with hypoacetylation of histones and with condensation of chromatin. Coffee et al. (2002) demonstrated that the degree of acetylation of histone H4 in the FMR1 region chromatin is proportional to the size of the CGG repeat. They also reported increased methylation of histone H3 at lysine 4 and lysine 9.

There is evidence that the permutation CGG repeat expansion in fragile X mental retardation carriers is transcribed but not properly translated. In permutation-carrying female carriers, the accumulation of untranslated FMR1 mRNA is likely responsible for premature ovarian failure. Recent studies indicate that it is the accumulated untranslated FMR1 mRNA that forms inclusions in neurons and glial cells in male carriers who have the FMR1 premutation (Chiurazzi et al. 2004). These inclusions, which accumulate particularly in the hippocampus and in the cerebral cortex, lead to cell damage and to a syndrome characterized by ataxia and other neurological manifestations. Jacquemont et al. (2003, 2004) first reported fragile X ataxia syndrome. Its manifestations include ataxia, gait disturbances, intention tremor, and speech difficulties. Other symptoms that patients may develop include short-term memory loss and symptoms of autonomic dysfunction (Willemsen et al. 2004).

Mutations in the *FMR1* gene, other than repeat expansion, have also been described. These include deletions and point mutations (Lugenbeel et al. 1995).

Fragile Site FRAXE

Repeat expansions over 200 in the fragile site in Xq28 lead to mild mental retardation or low normal intelligence, with IQ in the 50–85 range. Symptoms include delayed speech, learning disabilities, and poor writing skills (Mulley et al. 1995).

Mental Retardation Syndromes Associated with Dysmorphology and Disordered Chromatin Remodeling

In disorders associated with dysmorphology and chromatin remodeling, mutations in genes that encode enzymes or proteins that modulate chromatin structure lead to widespread deregulation of gene expression.

Chromatin is composed of a complex of DNA and its surrounding proteins. In interphase, chromatin is spread throughout the nucleus. During the metaphase of cell division, chromatin is condensed to give rise to chromosomes. Some chromosomal regions are more condensed than others, and the condensed chromatin, heterochromatin, stains darkly with nuclear staining reagents. Other regions of the chromosomes are less condensed and contain euchromatin, which stains less intensely.

High-magnification microscopy reveals that DNA strands are wound around the outside of bead-like structures that are composed of histone proteins. A helix comprised of approximately 165 bp of DNA is wound around a bead composed of eight subunits of histone. This structure forms the nucleosome. The histone octomer that forms nucleosome beads is comprised of two units each of different types of histone, including H2A, H2B, H3, and H4. Histone H1 binds to the nucleosome and to linker strands of DNA that lie between the nucleosomes (Felsenfeld and Groudine 2003) (Fig. 4–3).

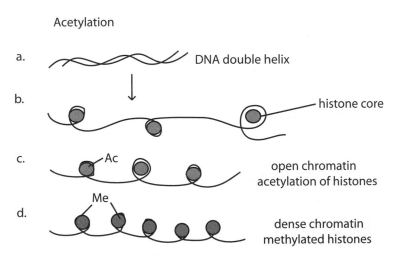

Figure 4–3. Histone modifications may activate or silence gene expression. The amino-terminal tails of the histone subunits that constitute the nucleosomes are accessible for modification. Lysine molecules in these tails may undergo acetylation or methylation.

There is abundant evidence that chromatin structure influences gene expression. Weintraub and Groudine (1976) demonstrated that nucleosomes associated with active genes have a more open, less condensed structure than those associated with inactive genes. Several factors play a role in altering chromatin structure. These will be discussed below.

Chromatin Remodeling and Gene Expression

Gene expression is controlled by the binding of transcription factors to DNA, particularly to promoter regions of genes and to control elements. Chromatin remodeling plays a key role in determining accessibility of DNA to transcription factors. In the process of chromatin remodeling, histone complexes (octomers) move a short distance along the DNA strand so that different DNA sequences lie in the open regions between beads. Chromatin remodeling complexes, such as members of the SW1/SNF family and RSF proteins, are required for this process. These complexes have ATPase activity to interact with ATP-rich compounds that provide energy for the remodeling process.

Histone modification plays a key role in the regulation of gene expression and in differentiation. Histone modifications may activate or silence gene expression. The amino terminal tails of the histone subunits that constitute the nucleosomes are accessible for modification. Lysine molecules in these tails may undergo acetylation, methylation, or coupling to the protein ubiquitin. Arginine residues in histone are sites of methylation, while serine residues within histone proteins may undergo phosphorylation. The modifications of different amino acids within histone are co-coordinated. Together these histone modifications affect gene expression and constitute a system sometimes referred to as " the histone code" (Felsenfeld and Groudine 2003) (Fig. 4–3).

Actively expressed genes are surrounded by acetylated histones. Enzymes responsible for histone deacetylation occur in the vicinity of repressed genes. Methylation of histone in some gene regions leads to gene expression, while in other gene regions it is associated with repression (Mermoud et al. 2002). At specific sites in the genome, variant forms of histone may substitute for core-specific histone subunits. Histone H3.3, a variant of histone H3, is incorporated in the chromatin in nondividing cells and is associated with expressing genes. In regions of reduced nucleosome stability, H2 histone is frequently replaced by H2AZ histone. The H2 variant H2AX is particularly susceptible to phosphorylation, and it occurs in regions where DNA breakages are being repaired. A very large form of histone H2A, macroH2A, occurs in chromatin of the inactive X chromosome. A variant of histone H3 occurs at centromeres.

DNA methylation and histone modification are closely associated. Following methylation of DNA at specific CpG dinucleotide sites, proteins bind to DNA at those sites. Bound proteins recruit histone deacetylases. Following deacetylation, DNA is silenced (Johnson 2000).

Syndromes Associated with Chromatin Defects

X-Linked Mental Retardation with α-Thalassemia and Variants

The syndrome of X-linked mental retardation with α-thalassemia (ATRX) occurs in male individuals and is characterized by mental retardation, microcephaly, growth problems, facial dysmorphology, urogenital malformations, and mild α-thalassemia leading to the presence of hemoglobin H inclusions in red blood cells. Gibbons et al. (1995) reported that this syndrome is due to mutations of an X-linked gene that maps to Xp13.3. At least five genetic syndromes associated with severe mental retardation in male individuals are due to deletions or mutations of this gene. These include ATRX syndrome, Carpenter syndrome, Juberg-Marsidi syndrome, Smith-Fineman-Myers syndrome, and X-linked mental retardation with spastic paraplegia.

The *ATRX* gene (sometimes referred to as *XNP*) contains several domains, including a specific domain with homology to homeotic genes, a helicase-like domain, and an ATPase domain. This gene regulates gene expression via its effects on chromatin structure and function.

McDowell et al. (1999) reported that ATRX protein is associated with pericentromeric heterochromatin during interphase. It associates with the short arms of acrocentric chromosomes during metaphase. This association occurs through binding of the protein to GC-rich DNA sequences that encode ribosomes. Gibbons et al. (2000) demonstrated that ATRX mutations lead to changes in the pattern of methylation of repeated sequence elements in the DNA in a number of different locations, including subtelomeric regions, ribosomal encoding regions, and the Y chromosome.

Immunodeficiency, Centromeric Instability, Facial Anomalies Syndrome

The immunodeficiency, centromeric instability, facial anomalies (ICF) syndrome, is associated with a variable degree of mental retardation, severe to mild; growth retardation; chronic infections; and malabsorption. Examination of chromosomes reveals that the centromeric regions of chromosomes 1, 9, and 16 are unstable.

The ICF syndrome is a recessive disorder caused by mutations in the enzyme DNA cytosine 5 methyltransferase (DNMT3B), which maps to chromosome 20q11.2. Mutations of DNMT3B in ICF patients usually occur in the catalytic domain. In these patients, DNA in general is not hypomethylated; however, pericentromeric of chromosomes 1, 2, and 16 is hypomethylated (Ausio et al. 2003).

There is evidence that DNMT3B is more active in embryonic life than during postnatal life. In human embryonic stem cells, DNMT3B localizes to pericentromeric heterochromatin (Bachman et al. 2001). Pradhan and

Esteve (2003) demonstrated that DNMT3B null mice have multiple developmental defects.

On one strand of DNA, DNMT3B methylates cytosine; maintenance methylase DNMT1 then methylates the cytosine on the opposite strand. Methyl CpG binding protein (MECP2) binds to symmetrically methylated CpG dinucleotides. Chromatin binding proteins are listed in Table 4–1.

Rubinstein-Taybi Syndrome

Rubinstein-Taybi syndrome is associated with mental retardation (IQ scores 25–80) and facial anomalies including wide nasal bridge, antimongoloid slant of the eyes, high arched palate, and widened terminal phalanges, particularly of the thumbs and great toes. Deletions of chromosome 16p13.3 are frequently found in patients with this syndrome. In all deletion patients, the gene encoding CREBBP is deleted. Heterozygous mutations in the gene encoding this protein occur in Rubinstein-Taybi patients who do not have deletions (Coupry et al. 2004).

The function of CREBBP is as a histone acetylase (HAT) that alters chromatin structure. Rubinstein-Taybi syndrome is therefore included in the category of chromatin remodeling disorders. The CREBBP protein is involved in the acetylation of a number of other proteins, including thyroid hormone receptor and bone morphogenic protein (BMP). This latter function of CREB

Table 4–1
Chromatin Binding Proteins

Symbol	Full Name and Function
Proteins that Bind to Chromatin of Centromeres, to Pericentromeric	
Regions, and to Other Heterochromatic Regions	
MECP2	Methyl CpG binding protein
MBD1	Methyl binding domain 1
MBD2	Methyl binding domain 2
ATRX	α-Thalassemia and X-linked mental retardation
HP1 alpha	
HDAC1	Histone deacetylase 1
HDAC2	Histone deacetylase 2
DNMT1	DNA methyltransferase 1
DNMT3B	DNA methyltransferase 3b
DNA Binding Transcription Factors that can Recruit Histone Deacetylases	
Directly to Promoters or Indirectly via Corepressors	
CTBP	
Sin3A	
Sin 3B	

may account for the skeletal anomalies observed in Rubinstein-Taybi syndrome (Hendrich and Bickmore 2001). Also, CREBBP functions as a platform for recruiting other components required for gene transcription and is a transcriptional coactivator in neurons, where it plays a critical role in memory consolidation (Korzus et al. 2004).

Coffin-Lowry Syndrome

Coffin-Lowry syndrome is included in the category of chromatin modification disorders because it is due to deficiency of the gene *RSK2*, a serine threonine kinase that plays a role in the phosphorylation of histone H3. The *RSK2* gene also participates in the RAS-dependent mitogen-activated protein kinase signaling cascade. It activates CREBBP. Coffin-Lowry syndrome maps to chromosome Xp22.2-Xp22.1 (Yntema 1999a).

Phenotypic features of Coffin-Lowry syndrome occur in male individuals and include mental retardation, seizures, hypotonia, microcephaly, coarse face with prominent brow and chin, short stature, spinal anomalies, and skeletal anomalies including short metacarpals with expanded terminal phalanges.

Rett Syndrome

Rett syndrome is included in the category of chromatin modification disorders because it is due to deficiency of MECP2, a protein that binds to chromatin and regulates transcription (Amir and Zoghbi 2000; Klose and Bird 2003). We will discuss Rett syndrome in Chapters 6 and 7 since it is not associated with dysmorphology.

Other Chromatin Effects: Position Effect

Analysis of genes in the vicinity of chromosomal translocations has revealed that some translocated genes are not expressed even though they are not interrupted as a result of the translocation. In these instances, disrupted expression may be due to position effect. A number of different factors may play a role in this (Kleinjan and van Heyningen 2005). A gene may be removed, through translocation, from its upstream elements such as the promoter or from upstream or downstream elements that influence gene expression.

Chromosomal rearrangements such as translocations or inversions may cause a gene to be moved from a *euchromatin* (decondensed chromatin) environment to a *heterochromatin* (condensed chromatin) environment. The specific chromatin environment in which the gene resides may influence expression. Specific DNA sequence elements known as "locus control regions" occur close to a number of genes whose expression in regulated in a tissue-specific or time-specific manner. Locus control elements play a role in "opening" or decondensing chromatin structure.

Chromosomal rearrangements may also cause genes to come under the influence of different enhancer elements so that genes that were previously silenced are actively transcribed following relocation.

Location of Transcriptional Regulators in Centromeric Heterochromatin

A number of transcriptional regulators are associated with centromeric heterochromatin. Francastel et al. (2001) reported that centromeric heterochromatin represents a default localization site for a number of transcriptional regulators, such as Ikaros and Kruppel-associated proteins. When required to induce gene expression, these factors are relocated to euchromatin components within cells.

It is interesting to consider the possibility that substantial expansion of pericentromeric heterochromatin regions may be associated with increased sequestration of proteins that bind to pericentromeric heterochromatin. Such expansions occur, e.g., in cases of 15q inverted duplication, where patients are tetrasomic for a pericentromeric region of chromosome 15.

Mental Retardation and Malformation Resulting from Metabolic Defects

Cholesterol Biosynthetic Defects: Smith-Lemli-Opitz Syndrome

Smith-Lemli-Opitz syndrome (SLOS) was first described in 1964. It was reported as a malformation syndrome that manifested an autosomal recessive pattern of inheritance. It is characterized by growth and mental retardation, microcephaly, and facial dysmorphology, including a small upturned nose and receding chin. Other congenital malformations that may be present include fusion of the toes, especially the second and third toes; the presence of extra digits; cleft palate; congenital heart disease; and intestinal malformation, such as pyloric stenosis and dilated colon due to absence of nerve ganglia. Genitourinary malformations may also be present. Brain MRI studies reveal the presence of structural brain abnormalities in 20%–35% of patients. Holoprosencephaly occurs in 5% of patients. A significant proportion of patients meet diagnostic criteria for autism.

Irons et al. (1993) first reported alterations in plasma cholesterol levels in patients with SLOS. Plasma cholesterol levels are decreased, and levels of 7-dehydrocholesterol are increased. Irons et al. postulated that these changes result from deficiency of the enzyme 7-dehydrocholesterol reductase (Fig. 4–4).

This syndrome was the first metabolic defect identified in the post-squalene biosynthetic pathway. Subsequently, other defects in this pathway have been described (Porter 2003).

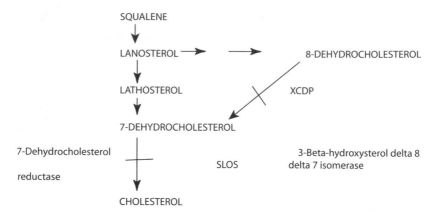

Figure 4–4. Cholesterol biosynthesis and position of metabolic block in Smith-Lemli-Opitz syndrome and in X-linked chondrodysplasia punctata (Conradi-Hünermann syndrome).

Treatment with high-cholesterol diets may be of some benefit to patients with SLOS (Herman 2003). This treatment does not improve central nervous system function. This observation is consistent with studies by King et al. (2002), who demonstrated that cholesterol required in the brain is synthesized in that organ. These investigators reported that the widespread formation of synapses that occurs during brain development requires cholesterol and is dependent upon the transfer of cholesterol from astrocytes. Adequate concentrations of cholesterol in the brain are required for the formation of synaptic vesicles. These organelles play a key role in the transport of neurotransmitters to synapses.

Cholesterol is a key component of cell membranes. It serves as a precursor for steroid hormones. Cholesterol plays a role in signaling pathways through modifications of proteins (Mann and Beachy, 2000). Figure 4–4 illustrates the positions of metabolic blocks in cholesterol biosynthesis.

X-Linked Chondrodysplasia Punctata (Conradi-Hünermann Syndrome)

The characteristic features of Conradi-Hünermann syndrome usually occur in heterozygous female individuals. They include skeletal abnormalities, particularly shortening of the upper segment of limbs (rhizomelia), and cartilage abnormalities, including defective development of nasal, laryngeal, and tracheal cartilage. X-ray reveals the presence of diffuse stippling in cartilage, bone epiphyses, and particularly the vertebral column. Sloughing of the upper layers of the epidermis may be present (ichthyosis), and in some cases baldness (alopecia) occurs.

Female individuals with this disorder do not usually manifest mental retardation. X-linked chondrodysplasia punctata was initially considered to be lethal in male individuals. However, live-born boys with this disorder have been described (Happle 1995, Milunsky et al. 2003). Male subjects manifest a different phenotype that more closely resembles that of SLOS. They have growth delay and developmental delay.

Kelley et al. (1999) found increased levels of 8-dehydrocholesterol in plasma and tissues of patients with Conradi-Hünermann syndrome. They also demonstrated reduced cholesterol synthesis in patients' cultured cells. On the basis of these findings, Kelley et al. (1999) postulated a deficiency in the enzyme that converts 8-dehydrocholesterol, which is derived from lanosterol, to 7-dehydrocholesterol, the immediate precursor of cholesterol. The gene encoding this enzyme maps to human chromosome Xp11.22-Xp11.23. Braverman et al. (1999) demonstrated mutations in this gene in all seven of the X-linked chondrodysplasia punctata patients they studied.

Lathosterolosis

Patients with lathosterolosis have severe psychomotor retardation and a phenotype that resembles that seen in SLOS (Brunetti-Pierri et al. 2002). Congenital malformations present in patients with lathosterolosis include microcephaly, receding forehead, upturned nose, prominent upper lip, high arched palate, thickened gums (alveolar ridges), extra digits, and fused digits. Liver disease often occurs due to intracellular and lysosomal lipid accumulation. Lathosterols accumulate in cells as a result of defective function of the enzyme 3β-hydroxysteroid-δ-5-desaturase, also known as sterol-C5-desaturase. The gene encoding this enzyme maps to chromosome 11q23.3. Gene mutations in sterol-C-desaturase have been reported by a number of investigators (Brunetti-Pierri et al. 2002; Krakowiak et al. 2003).

Zellweger Syndrome and Peroxisome Biogenesis Defects

Clinical manifestations of Zellweger syndrome include psychomotor retardation, craniofacial dysmorphology, malformations of the hands and feet, enlarged liver, and enlarged cystic kidneys. Features of the facial dysmorphism are high forehead, large fontanelle, and opacities in the lens of the eye. On X-rays, stippling in cartilage may be seen, especially in the patella. Neuronal defects in Zellweger syndrome include developmental defects and postnatal degenerative changes.

Zellweger syndrome was discussed in Chapter 3 in the context of brain malformations associated with mental retardation. This syndrome and other peroxisomal disorders will also be discussed in the context of mental retardation associated with postnatal degenerative changes due to abnormal storage of phospholipids.

Research between 1993 and 2004 has revealed that mutations in any one of at least six genes that play a role in peroxisome biosynthesis may lead to the Zellweger syndrome phenotype. These genes are the peroxins *PEX1*, *PEX2*, *PEX3*, *PEX5*, *PEX6*, and *PEX12*; each maps on a different chromosome (Steinberg et al. 2004).

Growth Abnormalities Associated with Mental Retardation

Growth Deficiency

Prenatal growth deficiency may be due to genetic or environmental causes. Genetic causes include chromosomal abnormalities and specific gene defects. Genetically determined growth deficiency syndromes provide insight into developmental processes related to growth.

X-linked Mental Retardation with Growth Hormone Deficiency

There are several reports in the literature of families with mental retardation and growth hormone deficiency where the phenotype follows an X-linked pattern of inheritance (Hamel et al. 1996; Raynaud et al. 1998). Through linkage studies, Hamel et al. (1996) demonstrated that this disorder maps to Xq24-q27.3.

Laumonnier et al. (2002) analyzed genes in the Xq26-Xq27 region in a family where mental retardation and isolated growth hormone deficiency mapped to that region of the X chromosome. They found mutations in the *SOX3* gene and demonstrated decreased gene expression. This is a transcription factor that is expressed at high levels in fetal brain and spinal cord. It is a homeobox gene. Rizzoti et al. (2004) demonstrated through studies in mice that *Sox3* gene expression is necessary for correct development of the hypothalamus and Rathke's pouch, the structure that gives rise to the pituitary gland.

Chromosome 2q37.3 Deletion Associated with Mental Retardation, Short Stature, Brachydactyly, and Osteodystrophy

There are numerous reports in the literature of patients with mental retardation, short stature, shortening of one or more metacarpal or metatarsal bones, and other skeletal abnormalities similar to those described in Albright's osteodystrophy. At least 10 of these reports document the presence of symptoms of autism in patients with this syndrome. Molecular genetic studies were carried out in some of the patients and revealed that chromosomal deletions encompassed between 1 and 3 Mb of DNA within the 2q37.3 region (Smith et al. 2002).

Giardino et al. (2003) described a male patient with mental retardation, short stature, vertebral abnormalities, lumbar lordosis, small feet, short fingers, and shortening of the fourth metacarpal bone. The patient's expressive speech was severely delayed, and his behaviors were abnormal; he was diagnosed as having a pervasive developmental disorder. Karyotype analysis revealed that the patient had an unbalanced chromosomal translocation that interrupted chromosome 2q37.3. The karyotype was 46XY,der(2) t2;6)(q37.3:q26). Giardino et al. used molecular cytogenetic techniques to define the position of the breakpoint in chromosome 2q37.3. Characterization of genes in this translocation breakpoint region will likely shed light on the precise etiology of this syndrome.

Overgrowth Syndromes Associated with Mental Retardation

Sotos Syndrome

In Sotos syndrome, pre- and postnatal overgrowth occurs and patients have macrocephaly, advanced bone age, variable degrees of mental retardation, and facial dysmorphology. Features of the latter include prominent forehead, receding hairline, and down-slanting palpebral fissures. Seizures, scoliosis, and strabismus may also occur. In some patients, cardiac and renal anomalies are present. Sotos syndrome patients may have an increased predisposition to development of tumors.

Kurotaki et al. (2002) reported a patient with Sotos syndrome in whom a chromosomal translocation occurred t 5:8(q35:q24.1). This finding led them to analyze genes in the translocation breakpoint region, and they discovered that a specific gene on chromosome 5 was disrupted. This gene, *NSD1* (nuclear receptor binding SET domain protein 1), encodes a protein that is localized in the nucleus and acts as a transcription factor that enhances transcription of androgen receptors (Huang et al. 1998; Rayasam et al. 2003; Turkmen et al. 2003). Further studies by Kurotaki et al. (2003) revealed *NSD1* microdeletions in 45% and point mutations in 14% of Japanese patients with Sotos syndrome. Douglas et al. (2003) reported that point mutations occurred in 70% of patients in their study, while microdeletions occurred in 5% of Sotos syndrome patients. Rio et al. (2003) reported that mental retardation was consistently more severe in patients with *NSD1* microdeletions.

The most common brain abnormality found on MRI in patients with Sotos syndrome is dilation of the ventricles, which occurs in 63% of patients (Cohen 2003b). Other brain malformations detected on MRI include absent corpus callosum and heterotopias, i.e., clusters of neurons that failed to complete neuronal migration.

Weaver Syndrome

Weaver syndrome is characterized by prenatal and postnatal overgrowth, mental retardation, and distinct facial features. The face is round, the chin is usually small and receding (micrognathia), and the eyes are widely spaced (hypertelorism) and slant down. The mouth is small with a long philtrum, the ears are large, and the voice is hoarse. Distal long bones are widened. Fingers may be abnormally curved, and finger pads are prominent. Brain abnormalities include dilation of the ventricles and evidence of regional hypervascularity. Rio et al. (2003) found mutations in the *NSD1* gene in three of six patients with Weaver syndrome. These findings indicate that Sotos syndrome and Weaver syndrome are allelic disorders due to heterozygous mutations that lead to haploinsufficiency of *NSD1*.

Bannayan-Riley-Ruvalcaba Syndrome

The features of Bannayan-Riley-Ruvalcaba syndrome are prenatal overgrowth, macrocephaly, presence of benign tumors including lipomas, intestinal polyps, hemangiomas, and vascular malformation. Other clinical features are hypotonia, gross motor delay, speech delay, and mild to moderate mental retardation. Other neurological features include seizures, ataxia, and tremors. Patients may develop thyroiditis and hypothyroidism or thyroid tumors. Pigmented lesions on the penis are a specific feature of this syndrome.

Overgrowth in height and weight is present at birth. During childhood, growth normalizes so that when patients reach adulthood they are frequently of average height and weight. Macrocephaly is a constant feature, present in childhood and in adult life.

This syndrome sometimes occurs in families and is transmitted as an autosomal dominant trait. In 1997, Zigman et al. discovered chromosome 10q23 microdeletions in two patients with Bannayan-Riley-Ruvalcaba syndrome. Marsh et al. (1997) identified mutations in the *PTEN* gene in patients with this syndrome. Mutations in *PTEN* are responsible for another tumor-associated syndrome known as Cowden syndrome (Dahia et al. 1997).

The *PTEN* gene contains both a tyrosine phosphatase domain and a tensin domain, and it preferentially dephosphorylates phosphoinositide substrates. It plays a role in negatively regulating the concentration of phosphatidylinositol-3,4,5-triphosphate in cells, and it negatively regulates the AKT/protein kinase B signaling pathway, thereby acting as a tumor-suppressor gene.

Simpson-Golabi-Behmel Syndrome

In Simpson-Golabi-Behmel syndrome, overgrowth begins in prenatal life and continues through to adult life. This is an X-linked disorder, and symptoms occur primarily in male subjects, though female carriers may manifest some of the features. Clinical features include macrocephaly, widely spaced eyes, short broad nose, cleft palate, and large tongue. Skeletal abnormalities may be present. These include defects of the ribs, sternum, vertebral column, and fingers, including extra fingers and fused fingers. Organ abnormalities may be present in patients with this syndrome; these include large cystic kidneys, intestinal malrotation, and cardiac defects. Some patients have mild mental retardation, while others have normal intellect.

Pilia et al. (1996) identified deletions in the Glypican 3 gene (*GPC3*) in patients with Simpson-Golabi-Behmel syndrome. Li et al. (2001) reported *GPC3* gene defects in 26 out of 65 patients with this syndrome. Approximately 30% of the gene defects are deletions. Deletions are frequently sporadic events, and in these cases there is no family history of the disorder.

Mental Retardation and Dysmorphology Due to Environmental Factors: Fetal Alcohol Syndrome

The clinical features of the syndrome that results from prenatal alcohol exposure are decreased growth in length and weight during prenatal life, microcephaly, hypotonia, mild to moderate mental retardation, and facial dysmorphology. Characteristic facial features include short palpebral fissures, epicanthal folds, flat midface, short nose, flat philtrum, thin upper lip, and small chin. Development of the facial features of fetal alcohol syndrome is dependent upon fetal exposure to alcohol early in pregnancy (Duerbeck 1997). Growth retardation and neurodevelopmental defects may occur even if alcohol exposure occurs only later in pregnancy. The typical facial features of fetal alcohol syndrome decrease over time. The central nervous system effects are, however, permanent.

Alcohol-induced developmental central nervous system defects in the absence of facial defects are referred to as *fetal alcohol effects* or *alcohol-related birth defects*. The incidence of alcohol-related birth defects in the population is approximately 8.3 per 1000. The incidence of fetal alcohol syndrome is 1.3–4.8 per 1000 (Sampson et al. 1997).

Neurological findings in fetal alcohol syndrome include impaired motor skills, ataxia, and sensorineural hearing loss. Neurocognitive and behavioral deficits in children with alcohol-related birth defects include learning difficulties, impulsivity, decreased social skills, deficits in expressive and receptive language, attention deficit, and difficulty in planning and in reasoning (Duerbeck 1997; Burd et al. 2003a–c).

Alcohol can induce loss of brain cells. In addition, MRI studies reveal that structural brain malformations occur more frequently in prenatal alcohol-exposed children. These include microcephaly, abnormalities of the size and shape of the corpus callosum, and cerebellar hypoplasia (Burd et al. 2003a–c).

5

Mental Retardation Associated with Other Neurological Defects

In this chapter, we discuss disorders that are due to a specific gene defect and where mental retardation occurs along with a striking neurological deficit. The neurological deficits described include epilepsy, episodes of acute illness, seizures and/or coma, movement disorders, and sensorineural abnormalities such as blindness, deafness, and muscle defects.

Mental Retardation Associated with Seizures

Mental retardation and seizures often occur together. In some cases, both may be due to the same underlying genetic defect. There is still considerable debate concerning the role that seizures play in directly damaging the brain. Two important questions arise then: Is there an underlying brain pathology that leads to mental retardation and seizures? Is mental retardation directly related to the effects of seizures on the developing brain?

Vasconcellos et al. (2001) studied 100 patients with intractable seizures, who on preoperative MRI each had a focal brain lesion limited to one lobe of the brain. Lesion resection resulted in a favorable outcome in 82% of cases. They analyzed cognitive development in all of these patients and found that mental retardation occurred more frequently in patients who developed seizures before 24 months of age than in patients who developed seizures later. Their results and the results of other investigators, including Seidenberg et al. (1986) and Bourgeois et al. (1983), indicate that compromised cognition is more severe in cases where seizures started early and occurred with high frequency. Vasconellos et al. (2001) noted that normally the brain triples in weight between birth and age 2 years due to extensive dendritic branching, synapse formation, and myelination. Dendritic branching, dendritic spine formation, and synaptogenesis are adversely affected by neuronal seizure activity (Collins et al. 1983). In addition, frequent seizure activity likely results in sensory deprivation.

112

Gene Mutations That Cause Idiopathic Epilepsy

Idiopathic epilepsy may be defined as epilepsy that occurs in the absence of underlying structural brain defects. It is generally considered to be genetically complex; in any one individual, a number of different genes interact to produce the phenotype. However, in a small percentage of cases, the genetics is simple rather than complex and, in each of these cases, mutation in a specific gene is responsible for the clinical phenotype. The discussion that follows is a description of phenotypes that include epilepsy and mental retardation due to specific gene mutations.

Generalized Epilepsy with Seizures During Episodes of Fever

This category of seizures includes various phenotypes and is genetically heterogeneous. In one subgroup, patients have severe epilepsy with seizures that are difficult to control therapeutically and cognitive impairment. Mutations in genes that encode voltage-gated sodium channels, *SCN1A*, *SCN2A*, or *SCN1B*, may lead to generalized epilepsy with febrile seizures. The exact mechanisms by which *SCN* mutations lead to epilepsy are not known. Meadows et al. (2002) studied the effects of *SCNB1* mutation C121W in vitro. Their data indicated that this mutation caused subtle effects on channel function and biased neurons toward hyperexcitability.

Febrile seizures may also occur in patients with mutations in the gene that encodes the γ2 subunit of the γ-aminobutyric acid (GABA) neurotransmitter receptor GABRG2 (Baulac et al. 2001).

Severe Myoclonic Epilepsy of Infancy

Myoclonic seizures are characterized by rapid contractions of one or more muscle groups. Myoclonic epilepsy in infancy is sometimes referred to as Dravet syndrome and is characterized by prolonged febrile and afebrile seizures that begin during the first year of life (Dravet 2000). Developmental delay and developmental regression may occur in these patients. Scheffer and Berkovic (2003) and Fujiwara et al. (2003) reported that mutations in the sodium channel gene *SCN1A* occurred in 30%–60% of Dravet syndrome patients they studied. The *SCN1A* mutations in their patients led to protein truncation or to formation of inactive proteins and haploinsufficiency.

Claes et al. (2003) reported that heterozygous *SCN1A* mutations occur in cases of generalized epilepsy with myoclonic episodes. In the patients they studied, missense mutations occurred most frequently.

Infantile Spasms

Infantile spasms begin during the first year of life. Spasms of the neck, trunk, and extremity muscles occur. West syndrome comprises a triad of manifestations:

infantile spasms, a seizure EEG pattern known as hypsarrhythmia and mental retardation. Infantile spasms frequently occur in patients with structural brain anomalies, including patients with tuberous sclerosis who have cortical tubers.

Most cases of infantile spasm present as sporadic cases with no family history of similar seizures. Familial infantile spasms sometimes follow an X-linked pattern of inheritance. Bienvenu et al. (2002) and Stromme et al. (2002) reported that *ARX* gene mutations occurred in a number of familial cases of infantile spasms that they studied. The phenotypes that arise in patients with *ARX* gene mutations will be described below.

Kalscheuer et al. (2003b) described two unrelated patients severely affected with West syndrome who had a translocation between the X chromosome and an autosome. In both cases, the translocation breakpoint occurred at Xp22.3. In one patient, the karyotype was 46Xt(X; 7)(p22.3; p15). In the second patient the karyotype was 46Xt(X; 6)(p22.3; q14). Molecular genetic analysis revealed that the break on the X chromosome disrupted the *STRK9* gene (serine threonine kinase 9).

Analysis of X-inactivation patterns revealed that in one patient the normal X was inactivated in 100% of cells studied. In the second patient, skewed X inactivation was found and, in most cells studied, the normal X was inactivated. *STRK9* gene expression was reduced in lymphoblast cell lines.

STRK9 is a protein kinase and a member of the mitogen-activated protein (MAP) kinase family of proteins that play a role in cell division. Kalscheuer et al. (2003b) noted that MAP kinases are important in the regulation of synaptic plasticity in neurons.

ARX Homeobox Gene Mutations: Diverse Phenotypes and Genotype–Phenotype Correlations

The aristaless-related homeobox gene, *ARX*, may lead to structural brain malformations such as lissencephaly and agenesis of the corpus callosum (discussed in Chapter 3). Stromme et al. (2002) reported that *ARX* mutations occurred in patients with mental retardation, seizures, and autism who had no structural brain anomalies. *ARX* mutations may also occur in patients with infantile spasms, myoclonic epilepsy, nonsyndromic mental retardation, or Partington syndrome characterized by mental retardation, ataxia, and dystonia.

Sherr (2003) reported that genotype–phenotype correlations are emerging in ARX syndrome. Mutations that lead to protein truncation or missense mutations in the conserved residues of the homeobox-encoding domain of ARX lead to structural brain malformation and a syndrome of X-linked lissencephaly with ambiguous genitalia. Patients with X-linked mental retardation and patients with the X-linked infantile spasm syndrome had duplication of a segment of DNA within the gene that resulted in an ARX protein with a polyalanine expansion.

Mental Retardation Associated with Episodes of Acute Illness, Coma, and Seizures

Inborn errors of metabolism that lead to accumulation of organic acids and to metabolic acidosis may be associated with failure to thrive, mental retardation, and recurrent episodes of vomiting and acute illness. Coma may occur during these episodes. It is important to recognize and accurately diagnose these disorders since appropriate treatment may prevent the long-term deleterious consequences to the central nervous system.

Disorders of Pyruvate Metabolism and of the Tricarboxylic Acid Cycle Leading to Accumulation of Lactate and Pyruvic Acid

Pyruvate Carboxylase Deficiency

Pyruvate carboxylase deficiency may present in the neonatal period with acidosis and seizures, and this neonatal form is usually fatal within the first few months of life. In cases that present later, developmental retardation, growth deficiency, spasticity, seizures, and acidosis are common. Brain MRI studies may reveal ventricular enlargement, periventricular cysts, and evidence of impaired myelination. In some cases, pyruvate carboxylase deficiency is characterized by mild neurological deficits and episodes of acidosis precipitated by infections or fasting (Robinson 1980; Robinson et al. 1983, 2001).

The key finding on clinical chemistry is a high lactate/pyruvate ratio. This occurs particularly when blood glucose is low. Blood ammonia levels may be increased, and ketosis may be present. An important part of the treatment of this disorder is avoidance of fasting and promotion of adequate intake of carbohydrate, especially before bedtime.

Pyruvate Dehydrogenase Complex Deficiency

Defects in the pyruvate dehydrogenase complex are a relatively common cause of primary lactic acidosis. Pyruvate dehydrogenase is composed of three subunits. The E1 subunit is encoded on the X chromosome at Xp22.3. The E1 subunit is most commonly defective in cases of pyruvate dehydrogenase deficiency (Lissens et al. 2000). This disorder is sometimes referred to as pyruvate decarboxylase deficiency. Manifestations occur in male and female individuals; however, the clinical features in the latter are more variable in severity. This variability is likely due to skewed X inactivation; in female individuals where the normal X chromosome is predominantly inactivated, the symptoms are likely to be more severe. Most cases of pyruvate decarboxylase deficiency represent new mutations.

The most common clinical manifestations are delayed development, seizures, and *ataxia* (difficulty in coordination of voluntary muscle activity).

Brain MRI studies may reveal evidence of basal ganglia injury and agenesis of the corpus callosum.

Blood lactate and pyruvate levels may be normal in these patients; cerebrospinal fluid lactate and pyruvate levels are frequently abnormal. Diagnosis may be made through analysis of pyruvate dehydrogenase levels and activity of the E1 subunit in cultured cells.

In these patients, it is important to minimize the amount of carbohydrate in the diet. Oral carbohydrate administration may increase blood lactate and pyruvate levels and exacerbate symptoms. Treatment with a ketogenic diet and additional administration of thiamine may be useful (Robinson et al. 1996).

The relationship of pyruvate metabolism to the tricarboxylic acid cycle and the position of the metabolic block in pyruvate carboxylase and pyruvate dehydrogenase metabolism are illustrated in Figure 5–1.

Leigh Encephalopathy (Leigh Disease)

Altered muscle tone, spasticity or hypotonia, developmental delay or developmental regression, optic atrophy, abnormal eye movements such as nys-

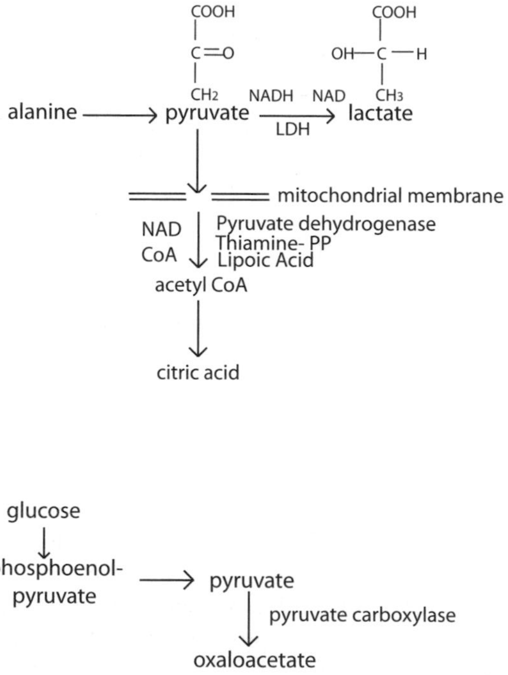

Figure 5–1. Pyruvate metabolism and the tricarboxylic acid cycle. LDH, lactate dehydrogenase; CoA, coenzyme A; NAD, nicotinamide adenine dinucleotide; NADH, reduced NAD; PP, pyrophosphate.

tagmus, ophthalmoplegia, and a history of worsening symptoms during acute illness characterize Leigh disease. Brain MRI studies reveal evidence of demyelination and basal ganglia injury.

Leigh encephalopathy may occur as a result of mutations in pyruvate dehydrogenase genes or pyruvate carboxylase–encoding genes. It may also occur as a result of mutations in the mitochondrial DNA or the nuclear DNA that encodes the respiratory complex enzymes (Dahl 1998).

The Mitochondrial Respiratory Chain

Five complexes that are embedded in the inner mitochondrial membrane form the mitochondrial respiratory chain. These complexes catalyze the translocation of protons [H$^+$] from reduced nicotinamide adenine dinucleotide (NADH) and reduced flavin adenine dinucleotide (FADH) and the parallel transduction of energy to ATP (adenosine triphosphate). Each complex is composed of multiple polypeptides. Some of these are encoded by the mitochondrial genome; most are encoded by the nuclear genome. The mitochondrial respiratory chain and oxidative phosphorylation are illustrated in Figure 5–2. The five complexes and their functions are as follows:

Complex I: NADH coenzyme Q reductase transfers protons to coenzyme Q and is composed of 28 different polypeptides, seven of which are mitochondrially encoded.

Complex II: Succinate coenzyme Q reductase carries protons from the reduced form of flavin adenine dinucleotide (FADH) to coenzyme Q. This complex contains five polypeptides, including flavin-dependent succinate dehydrogenase and iron–sulfur complexes.

Complex III: Reduced coenzyme Q cytochrome *c* reductase facilitates the transfer of H$^+$ protons from reduced coenzyme Q to cytochrome *c* and is composed of 11 subunits.

Complex IV: Cytochrome *c* oxidase is involved in the transfer of protons from cytochrome *c* to molecular oxygen. (Through the activity of complexes I, II and IV, protons pass into the space between the inner and outer mitochondrial membranes.)

Complex V: Adenosine triphosphate synthase mediates the transfer back across the mitochondrial membrane and provides energy for the synthesis of ATP.

The mitochondrial respiratory complex is also known as the oxidative phosphorylation system. It carries out the transfer of protons, and the free energy derived from the transfer of protons from NADH and FADH2 to oxygen is coupled to ATP synthesis (Hatefi 1985; Lodish et al. 1995).

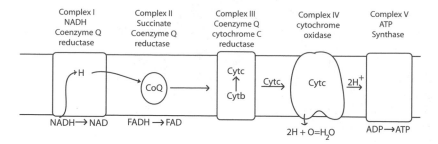

Figure 5–2. The mitochondrial respiratory chain and oxidative phosphorylation. NAD, nicotinamide adenine dinucleotide; ATP, adenosine triphosphate; FAD, flavin adenine dinucleotide; ADP, adenosine diphosphate; NADH, reduced NAD; FADH, reduced FAD.

Mitochondrial Respiratory Chain Defects

The mitochondrial respiratory chain is active in most cells. Patients with defects in one of the genes that form this complex may manifest symptoms in a number of different organs, and different symptoms may occur at different times. These disorders tend to get worse over time (Shoffner 2001; Scaglia et al. 2004; Sacconi et al. 2003).

In a particular patient, the disorder may present in the neonatal period with ketoacidosis, seizures, cardiomyopathy, hypotonia, anemia, or coma. It may present later in infancy with failure to thrive, growth retardation, and psychomotor regression. Neuromuscular deficits are often present. These include muscle weakness, muscle spasms (myoclonus), and ataxia. Histological studies on muscle may reveal abnormal muscle fibers known as ragged red fibers. Ophthalmological symptoms may occur. These include abnormal or reduced eye movements and pigmentary retinal degeneration. The latter symptoms are features of one particular mitochondrial respiratory chain defect, the Kearns-Sayre syndrome. Optic neuroretinopathy with loss of central vision is a frequent finding in another mitochondrial respiratory chain defect, Leber's optic neuroretinopathy.

Encephalopathy leading to coma may occur during episodes of lactic acidosis. In some cases, stroke-like episodes occur, leading to headache, vomiting, and limb weakness. Stroke-like episodes are common in the mitochondrial encephalopathy, lactic acidosis, and stroke-like episodes (MELAS) syndrome.

Neurogenic symptoms, including mental retardation and loss of previously developed skills, may occur in association with retinitis pigmentosa in the neuropathy, ataxia, and retinitis pigmentosa (NARP) syndrome.

In some cases, mitochondrial respiratory pathway defects are associated with gastro-intestinal symptoms, liver failure, or diabetes.

Clinical chemistry screening tests include determination of lactate/pyruvate ratios, assessment of ketones including β-hydroxybutyrate/acetoacetate ratios, urinary organic acid analysis, enzyme assays of specific complexes, and mitochondrial DNA analysis.

In mitochondrial respiratory chain defect and oxidative phosphorylation defects, it is often difficult to make a definitive diagnosis at the gene level. Many of the genes that are located on chromosomes in the nucleus and encode subunits in these complexes that function in the mitochondria are not fully characterized. Several nucleus-encoded genes important in mitochondrial respiratory complexes have been cloned. These include the Surfeit genes and succinate dehydrogenase.

The mitochondria present in a particular cell differ in their DNA sequence, a condition referred to as *heteroplasmy*. In some cells, mutant mitochondria may predominate, while in other cells, normal mitochondria predominate. Cell sampling influences results of mitochondrial DNA sequencing. Also, if tissue samples are cultured, normal cells may preferentially survive so that mutant mitochondrial DNA that is present in the patient may not be represented in the sample of cultured cells used for DNA analysis.

Treatment of oxidative phosphorylation defects includes administration of succinate, coenzyme Q, and carnitine and symptomatic treatment of acidosis.

Other Forms of Organic Acidemia where Episodes of Metabolic Acidosis and Coma may Occur

Organic acidemias are sometimes referred to as organic "acidurias" since abnormal concentrations of organic acids occur in blood and in urine. These disorders are most commonly inherited as autosomal recessive traits. They include branched chain aminoaciduria, isovaleric aciduria, propionic aciduria, and methylmalonic aciduria (see Fig. 5–3).

Branched Chain Aminoaciduria

Branched chain aminoaciduria is also known as maple syrup urine disease because the urine of affected individuals has a smell similar to that of maple syrup (Menkes et al. 1954). It results from deficiency of branched chain keto acid dehydrogenase (Chuang and Shih 2001). Deficiency of isovaleryl coenzyme A (CoA) dehydrogenase leads to isovaleric aciduria. Propionic aciduria is due to deficiency of propionyl-CoA carboxylase (Ogier de Baulny and Saudubray 2002).

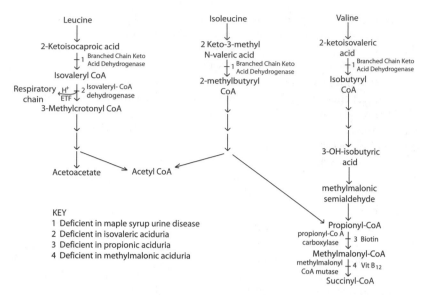

Figure 5–3. Branched chain amino acid metabolism and the position of metabolic blocks in maple syrup urine disease and three types of organic aciduria. CoA, coenzyme A; ETF, electron transport flavo-protein.

Methylmalonicaciduria

Methylmalonicaciduria is due to deficiency of methylmalonyl-CoA mutase. Activity of this enzyme can be impaired by defects at a number of different gene loci. In some cases, there are defects in the gene that encodes methylmalonyl-CoA mutase. In other cases, synthesis of the coenzyme required by methylmalonyl-CoA mutase, adenosine cobalamin (AdoCbl), is defective. This coenzyme is derived from cobalamin (vitamin B_{12}), a cobalt-containing, water-soluble vitamin that has an intricate absorption and transportation system in vertebrates. Cobalamin undergoes intracellular transformations. One of these transformations involves coupling to deoxyadenosine to generate the coenzyme (Fenton and Rosenblatt 2001).

Diagnosis and Treatment of Organic Acidemias

In all of the disorders characterized by organic aciduria, children may have developmental delay and hypotonia. They have intermittent episodes of vomiting and lethargy that may lead to acidosis and coma. Appropriate treatment of these disorders may minimize their neurological complications. In each of the organic acidemias, symptoms may present in the neonatal period or later in childhood. Symptoms may be precipitated by infections, fever, or fasting.

Diagnosis may be made on the basis of a specific abnormal profile of urinary organic acid excretion. Plasma total carnitine levels and particularly levels of free carnitine may be reduced. Specialized diagnostic laboratories may confirm diagnosis through assay of specific enzymes.

Treatment is based on administration of specific formulas, e.g., formulas free of branched chain amino acids in branched chain ketoacidosis. Patients with an inborn error of valine metabolism, isovalericacidemia, may benefit from addition of glycine to their diet.

Methylmalonicaciduria may be responsive to administration of vitamin B_{12} in quantities that exceed the normal recommended daily allowance (RDA). Carnitine administration is also an important part of the therapy. Increased levels of organic acids frequently lead to increased levels of acylcarnitine and to a relative deficiency of free carnitine and free CoA (Wajner et al. 2004). Carnitine deficiency may also be exacerbated by the fact that the acyl form is not reabsorbed in the renal tubules but excreted in the urine. Carnitine transfers long chain fatty acids into the mitochondria for use in energy metabolism. Deficiency of free carnitine leads to impaired mitochondrial energy metabolism (see Fig. 5–4).

Inborn Error of Metabolism of Leucine Responsive to Biotin

An inborn error of leucine metabolism due to deficiency of 3-methylcrotonyl-CoA carboxylase leads to excretion of excessive quantities of organic acids, including 3-methylcrotonylglycine and 3-hydroxyvaleric acid. The 3-methylcrotonyl-CoA carboxylase protein is composed of two subunits, an α subunit encoded by the *MCCA* gene and a β subunit encoded by *MCCB*. The α subunit binds to biotin. Baumgartner et al. (2004) described two patients with this disorder who responded favorably to biotin therapy. The first patient presented with psychomotor retardation and seizures. Biotin therapy led to seizure reduction and to decreased excretion of organic acids. In the second patient, Baumgartner et al. diagnosed 3-methylcrotonyl-CoA carboxylase deficiency shortly after birth. They initiated therapy with biotin in the early postnatal period, and this resulted in the patient being asymptomatic.

Interestingly, both of the patients described above were found to be heterozygous for an *MCCA* mutation, R85S. No other mutations in the *MCCA* gene were found. This finding implies that *MCCA* deficiency may be inherited as a dominant condition. This is an unusual form of inheritance for inborn errors leading to organic acid accumulation; most are inherited as autosomal recessive conditions. Baumgartner et al. (2004) demonstrated that transfection of the mutant gene into normal cells led to reduced activity of *MCCA* in those cells. Their findings support the conclusion that R85S is an example of a dominant negative mutation. The mutant allele reduced the activity of the normal allele.

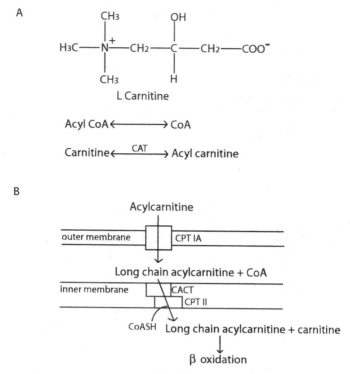

Figure 5–4. Carnitine shuttle: transport of acyl carnitine across the mitochondrial membrane to undergo β-oxidation. CoA, coenzyme A; CoASH, uncombined CoA; CPT, carnitine palmitoyltransferase; CAT, carnitine acyltransferease; CACT, carnitine acylearnitine translocase.

Inborn Errors of Biotin Metabolism

Biotin is a water-soluble enzyme that acts as a coenzyme for carboxylases involved in gluconeogenesis, fatty acid synthesis, and synthesis of amino acids. These carboxylases are inactive in the absence of covalently linked biotin. Activation requires a specific enzyme, holocarboxylase synthase, to couple biotin to carboxylases. In body tissues, biotin is stored bound to protein or to peptides and is released from biotinylated proteins and peptides to be used in enzyme activation. This release requires an enzyme, biotinidase (see Fig. 5–5).

Two genetic abnormalities of biotin metabolism are known: holocarboxylase synthase deficiency (Burri et al. 1981) and biotinidase deficiency (Hymes and Wolf 1996). These deficiencies can be effectively treated if recognized early, and in a number of countries and states in the United States newborns are screened for these disorders. Holocarboxylase synthase deficiency and biotinidase deficiency are inherited as autosomal recessive traits. The

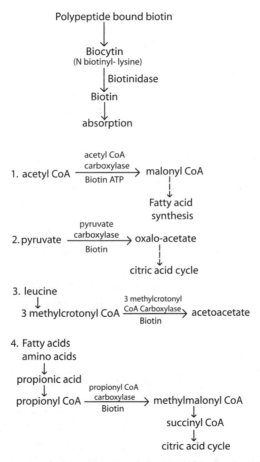

Figure 5–5. Biotin metabolism. Polypeptide-bound biotin is released by biotinidase. Carboxylases are activated by attachment of biotin through the activity of holocarboxylase synthase. CoA, coenzyme A; ATP, adenosine triphosphate.

frequency of biotinidase deficiency is 1:120,000 and it occurs more commonly than holocarboxylase synthase deficiency.

Holocarboxylase Synthase Deficiency

In approximately 50% of patients with holocarboxylase deficiency, symptoms occur in early infancy. Infants develop lethargy, vomiting, seizures, and severe acidosis; and they may lapse into coma. Patients with a less severe enzyme deficiency may present with psychomotor retardation, hair loss (*alopecia*), and a red scaly eczematous skin rash. The skin lesions often become infected, particularly with fungus of the *Candida* type. Infections, fever, or high protein intake may precipitate symptoms.

In patients with holocarboxylase synthase deficiency, there may be nonspecific elevation of organic acids in the urine. Biotin concentration in the plasma is normal. In lymphocytes, levels of holocarboxylase synthase are decreased. Levels of this enzyme in cultured cells may be normal if the culture medium contains sufficient biotin.

Treatment includes administration of biotin in quantities exceeding the RDA, vigorous and early treatment of infections, and avoidance of a high-protein diet (Wolf 2001).

Biotinidase Deficiency

Neurological symptoms are particularly prominent in biotinidase deficiency. These include lethargy, hypotonia, ataxia, and myoclonic seizures. If diagnosis is not made early and if treatment is not initiated within the first year of life, psychomotor retardation, deafness, and blindness due to optic atrophy may result. Patients with biotinidase deficiency may have eczematous skin rashes and hair loss (Moslinger et al. 2003).

Levels of free biotin in the plasma and urine are decreased. Urinary excretion of biocytin (biotin coupled to peptides) is increased. Biotinidase activity in lymphocytes and cultured cells is decreased.

Homocystinuria

Homocystinuria results from a defect in the conversion of methionine to cysteine. The most common cause of this disorder is deficiency of the enzyme cystathionine β-synthase. (see Fig. 5–6). Four organ systems are affected: the brain, eye, skeleton, and vascular system (Mudd et al. 1985). Developmental delay and mental retardation occur in 60% of cases. Approximately 60% of adults with this disorder have psychiatric symptoms. Thromboembolic episodes are common in this disorder, and these episodes may contribute to the central nervous system defects. Patients often have visual impairment, due in part to lens dislocation. Osteoporosis is often a significant problem. The high levels of homocysteine are thought to induce these problems.

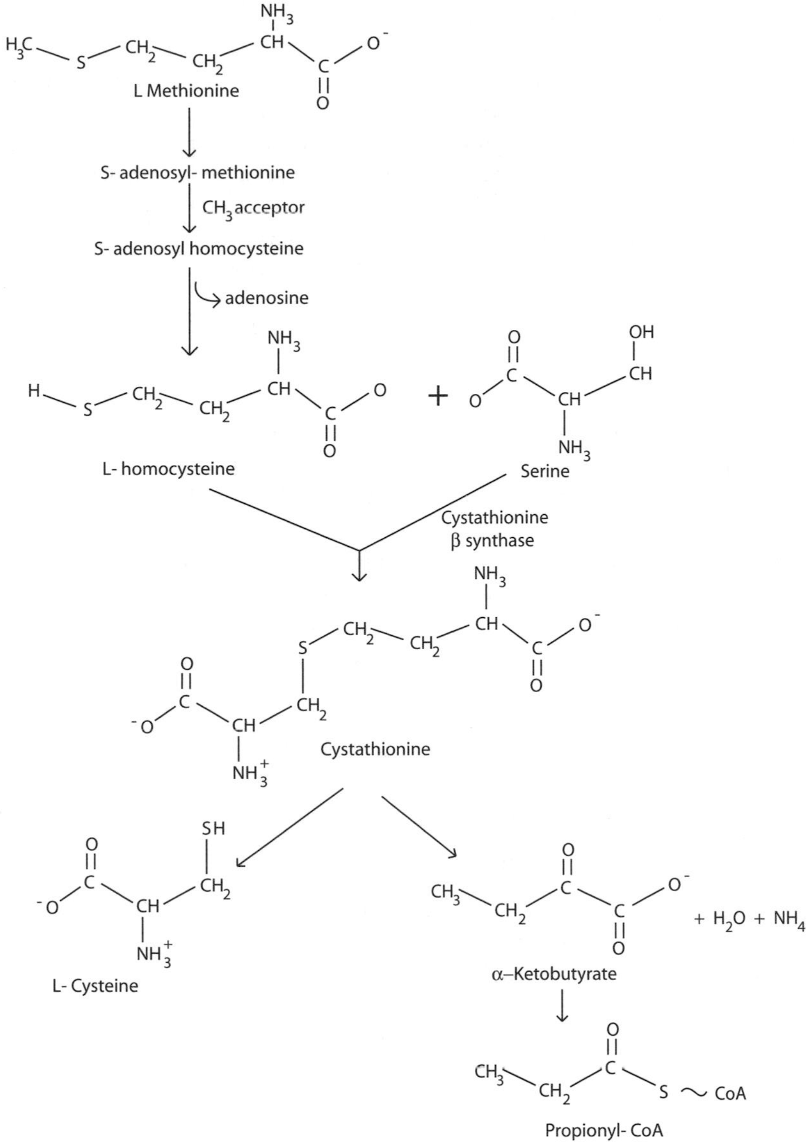

Figure 5–6. Metabolism of methionine and homocysteine. CoA, coenzyme A.

Therapy includes administration of a diet that is low in methionine and high in cystine. Some forms of the disorder are responsive to high doses of vitamin B_6. Intake of calcium and vitamin C must be adequate. Administration of betaine is useful in cases that are not vitamin B_6-responsive. Betaine (trimethylglycine) acts as a donor of methyl groups and promotes the methylation of homocysteine to methionine. This causes a reduction in the levels of homocysteine.

It is important to note that abnormally high levels of homocysteine may occur in patients who have defects in folate or vitamin B_{12} metabolism (see Fig. 5–7).

Urea Cycle Defects

The urea cycle is illustrated in Figure 5–8. Deficiency of any one of the enzymes that are involved in the synthesis of urea and disposal of excess ammonia nitrogen may lead to acute illness in the newborn period. Acute illness may occur later in infancy, particularly when larger quantities of protein are added to the diet. Other forms of stress, including infections and fever, may lead to acute episodes of lethargy and even to coma. Urea cycle defects are frequently lethal early in life. Urea cycle enzyme deficiencies are most commonly inherited as autosomal recessive traits. Ornithine transcarbamylase (OTC) deficiency is an X-linked condition (Brusilow and Horwich 2001). The gene encoding OTC maps to Xp21.1. Deficiency of OTC in male individuals is characterized by severe hyperammonemia, frequently with onset in the neonatal period. Female carriers of this disorder may be asymptomatic. They may, however, have symptoms and present with episodes of cyclic vomiting and lethargy, particularly when dietary protein intake is high. Female carriers of OTC deficiency frequently have chronic low-grade hyperammonemia. Maestri et al. (1996) and Gropman and Batshaw (2004) reported that chronic low-grade hyperammonemia and episodes of more severe hyperammonemia lead to lower intelligence quotient (IQ) scores.

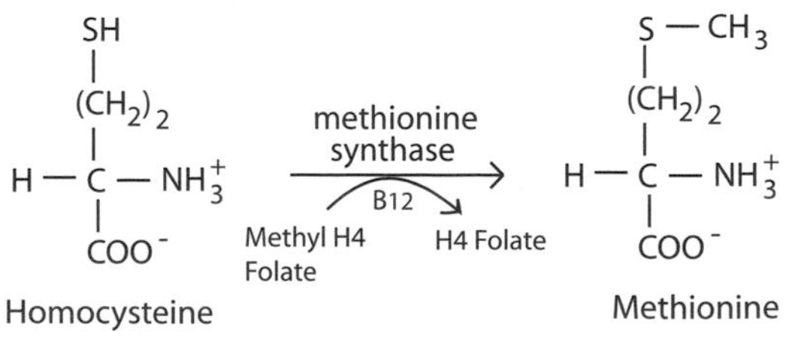

Figure 5–7. Homocysteine metabolism requires vitamin B_{12}. Deficiency of this vitamin and defects in the function of methionine synthase lead to elevated levels of homocysteine, and folate remains trapped as methyltetrahydrofolate.

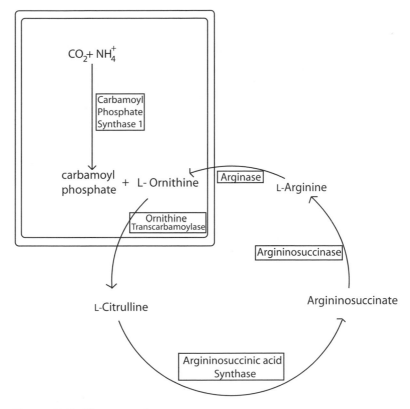

Figure 5–8. The urea cycle.

Urea cycle defects may be diagnosed by determination of blood ammonia levels and amino acid analysis of the plasma and urine. In OTC deficiency, urinary excretion of orotic acid is increased.

Treatment of urea cycle defects includes protein restriction and administration of specific amino acids and of compounds that facilitate nitrogen excretion, such as sodium benzoate or phenylacetate. Benzoate conjugates with glycine, and phenylacetate conjugates with glutamine (Endo et al. 2004).

Nonketotic Hyperglycinemia

Nonketotic hyperglycinemia disorder results from deficiency in the glycine cleavage system. This system is present in mitochondria; however, the enzymes that comprise the system are nucleus-encoded. Four proteins are involved: P protein, which is glycine decarboxylase coupled to pyridoxal phosphate (GLDC); lipoic acid–containing protein or H protein; T protein, tetrahydrofolate-requiring aminomethyltransferase (AMT); and L protein, lipoamide dehydrogenase. The first two steps in glycine catabolism involve decarboxylation and require P protein and H protein. In the third step, catalyzed by T protein, the amino group of glycine is released as ammonia and the carbon of glycine is transferred to a tetrahydrofolate cofactor. In the final step, H factor is reoxidized in a reaction that requires lipoamide dehydrogenase (Hamosh and Johnston 2001).

Nonketotic hyperglycinemia is a recessively inherited condition that occurs with a frequency of 1:55,000 newborns in Finland and 1:63,000 newborns in Canada.

In 80% of patients, nonketotic hyperglycinemia is due to mutation in the gene encoding P protein. Although the gene for P protein has been cloned and sequenced, mutation analysis is not useful for diagnosis of nonketotic hyperglycinemia except in certain population isolates. In the Finnish population, two common mutations occur. In other populations, most mutations are unique to a specific family.

In 15% of patients, this disorder is due to mutations in the gene encoding T protein.

L protein is required not only for glycine cleavage but also for activity of branched chain ketoacid dehydrogenase and pyruvate dehydrogenase. In patients with defects in the gene encoding lipoamide dehydrogenase, plasma levels of glycine and branched chain amino acids are elevated.

Patients with nonketotic hyperglycinemia usually develop symptoms during infancy. These include feeding difficulties, hypotonia, and seizures. Uncontrolled seizures may lead to respiratory failure. Diagnosis is based on finding high glycine levels in plasma, urine, and cerebrospinal fluid in patients who do not have acidosis or ketosis and who have normal urinary organic acids. Hyperglycinemia may occur secondarily in organic acidemias that are associated with acidosis and ketosis (Hamosh and Johnston 2001). Several authors have reported a transient neonatal form of hyperglycinemia associated with seizures, which resolves after the newborn period (Applegarth and Toone 2001). Nonketotic hyperglycinemia may present in childhood with developmental delay, mental retardation, and seizures (Hoover-Fong et al. 2004).

There is no treatment that prevents the neurological complications of this disorder. Dietary therapies that may decrease symptoms to some degree include low-protein diet, sodium benzoate, and administration Dextromethorphan, which apparently decreases seizures. This drug suppresses N-methyl-D-aspartate (NMDA) glutamate receptors, which are apparently stimulated by high levels of glycine (Hamosh et al. 1998). Figure 5–9 illustrates the metabolic effect of benzoate in the treatment of hyperglycinemia; glycine conjugates with activated benzoate and is excreted as hippuric acid.

Serine Biosynthetic Defects

Serine is classified as a nonessential amino acid since it is synthesized in the body (see Fig. 5–10). Jaeken (2000) reported that in certain patients adequate

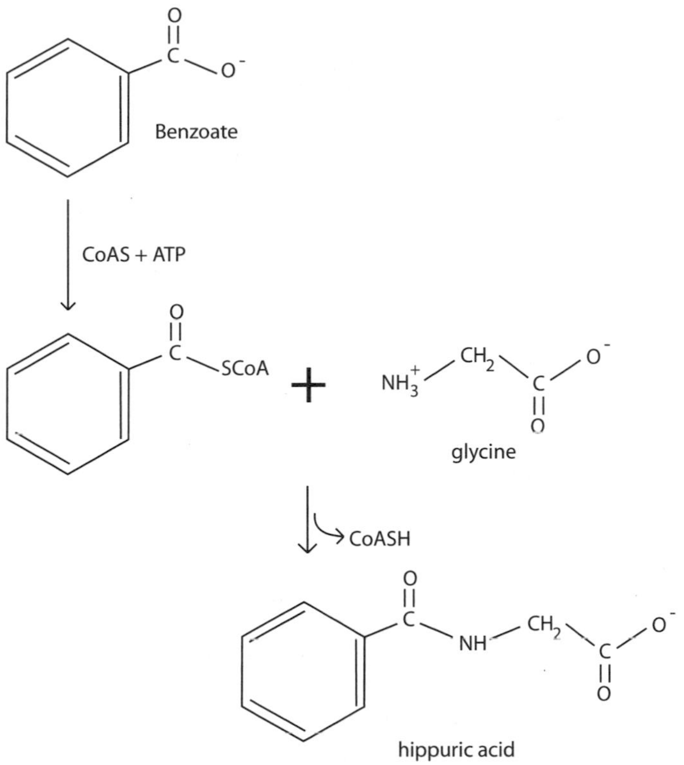

Figure 5–9. Sodium benzoate is used in the treatment of nonketotic hyperglycinemia. Activated benzoate conjugates with glycine and is excreted as hippuric acid. ATP, adenosine triphosphate; CoA, coenzyme A; CoAS, non-reduced form; CoASH, reduced form; SCoA, coenzyme A bound via sulfhydryl group.

serine biosynthesis does not occur and serine deficit leads to neurological symptoms. Defective serine biosynthesis may occur due to defects in the gene encoding 3-phosphoglycerate dehydrogenase (Pind et al. 2002) or in cases where the gene encoding phosphoserine phosphatase is deficient (de Koning et al. 2003).

In the biosynthesis of serine and glycine, 3-phosphoglycerate is converted to phosphohydroxypyruvate, which is then converted to phosphoserine. The latter is converted to L- serine, which in turn is converted to glycine. Serine is synthesized by astrocytes and supplied to neurons. Glycine and serine are activating ligands of the NMDA neuroreceptor complex, and they modulate neurotransmission. They participate differently in different parts of the brain. (see Fig. 5–11).

Patients with 3-phosphoglycerate dehydrogenase deficiency develop severe psychomotor retardation, seizures, and microcephaly. On brain MRI

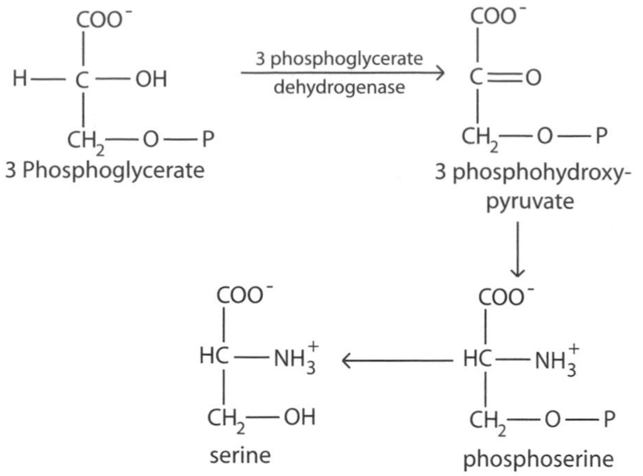

Figure 5–10. Biosynthesis of serine.

there is evidence of hypomyelination and white matter attenuation. Diagnosis is made on the basis of amino acid analysis in the fasting state. Glycine and serine levels are low in plasma and cerebrospinal fluid. Diagnosis may be confirmed by enzyme assays in cultured fibroblasts. These assays reveal deficient activity of 3-phosphoglycerate dehydrogenase. Seizures may be controlled by administration of serine (Hausler et al. 2001).

Phosphoserine phosphatase deficiency is a very rare condition. Seizures that occur in this condition may be controlled by serine administration.

Mental Retardation Associated with Spasticity and Movement Disorders

Pelizaeus-Merzbacher Disease and Spastic Paraplegia Type 2

Pelizaeus-Merzbacher disease and spastic paraplegia type 2 are characterized by the inability to form normal myelin (Hudson 2003). Myelination begins in prenatal life and continues during postnatal life, primarily during the first 2 years. Myelination is, however, not complete until the second decade of life. Myelin sheaths are formed from the cell membranes of oligodendrocytes. Sensory pathways develop myelin sheaths before motor pathways.

The first signs of classical Pelizaeus-Merzbacher disease appear in early infancy and include wandering, undirected, or rhythmical eye movements. Infants have very poor head control. Later, abnormal limb movements and limb spasticity develop. Intellectual handicap is present, though the extent of this is difficult to evaluate given the motor deficits and delayed speech. Patients may survive through the second decade of life.

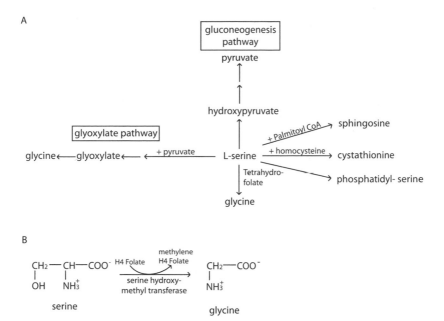

Figure 5–11. Key metabolic roles of L-serine. CoA, coenzyme A.

Type II Pelizaeus-Merzbacher disease, sometimes referred to as the connatal form, is a severer form of the disorder characterized by abnormal eye movements, breathing difficulties, jerky and uncoordinated movements of the extremities, and rapidly progressing spasticity. Children with this disorder usually die before the age of 10 years.

A form of the disease that is milder than the classical form also occurs. In this disorder, abnormal eye and limb movements occur, spasticity is less severe, and mental development is not impaired.

Spastic paraplegia type 2 is a related disorder in which patients manifest abnormal eye movements and ataxia; spasticity of the lower limbs develops more slowly than in Pelizaeus-Merzbacher disease. Mental retardation is usually mild, and in some patients there is no evidence of intellectual impairment.

Electrophysiological studies reveal reduced visual and auditory evoked potentials. Central nervous system MRI shows hypomyelination. Histopathology of the brain in the severest form of Pelizaeus-Merzbacher disease reveals an absence of myelin. Central nervous system myelin is reduced in the less severe form of the disease and in spastic paraplegia type 2. Oligodendrocytes may be reduced in number.

Genetics

The earliest description of Pelizaeus-Merzbacher disease noted that this disorder is inherited as an X-linked trait, symptoms occur in male individuals, and the disease is passed on by female carriers who themselves have no manifestations of the disease. In a few reports, female individuals were noted to have symptoms. Development of symptoms in these female subjects may have been due to nonrandom X inactivation that resulted in inactivation of X chromosomes that carry the normal allele so that the X chromosome that carried the disease gene locus was expressed.

In 1994, Boespflug-Tanguy et al. reported that the Pelizaeus-Merzbacher disease gene mapped to the proteolipid protein (PLP) gene locus on Xq22-q23. Discovery of the PLP defect in Pelizaeus-Merzbacher disease was in part facilitated by the discovery that the PLP gene is mutated in "jimpy" mice. Mice in this mutant strain have a neurological disease with some of the same manifestations as Pelizaeus-Merzbacher disease.

The PLP gene in humans is subject to duplication and deletion. Approximately 50% of reported patients with Pelizaeus-Merzbacher disease have PLP gene duplications (Woodward et al. 1998; Woodward and Malcolm 1999). One extra copy of the gene leads to the classical form of the disease; triplication of the gene locus results in severe disease. Cailloux et al. (2000) reported that mutations leading to single amino acid changes in regions of the PLP gene that are evolutionarily highly conserved occur in patients with the most severe form of Pelizaeus-Merzbacher disease. Point mutations and splice site mutations in the less highly conserved gene regions are usually associated with less severe disease. In a number of families with Pelizaeus-Merzbacher disease the disorder mapped to Xp22 but no mutations in the PLP gene were found. It is possible that in these cases disease results from mutations in upstream or downstream loci that control expression of the PLP gene.

Mental Retardation Associated with Involuntary Abnormal Movements, Dystonia, and Athetosis

Glutaric Acidemia Type 1

Glutaric acidemia type 1 is due to deficiency of the enzyme glutaryl-CoA dehydrogenase. As many as 60 different disease-causing mutations have been identified, and patients may be homozygous for a particular mutation. Some patients are compound heterozygotes; they inherit a different glutaryl-CoA dehydrogenase gene mutation from each parent. The metabolism of lysine and tryptophan and the functions of glutaryl-CoA dehydrogenase are illustrated in Figure 5–12.

Patients with this inborn error of metabolism develop movement disorder, athetosis, and hypotonia during the first year of life. *Athetosis* is a condition in which slow, writhing involuntary movements of flexion, extension, pronation, and supination occur. Abnormal movements and decreased muscle tone frequently begin after an episode of acute illness associated with acido-

A.

Lysine metabolism and glutaric aciduria Type 1

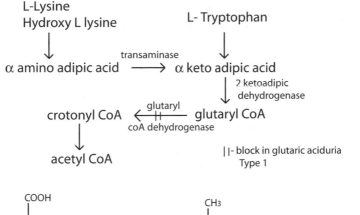

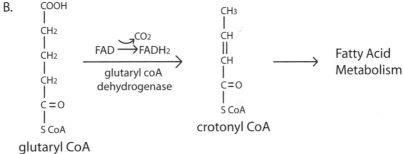

Figure 5–12. Metabolic defect in glutaric aciduria. CoA, coenzyme A; FAD, flavin adenine dinucleotide; FADH, reduced FAD; SCoA, coenzyme A bound through sulfhydryl group.

sis. Progressive cerebral atrophy occurs in untreated patients. Fronto-temporal atrophy occurs, and in many cases neuronal degeneration is detectable in the caudate nucleus and putamen.

It is important to recognize this disorder because it is responsive to treatment with protein restriction and carnitine administration (Hoffman et al. 1996). This disorder may be missed on organic acid analysis. Analysis of plasma and urine carnitine is important. Free carnitine is reduced and glutaryl carnitine is increased in plasma samples from patients.

In certain population isolates, including the Old Order Amish, glutaric acidemia type 1 occurs with a higher frequency than in the general population (Strauss et al. 2003).

N-Glycan Synthesis Defects

Many proteins undergo posttranslational modification that involves glycosylation and addition of chains composed of oligosaccharides. Following translation, oligosaccharides are attached to proteins through *O* or *N* linkages. *O*-Linked glycosylation defects were discussed in Chapter 3 (see Muscle-Eye Brain MEB disease). In *N*-linked glycan synthesis, oligosaccharides are bound to the amino acid asparagine.

Glycan synthesis is dependent upon the activity of glycosyl transferases and sugar donors including nucleotide sugars or dolichol phosphate-linked sugars. Degradation of glycan chains occurs through the activity of glycosidases. *N*-Glycan synthesis and protein glycosylation takes place in the endoplasmic reticulum, Golgi apparatus, and cytoplasm of the cell. It involves at least 40 steps (Grunewald et al. 2002). *N*-Linked glycoproteins may be secreted from cells. They are also constituents of cell membranes.

Jaeken et al. (1997) discovered the first genetic disorder of *N*-glycan synthesis in monozygotic twins with seizures, abnormal muscle tone, and developmental delay. They noted that when serum from these patients was electrophoresed, a number of different serum proteins showed abnormal electrophoretic mobility compared with serum from controls. At least 20 disorders involving *N*-glycans are known (Jaeken and Carchon 2004).

Phosphomannomutase Deficiency: Congenital Defect in Glycan Synthesis Type 1A

Congenital defect in glycan synthesis type 1A (CDGS1A) is the most common congenital disorder of glycan synthesis. It has a worldwide distribution (reviewed by Jaeken 2003). Patients often present during infancy with abnormal head and eye movements, including eye rolling and abnormal horizontal or vertical movements. Later mental retardation manifests. In affected children, IQ usually ranges 40–60. There is no progressive loss of IQ. Patients are usually not able to walk unaided. Patients usually do not have dysmorphic features. Some patients have large, somewhat abnormally shaped ears. In others, abnormal fat distribution and nipple retraction have been noted. Patients may have episodes of thrombosis and stroke-like episodes.

Biochemical findings include electrophoretic and functional abnormalities of many glycoproteins including enzymes, hormones, and transport proteins. Serum levels of many proteins, including thyroid hormones, may be reduced due to the fact that inadequately glycosylated proteins are more rapidly cleared from the circulation than normally glycosylated proteins.

Postmortem studies on brains from patients with CDGS1A have revealed neuronal loss and gliosis that involves the cortex, basal ganglia, and spinal cord. The olivopontocerebellar regions of the brain are frequently hypoplastic.

Rett Syndrome

Rett syndrome represents a category of mental retardation that is associated with abnormal hand movements. This syndrome is discussed in Chapters 4 and 7.

Mental Retardation Associated with Sensorineural Abnormalities Such as Blindness and/or Deafness

Sensorineural deficit and impaired intellectual function may be due to the same underlying biochemical or developmental defect. However, sensorineural deficit may in and of itself impact learning and adaptation. Fazzi et al. (2003) emphasized the risk of overestimating the frequency of mental retardation in cases of congenital blindness because of the use of tests that are not adequate to evaluate intellect in such children.

Evenhuis et al. (2001) carried out screening of hearing and visual function in institutionalized patients with intellectual disability. They reported that the prevalence of hearing and visual impairment was considerably increased in all groups, including mildly, moderately, and severely impaired individuals. In patients younger than 50 years with mild to moderate intellectual disability, they determined that hearing impairment was present in 21% and visual impairment was present in 4% of cases. In the general Dutch population in the same age group, hearing impairment is present in 2%–7% and visual impairment is present in 0.2%–1.9%.

Leber Amaurosis

Leber amaurosis is a form of retinal dystrophy. Diagnosis of blindness is usually made shortly after birth or in the first few months of life. Retinal examination reveals atrophy of the retina and macula; optic disc pallor and pigment spicules may be present at the periphery of the retina. Vision is greatly impaired, and there is an absence of activity on the electroretinogram. Mental retardation occurs in approximately 20% of cases of Leber amaurosis. Children with this disorder and children with other forms of blindness often manifest stereotypic behaviors, including head rocking, finger movements such as eye poking, and facial grimacing. Language is reported to be peculiar; although vocabulary is rich, it seems that language is not used for interactive communication (Fazzi et al. 2003).

Leber amaurosis is genetically heterogeneous. At least 10 gene loci play a role in this disorder, and specific gene mutations have been identified at seven of these loci. There are three mapped loci that determine Leber amaurosis, where at the time of writing no specific disease-determining gene was yet identified. These loci are LCA3 on 14q24, LCA5 on 6q11-q16, and LCA9 on 1p36.

Table 5–1
Gene Defects Leading to Visual Impairment

Gene Symbol	Name, Function	Map Location	% of Cases
GUCY2D	Retina-specific	LCA1	21%
RetGC1	Guanylate kinase	17p13.1	
CRB1	Homolog of Drosophila Crumbs gene	CRB1 1q31	10%
RPE65	Retinal pigment, epithelium protein 65	LCA2 1p31	6.1%
RPGP1P1	Retinal pigment quanine triphosphatase– interacting protein	LCA6 14q11	4.5%
AIPL1	Arylhydrocarbon receptor–interacting protein-like	LCA4 17p13.3	3.4%
TULP1	Tubby-like protein	6q21.3	1.7%
CRX	Cone rod homeobox gene	19q13.3	0.6%

Specific genes involved in this disorder are summarized in the Table 5–1. Leber amaurosis is usually inherited as an autosomal recessive condition; for the disorder to manifest, each parent must transmit a mutation in the same gene. However, in the case of the CRX gene, deleterious heterozygous mutations can give rise to the phenotype (Perrault et al. 2003).

Hanein et al. (2004) reported that the seven genes identified as playing a role in this disorder are preferentially expressed in retinal photoreceptor cells or in the retinal pigment epithelium. Each of these genes is, however, involved in a different pathophysiological pathway. Hainen et al. (2004) reported that 38% of their Leber amaurosis patients originated in Mediterranean countries and that in 40% of these patients GUCY2D gene mutations led to the disease.

It is not clear at the time of writing whether or not specific gene mutations that lead to Leber amaurosis are likely to lead to mental retardation. Schuil et al. (1998) proposed that mental retardation was a variable expression of Leber amaurosis. In a study of 229 cases, they identified 11 siblings who were concordant for Leber amaurosis and discordant for intellectual impairment.

Leber Hereditary Optic Neuropathy

Leber hereditary optic neuropathy is different from Leber amaurosis. It is characterized by loss of central vision that is acute in onset and rapidly affects both eyes. The age at onset is between 15 and 35 years. Loss of vision is caused by degenerative changes in the optic nerve and in retinal ganglion cells. Other neurodegenerative changes may occur and lead to dystonia, rigidity of muscles, and intellectual impairment.

Leber hereditary optic neuropathy is caused by missense mutations in mitochondrial DNA. Four specific mitochondrial DNA mutations lead to this disorder in the majority of cases. Each patient will have one of these mutations. Deleterious mitochondrial DNA mutations affect both male and female individuals and are transmitted by female individuals. Nucleus gene defects that lead to visual impairment are listed in Table 5–1.

Usher Syndrome

Usher syndrome is characterized by progressive retinitis pigmentosa leading to blindness and sensorineural deafness with or without vestibular abnormality. There is evidence that Usher syndrome results from a defect in ciliary structures or in ciliary progenitor cells. Ciliated progenitor cells give rise to retinal photoreceptor cells, auditory hair cells, and vestibular hair cells. Retinitis pigmentosa results from degeneration of the retinal photoreceptor cells, and this in turn leads to loss of visual function. The retinal photoreceptor cells carry out the first step in the visual process, namely absorption of light and conversion of vitamin A–derived chromophores to the activated visual pigment rhodopsin. This in turn participates in transduction of the visual signal. Retinal pigment epithelium also participates in regeneration of photopigments.

Hallgren (1959) published a study on 177 cases of Usher syndrome in 102 families. He reported that mental deficiency and/or psychosis occurred in 25% of cases. Schaefer et al. (1998) reported results of brain MRI studies on 19 patients with Usher syndrome. The size of the brain and of the cerebellum was decreased and that of the subarachnoid space was increased. Schaefer et al. (1998) concluded that the disease process in Usher syndrome affects the whole brain.

Usher syndrome displays clinical heterogeneity. Patients with Usher syndrome type 1 (USH1) have retinitis pigmentosa, marked hearing loss, and vestibular dysfunction. Their disease manifests shortly after birth. Type 2 (USH2) patients have retinitis pigmentosa, less severe hearing loss, and normal vestibular function. Type 3 (USH3) occurs primarily in Finland and is characterized by retinitis pigmentosa and hearing loss that progresses over time; vestibular function is variable.

Ahmed et al. (2003) reviewed linkage studies and molecular genetic analyses in Usher syndrome. The gene loci involved, the proteins they encode, and the frequency of mutations at these loci in the Usher syndrome population are listed in Table 5–2. Data for this table are compiled from information published by Ahmed et al. (2003) and Keats and Savas (2004).

At least eight different loci play a role in USH1. Specific genes at five of these loci have been identified, and mutations that lead to USH1 have been characterized. In schools for the deaf in a number of different countries, USH1 occurs in approximately 10% of cases; half of these cases are USH1B that are due to mutations in the *Myo7a* gene, which maps to chromosome 11q13.5.

Table 5–2
Gene Defects in Usher Syndrome

Syndrome	Map Position	Gene	Protein	% of Usher Patients
USH1B	11q13.5	*Myo7a*	Myosin7a	49%
USH1C	11p15.1	*USH1C*	Harmonin	>2%
USH1D	10q22.1	*CDH23*	Cadherin 23	USH1D + USH1F 33%
USH1F	10q21.1	*PCDH15*	Protocadherin 15	
USH1G	17q24-q25	*SANS*	Sans	
USH1		Unknown		16%
USH2A	1q41	*USH2a*	Usherin	70% of USH2
USH3A	3q25.1	*USH3*	Clarin	

USH1F is due to mutations in Protocadherin 15. A particular mutation, R245X, is common in the Ashkenazi Jewish population. Brownstein et al. (2004) determined that the carrier rate for this mutation in the hearing population in Israel is 1%. These investigators noted that Usher syndrome mutations, such as R245X, lead to early deafness and later to retinitis pigmentosa and blindness. Early restoration of hearing can then be implemented through cochlear implants before the onset of visual loss. By enabling these children to hear, they are rescued from dual neurosensory deficit.

The USH2 phenotype is linked to four different loci. Mutations in usherin account for 70% of cases of USH2. The most common form is USH2A. A specific USH2A mutation, 2299delG, is common in the United States, Europe, South Africa, and China (Ahmed et al. 2003).

Type 3 Usher syndrome is linked to two different gene loci. Mutations in the Clarin gene lead to USH3A. Gene defects in Usher syndrome are listed in Table 5–2.

Many of the Usher syndrome loci overlap with loci that are linked to nonsyndromic deafness. Mutations in myosin7a occur not only in USH1 but also in two different forms of inherited nonsyndromic deafness, DFNA11 and DFNB2. Most of the mutations that cause USH1B are located in the motor domain of myosin7a. Mutations in the gene that encodes the protein Harmonin occur in USH1C and in nonsyndromic deafness DFNB18.

A specific mutation in the USH2A encoded protein Usherin is present in 4.5% of cases of recessively inherited retinitis pigmentosum without deafness.

There is evidence that myosin7a, harmonin, cadherin 23, and sans interact through PDZ domains present in harmonin (Siemens et al. 2002). The motor domain in myosin is linked to actin bundles (see Fig. 5–13). The interaction of these proteins leads to a transmembrane complex that stabilizes stereocilia in the inner ear (Boeda et al. 2002; Delprat et al. 2004). Disorganized stereocilia occur as a result of mutations in myosin or cadherin (Di Palma et al. 2001) (see Fig. 5–14).

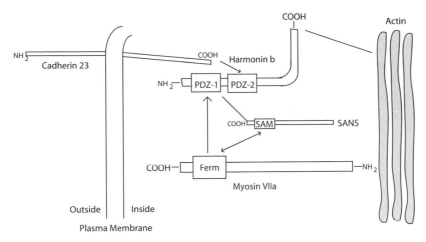

Figure 5–13. The interactions of proteins that play a role in hearing (illustration based on Ahmed et al. 2003; Weil et al. 2003; DePrat et al. 2004).

Protocadherin 15, the protein that is defective in USH1F, is expressed in a number of different tissues and is particularly abundant in the inner and outer hair cells of the inner ear.

Usherin, the protein that is mutated in USH2A, is a critical component of the basement membrane in the cochlea and in the retina. Clarin, the protein that is mutated in USH3A, is present in hair cells and in the cochlear ganglia (see Fig. 5-15).

Norrie Disease

Norrie disease occurs in male individuals and is characterized by congenital blindness due to degenerative and proliferative processes in the neuroretina. It

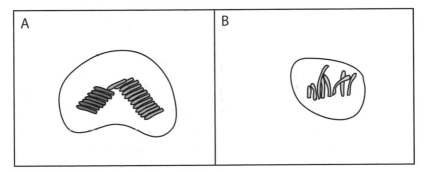

Figure 5–14. *A*: The normal organization of stereocilia. *B*: Disorganized stereocilia associated with mutations in myosin7a or mutations in cadherin 23 (based on Adato et al. 2002).

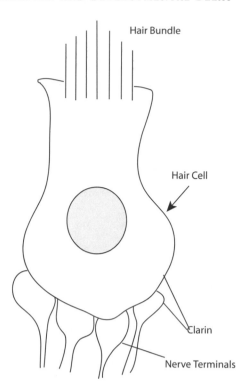

Figure 5–15. Hair cell, hair bundles, cochlear nerve cell terminals, and location of Clarin protein. Clarin is mutated in Usher syndrome type 3A (USH3A).

is often associated with microphthalmia. Ophthalmoscopy shortly after birth frequently reveals an intraocular mass that may be mistaken for retinoblastoma. Histological analysis of the intraocular mass proves that it is composed of immature retinal cells, vascular connective tissue, and ocular vitreous material.

A number of authors have reported that deafness and mental retardation sometimes occur in patients with Norrie disease. Royer et al. (2003) reported results of clinical and molecular studies in patients with Norrie disease. They examined 16 patients and determined that 10 of them were mentally retarded and six patients suffered progressive hearing loss. Progressive hearing loss and mental retardation occurred in 3 of the 16 patients.

Berger et al. (1992) and Chen et al. (1992) identified mutations in a gene in Xp11.2. They designated the gene *NDP*, for Norrie disease protein. Royer et al. (2003) reported that in 7 of the 22 families they studied there was no evidence of *NDP* sequence changes. They proposed that other gene loci play a role in generating a phenotype similar to that of Norrie disease.

Xu et al. (2004) reported that incomplete retinal vascularization occurs in Norrie disease and in familial exudative vitreoretinopathy. The latter condition is due to mutations in the human homolog of the *Drosophila* gene Frizzled 4, which functions as a receptor for the *WNT* gene. Xu et al. (2004) determined that the protein encoded by the NDP locus, Norrin, interacts with FZ4. They proposed that the Norrin FZ4 signaling system plays a central role in vascular development in the eye and ear.

Mental Retardation Associated with Sensorimotor Neuropathy (Anderman Syndrome)

Anderman syndrome is transmitted as an autosomal recessive trait. It occurs with a frequency of 1:2117 in Quebec Province, Canada, and has been reported in Spain, Italy, Austria, and the Middle East. During the first years of life, infants with this disorder are hypotonic and their developmental milestones are delayed. Children may develop the ability to walk by 6 years of age. In adolescence, there is frequently a loss of previously attained motor skills. Seizures commonly occur. Brain MRI frequently reveals agenesis of the corpus callosum.

The gene determining this disorder was mapped to chromosome 15 through linkage analysis in extended pedigrees with multiple affected individuals (Casaubon et al. 1996). Howard et al. (2002) achieved fine mapping of the disorder through linkage disequilibrium analysis. They subsequently identified mutations in the gene that encodes the potassium and chloride cotransporter *SLC12A6*. They identified a mutation in exon 18 of this gene in all French Canadian individuals affected with this disorder. Howard et al. (2002) disrupted the *Slc12A6* gene in mice. The *Slc12A6*$^{-/-}$ mutants showed locomotor deficits that manifested as limb weakness and disorganized limb movements. Exploratory activity was also significantly reduced in these mice. Histological studies revealed hypomyelination, demyelination, axon swelling, and axon fiber degeneration.

The *SLC12A6* gene is expressed in most areas of the brain and in white matter tracts in the spinal cord. Very low levels of SLC12A6 protein are detected in the dorsal root ganglia in the spinal cord.

Howard et al. (2002) noted that Anderman syndrome represents the first known neurodevelopmental disorder of the central nervous system caused by an ion transporter defect. They postulated that the KCl cotransporter encoded by *SLC12A6* participates in the regulation of cell volume in neurons, oligodendrocytes, and Schwann cells that constitute nerve sheaths.

Canavan Disease

Key features of Canavan disease are abnormal muscle tone, macrocephaly, and visual loss. The latter occurs later in the course of the disease. Canavan disease is rare in most populations; however, in the Ashkenazi Jewish population, the carrier frequency is approximately 1 in 40. Developmental delay and abnormal muscle tone frequently occur by 4 months of age. Infants are hypotonic, and head control is poor. By 6 months of age, they have an abnormal increase in head circumference and the fontanelle size is larger than expected for age.

Later in the course of the disease, muscle tone is increased, tendon reflexes are brisk, and the plantar reflex is abnormal (Babinski's sign is positive). Opisthotonic posturing may occur. Infants may become blind. Death frequently occurs by 3 years of age; some children survive longer.

Brain neuropathology reveals that Canavan disease is a leukodystrophy that leads to spongiform degeneration in the brain.

Kvittingen et al. (1986) reported that elevated levels of N-acetylaspartic acid occur in the urine of patients with Canavan disease. Matalon et al. (1988) and Diory et al. (1988) reported that deficiency of the enzyme aspartoacylase occurs in this disorder. N-acetylaspartic acid occurs predominantly in the nervous system. It can be readily imaged in normal brain by proton nuclear magnetic resonance spectroscopy. Aspartoacylase is expressed primarily in glial cells, particularly in oligodendrocytes (Gordon 2001). In the absence of normal enzyme, N-acetylaspartic acid accumulates in glial cells. This promotes swelling of the cells and subsequent vacuolization. This interferes with the function of oligodendrocytes, namely provision of a stable myelin sheath.

Many of the clinical findings in Canavan disease resemble those in Tay-Sachs disease and glutaric aciduria; it is important to distinguish these disorders. Diagnosis of Canavan disease may be made through finding elevated levels of N-acetylaspartate in urine, blood, and cerebrospinal fluid.

DNA analysis is useful for carrier screening. Two mutations commonly occur in the aspartoacylase-encoding gene in Ashkenazi Jewish carriers. In 83% of carriers, an E285A amino acid substitution occurs, and a Y231X substitution is present in 15% of cases (Matalon and Matalon 2002). In non-Jewish patients, the mutation range is broader; however, A305E mutations occur in 60% of cases.

Canavan disease is not rare in Turkish communities. The most common mutation in this community is a deletion mutation in exon 4 (Sistermans et al. 2000). This mutation is rare in other population groups, indicating a founder effect for Canavan disease in Turkey.

Mental Retardation Associated with Muscle Defects

Duchenne Muscular Dystrophy

Duchenne muscular dystrophy results from deletions or mutations in the gene that encodes the protein dystrophin. Intragenic deletions constitute the most common form of mutation. The dystrophin-encoding gene is the largest known gene in humans. This gene is located at Xp21.2 and comprises 1.5% of the X chromosome. It includes sequence for 79 coding exons and 7 promoters. Dystrophin is expressed primarily in muscle. There are, however, a number of different tissue-specific isoforms of dystrophin. Several of these are expressed in brain or in retina. Mutations or deletions that affect the structure or expression of the brain-specific isoforms of dystrophin are associated with central nervous system manifestations.

There are three upstream promoters that give rise to three different full-length transcripts, each with a different first exon. The full-length transcripts are approximately 14,000 bp in length. Within the dystrophin-encoding gene, there are four internal promoters; and these give rise to short forms of dystrophin, DP260, DP140, DP116, and DP71. These short forms lack the actin-binding domain but retain the domains that bind dystroglycan, dystrobrevin, and syntrophin. DP260 is expressed at high concentrations in the retina; DP140 is expressed in the brain; DP71 is expressed in the brain and retina; DP116 is expressed only in peripheral nerves (Muntoni et al. 2003).

There is considerable variation in IQ in Duchenne muscular dystrophy patients (Giliberto et al. 2004). Deletion mutations or exon-skipping mutations that disrupt the shorter isoforms of dystrophin are correlated with IQ deficits in Duchenne and Becker muscular dystrophy patients (Muntoni et al. 2003). Patients with mutations that lead to loss of exons 3' of exon 63, i.e., loss of the DP71 isoform of dystrophin, have severe mental retardation. Some of these patients have autistic manifestations (Felisare et al. 2000).

Dystrophin is expressed primarily in postsynaptic neurons in the cerebral cortex, hippocampus, and cerebellum. Brunig et al. (2002) reported that dystrophin colocalizes with $GABA_A$ receptor subunits. Knusel et al. (1999) proposed that dystrophin plays an important role in the clustering and stabilization of GABA-type receptors.

Although altered vision is not a symptom of Duchenne muscular dystrophy, abnormal electroretinography analyses occur in some patients. This phenotype occurs more commonly in patients with mutations in the central or 3' Dystrophin gene regions.

Facioscapulohumeral Muscular Dystrophy

Facioscapulohumeral muscular dystrophy (FSHD) is characterized by weakness and atrophy of the muscles of the face, shoulders, and upper arms. Early-onset cases of FSHD may display mental retardation and epilepsy. Funakoshi et al. (1998) reported that mental retardation occurred in eight out of nine patients with early-onset FSHD. Miura et al. (1998) described two patients with early-onset FSHD and seizures. One patient had infantile spasms; the other had localized seizures. In one patient, the IQ score was 33; in the other, it was 45.

In 1992, Wijmenga et al. reported that FSHD is linked to polymorphic marker D4Z4. Detailed analysis of this locus revealed that it is comprised of tandem copies of a 3.3 kb dispersed repeat. In normal individuals, between 10 and 100 tandem copies of this repeat are present. Deletions of this locus that leave between 1 and 8 copies of the repeat result in FSHD. Severity of the disease is correlated with the number of repeats that remain; the fewer repeats that remain, the more severe the disease (Padberg et al. 1995). Ding et al. (1998) and Gabriels et al. (1999) analyzed the sequence of the 3.3 kb repeat and determined that it included an open reading frame that encoded the protein DUX4, with two homeodomains.

The subtelomeric region of chromosome 10q contains sequences that are highly homologous to D4Z4. A series of different restriction endonuclease digestions must be carried out to distinguish 4q-derived repeats from 10q repeats.

Gabellini et al. (2002) reported that an element within the D4Z4 repeat binds to a multiprotein complex. This complex includes a transcriptional repressor, HMGB2; an architectural protein; and a nucleolin protein. They demonstrated that binding of this multiprotein complex to D4Z4 leads to transcriptional repression of a number of genes in 4q35. Gabellini et al. (2002) proposed that when quantities of the D4Z4 element are insufficient or when sequence is altered so that binding of the multiprotein complex to D4Z4 is insufficient, there is inadequate transcription repression and overexpression of 4q35 genes. Symptoms of FSHD result from overexpression of genes in 4q35. The FSHD locus is therefore not a protein-producing locus; it is a regulatory locus (Tupler and Gabellini 2004).

Lemmers et al. (2002, 2004) described a polymorphic segment of 10 kb distal to D4Z4 on 4q35. They reported that this polymorphic segment occurs in two size forms, designated 4qA and 4qB, that occur at approximately equal frequencies in the normal population. In 80 unrelated cases of FSHD, only the 4qA polymorphism occurred. Lemmers et al. proposed that the inadequate transcription repression that is characteristic of FSHD must be associated with the 4qA allele or that the 4qB allele protects against transcriptional derepression. They proposed that 4qA is a benign polymorphism that influences development of a genetic disease.

6

Mental Retardation That Develops after a Period of Normal Cognition

In this chapter, we will review disorders that disrupt development and the maturation of cognition in children with no previous evidence of delay. We will focus primarily on genetic diseases that are associated with abnormal storage of normal substances, i.e., lysosomal storage diseases, peroxisomal disorders, and copper storage disease. We include a discussion of Rett syndrome since in this condition girls who have developed normally for 1 or more years undergo regressive changes. There are also environmental conditions that lead to disruption of normal development. We will review neurodevelopmental effects of malnutrition in early childhood and neurocognitive deficits in children exposed to certain pesticides and heavy metals.

Lysosomal Storage Diseases That Lead to Mental Retardation

It is extremely important to recognize those patients where lysosomal storage disease leads to developmental delay or mental retardation. Accurate diagnosis is necessary for patient management and for appropriate counseling of the family. At the end of this section, recent advances in the treatment of lysosomal storage diseases are discussed.

Lysosomal storage diseases are most often, but not always, inherited as autosomal recessive traits. They result from genetic defects that impact the function of enzymes that are active in lysosomes. These disorders may also result from defective function of proteins that are expressed outside of lysosomes but are involved in the posttranslational modification of lysosomal enzymes and their targeting to lysosomes. Deficiency of a single lysosomal enzyme results in inability to catabolize compounds that serve as a substrate for that enzyme. Mutations in specific enzymes involved in the posttranslational modification of lysosomal enzymes results in the deficiency of multiple lysosomal enzymes because they are not appropriately targeted to lysosomes.

De Duve discovered lysosomes in 1949 (see De Duve 1963). Lysosomal membranes serve to segregate a series of hydrolytic enzymes that function optimally under acidic conditions, between pH 3.0 and 6.0. These enzymes degrade complex macromolecules that are taken up into the lysosomes from the cytoplasm or from outside the cell. Macromolecules digested by lysosomes include polysaccharides, lipids, glycoproteins, and glycolipids. There are within lysosomes specific enzymes that are capable of cleaving specific linkages.

In Hunter syndrome, e.g., where there is a deficiency of α-iduronidase, the mucopolysaccharide dermatan sulfate accumulates along with partially degraded forms of dermatan sulfate. These compounds accumulate in lysosomes, cells, and tissues and may be excreted in the urine. Different tissues vary with respect to the quantity of partially degraded mucopolysaccharide that they accumulate. Furthermore, the degree of mucopolysaccharide accumulation depends upon the quantity of residual or partially active enzyme that is present in the patient.

Different patients with the same type of lysosomal storage disease, e.g., Hunter syndrome, vary in their clinical phenotype and in their age at onset of symptoms. Thus, in a specific lysosomal storage disease, there are different groups of patients: those with onset of symptoms in the neonatal period, another group with onset of symptoms in childhood, and a third group whose symptoms may first develop during adult life.

Targeting of Proteins Synthesized in the Endoplasmic Reticulum to Organelles

Lysosomal enzymes and other proteins that are destined for secretion have a specific segment of their amino acid sequence (signal peptide) that acts as a signal for binding with a specific particle known as a signal recognition particle (SRP) or docking protein. The interaction between signal peptide and docking protein facilitates translocation of proteins destined for secretion to the lumen of the endoplasmic reticulum. There, the SRP is cleaved from the enzyme or protein. Within the lumen of the endoplasmic reticulum, lysosomal enzymes are modified by addition of oligosaccharides. In the endoplasmic reticulum, oligosaccharides rich in mannose are added to lysosomal enzymes and to other glycoproteins. In the Golgi apparatus, trimming of the oligosaccharide side chains occurs and a modification takes place that is specific to lysosomal enzymes. In the first step in this modification, a phosphotransferase enzyme, uridine diphosphate (UDP) N-acetylglucosamine-1-phosphotransferase, adds N-acetylglucosamine-1-phosphate is added to position 6 of the mannose oligosaccharide that is bound to the lysosomal enzyme. The second reaction is catalyzed by an N-acetylglucosaminidase. This process results in the generation of an exposed mannose-6-phosphate on the lysosomal enzyme (see Fig 6–1).

One enzyme acts as a phosphotransferase; the second enzyme is a phosphodiesterase (Reitman and Kornfeld 1981; Waheed et al. 1982; Kornfeld

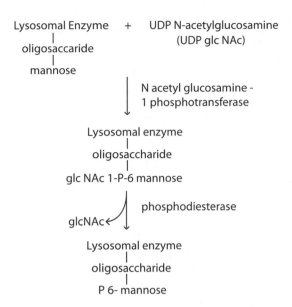

Figure 6.1. Generation of the mannose-6-phosphate target on lysosomal enzymes. UPD, uridine diphosphate; P, phosphate.

and Sly 2001) (see Fig. 6–1). The phosphotransferase is particularly important in the targeting of lysosomal enzymes. Its affinity for lysosomal enzymes is approximately 100 times greater than its affinity for other proteins. Lysine residues that are spaced at specific intervals within the lysosomal enzymes serve as the recognition sequence for the phosphotransferase enzymes (Kornfeld and Sly 2002).

The phosphotransferase enzyme is composed of three subunits. Two subunits, α and β, are the products of a single gene located on chromosome 4q21. A precursor protein produced from this gene undergoes cleavage to produce the α and β subunits. A gene on chromosome 16p encodes the γ subunit. Deficiency of α and β subunits occurs in patients with mucolipidosis type II (I cell disease) and in some patients with mucolipidosis type III. Deficiency of the γ subunit occurs in a subgroup of mucolipidosis type III patients.

The Endosome–Lysosome Pathway: Uptake of Lysosomal Enzymes

Current research indicates that newly synthesized mannose-6-phosphate-tagged acid hydrolases are transferred along the trans-Golgi network and taken up by vesicular structures, the endosomes, via the mannose-6-phosphate receptors that are present on them. Two receptors on the endosome surface recognize mannose-6-phosphate modified lysosomal enzymes. One is a

46 kDa cation-dependent mannose-6-phosphate receptor. The second is a 300 kDA cation-independent receptor.

Following binding to the receptors, lysosomal enzymes are ingested into endosomes. Endosomes then fuse with lysosomes, resulting in transfer of hydrolases to lysosomes. There, primarily due to the low pH in the interior of the lysosome, the enzyme is freed from the receptor protein. The receptor is then recycled to the Golgi network.

There are a number of different cell types, including hepatocytes and Kupffer's cells, in the liver that are capable of ingesting lysosomal enzymes through a mechanism that does not involve mannose-6-phosphate receptors.

Uptake of Macromolecules

The uptake of extracellular macromolecules (mucopolysaccharides, glyco-lipids, glycosphingolipids) occurs by several mechanisms that each result in the generation of a vesicular structure, the endosome. This structure fuses with lysosomes. Lysosomes may also fuse with the plasma membrane of the cell. This occurs particularly in response to damage of the cell membrane and a rise in intracellular calcium. Lysosomal membranes contain many different glycoproteins, including lysosome-associated membrane proteins (Lamps), lysosomal integral membrane proteins (Limps), and lysosomal glycoproteins (LGPs). Deficiency of Lamp2 results in a rare lysosomal storage disease, Danon disease, that leads to myopathy, cardiomyopathy, and variable mental retar-dation (Winchester 2001; Horvath et al. 2003).

Disorders Characterized by Deficiency of Multiple Lysosomal Enzymes

There are at least two disorders, mucolipidosis II and mucolipidosis III, where multiple lysosomal enzymes are deficient in cells as a result of defects in posttranslational processing of lysosomal enzymes. When the activity of N-acetylglucosamine phosphotransferase is deficient, lysosomal enzymes do not acquire the phosphomannosyl tag that is required for their uptake into endosomes and lysosomes. In both of these disorders, lysosomal enzymes are present in the cytoplasm of cells and in the extracellular fluids and levels of lysosomal enzymes in serum are increased. Lysosomes are deficient in lysosomal enzymes.

I Cell Disease (Mucolipidosis II)

The term *I cell disease* stems from the observation that in mucolipido-sis II particularly cells from the patient have prominent inclusions that are readily seen on microscopy (Leroy et al. 1972). These inclusions are lyso-somes that are filled with mucopolysaccharides and glycolipids that are not digested. In 1981, Varki and Kornfeld demonstrated deficiency of N-acetylglucosaminylphosphotransferase in patients with this disorder.

I cell disease manifests during infancy. Infants present with developmental delay and failure to thrive. Initially, motor delay is particularly prominent. In early childhood, there is evidence of loss of previously attained skills; and later, children manifest severe psychomotor retardation. In addition, significant storage occurs in soft tissues and in the skeletal system. This results in facial coarsening and skeletal abnormalities, including kyphoscoliosis. Widening of the ribs and thickening of the metacarpals occurs. Cardiomegaly and hepatomegaly are prominent features. Death frequently occurs before adolescence and is due to cardiorespiratory failure.

Mucolipidosis III (Pseudo-Hurler Polydystrophy)

Mucolipidosis III is a milder disease than I cell disease. Some patients survive to adulthood. Joint immobility and development of claw hand deformity may be the presenting symptoms. Abnormal storage in the skeleton and consequent bone destruction may lead to destruction of the hip joints, reduced mobility, and short stature. Approximately 50% of patients have learning disabilities or mental retardation. Corneal clouding may develop. After the first decade of life, symptoms of cardiac insufficiency occur due to thickening and reduced mobility of the heart valves (Varki et al. 1981).

Mucopolysaccharidoses, Each Due to Deficiency of a Specific Lysosomal Enzyme

Mucopolysaccharidoses (MPS) are characterized by the accumulation of mucopolysaccharides, also known as glycosaminoglycans, in tissues and organs. This abnormal storage is due to a deficiency of specific lysosomal hydrolases that normally cleave and degrade glycosaminoglycans through cleavage of a terminal saccharide. We will review three forms of MPS that lead to mental retardation, Hurler syndrome, Hunter syndrome, and Sanfilippo syndrome. Hurler and Sanfilippo syndromes follow an autosomal recessive pattern of inheritance; Hunter syndrome is X-linked. Excessive mucopolysaccharides are excreted in the urine. In Hurler and Hunter syndromes, increased quantities of dermatan sulfate and heparan sulfate are excreted. In Sanfilippo syndrome, urinary excretion of heparan sulfate is increased.

Diagnosis

Analysis of urine mucopolysaccharides is useful in establishing a preliminary diagnosis. Definitive diagnosis requires enzyme assays that can be performed on serum, white blood cells, or cultured cells, including fibroblasts and amniocytes. Carrier testing by enzyme analysis is often not reliable, particularly in Hunter syndrome.

Molecular diagnosis using deoxyribonucleic acid (DNA) analysis is difficult because a large number of different mutations can lead to each of these disorders. Furthermore, in Hurler and Sanfilippo syndromes, which are inherited as autosomal recessive conditions, many patients are compound heterozygotes. They inherit a different mutation from each parent.

Hurler Syndrome (MPS1)

In Hurler syndrome, deficiency of the enzyme α-L-iduronidase leads to accumulation of the mucopolysaccharide dermatan sulfate in many tissues, including soft tissues, bones, organs, and brain (Yamagishi et al. 1996). The structure of dermatan sulfate is illustrated in Figure 6–2. Delayed motor and mental development and frequent upper respiratory tract infections may be the first symptoms of this disorder. Within the first few years of life, patients develop coarse facial features, skeletal deformities, and corneal clouding. X-ray surveys of the skeleton reveal dysplasia and shortening of the long bones as well as deformed, hook-shaped vertebrae, particularly in the thoracic and lumbar regions of the spine. The skeletal abnormalities seen on X-ray are sometimes referred to as dysostosis multiplex syndrome. Storage of glycosaminoglycans in the heart valves and major blood vessels leads to cardiac failure. In some patients, deficiency of α-L-iduronidase is less severe and the phenotype may be milder (Neufeld and Muenzer 2001).

Hunter Syndrome (MPSII)

Hunter syndrome is due to deficiency of iduronate sulfatase, an enzyme encoded by a gene on the X chromosome. It often results from large deletions or rearrangements in this gene (Hopwood et al. 1993). Disease manifestations occur in male individuals. The glycosaminoglycan dermatan accumulates in soft tissues, bone, and many organs, including the brain. The clinical manifestations in Hunter syndrome closely resemble those in Hurler syndrome. The clinical phenotype is much more variable than in Hurler syndrome. In some patients, mental retardation may be mild or moderate, while in other patients it may be severe (Young et al. 1982a,b; Neufeld and Muenzer 2001).

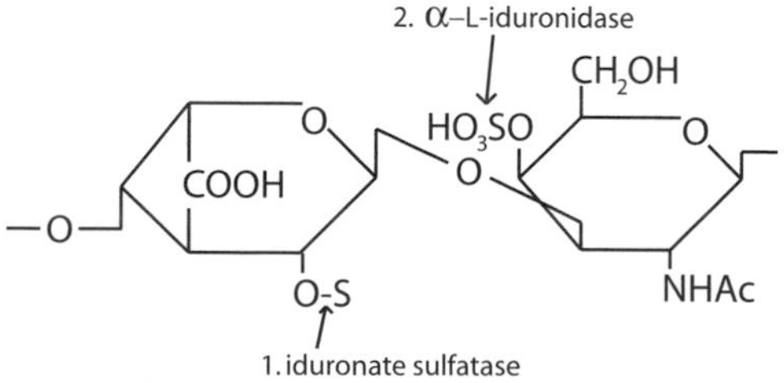

Figure 6.2. Dermatan sulfate and sites of cleavage by α-L-iduronidase (deficient in Hurler syndrome) and iduronate sulfatase (deficient in Hunter syndrome).

Sanfilippo Syndrome (MPS III)

Patients frequently manifest developmental regression after the first 3–4 years of life. They may become hyperactive and aggressive. Bone changes are not prominent in Sanfilippo syndrome, and height is frequently normal. Hair is often coarse, and hirsutism may be present. By 6–10 years of age, marked cognitive and behavioral deterioration occurs.

Deficiency in any one of four different enzymes involved in the degradation of intra-cellular heparan sulfate may lead to Sanfilippo syndrome. Patients may be deficient in heparan *N*-sulfatase, α-*N*-acetylglucosaminidase, acetyl-coenzyme A (CoA)-glucosaminide acetyltransferase, or *N*-acetlyglucosamine-6-sulfatase (Yogalingam and Hopwood 2001).

Oligosaccharidoses Characterized by Mental Retardation

Oligosaccharidoses are due to deficiency of lysosomal enzymes involved in the breakdown of glycoproteins and oligosaccharides. These disorders result from impaired cleavage within the glycoprotein or oligosaccharide. Abnormal storage of oligosaccharide glycoproteins usually leads to symptoms that are milder than those that occur in mucopolysaccharide storage diseases. Oligosaccharides are excreted in excessive quantities in the urine (Beck 2000; Thomas 2001).

α-Mannosidosis

Deficiency of α-mannosidase leads to urinary excretion of mannose-rich oligosaccharides. Early-onset and late-onset forms of this disorder occur. Both forms are characterized by mental retardation, hepatosplenomegaly, and skeletal abnormalities similar to those found in mucopolysaccharidosis.

β-Mannosidosis

In β-mannosidase deficiency, patients may present with seizures and severe neurological symptoms. They may present with a milder disorder characterized by speech difficulties, learning disabilities, and skin lesions known as *angiokeratoma*, which are punctate red skin lesions that blanch on compression.

Fucosidosis

In fucosidase deficiency, symptoms may be severe or mild. Severely affected patients show developmental delay, growth retardation, and soft tissue swelling, leading to coarse face. In mildly affected patients, skin lesions (angiokeratoma) may predominate.

Sialidosis

Sialidosis type 1 is characterized by myoclonic seizures, difficulties in walking, visual problems, and development of a cherry red spot in the optic fundus. These symptoms follow a period of several years of normal development. It is due to deficiency of the enzyme sialidase, also known as neuraminidase. This enzyme cleaves terminal sialic acid residues from glycoproteins and glycolipids. The gene that encodes sialidase, *NEU1*, maps on chromosome 6p21.3 between the histocompatibility gene loci in the major histocompatibility complex (MHC). There is evidence that sialidase plays a role in the immune response. Sialidase is expressed in greater quantities in activated T and B cells than in the resting forms of these cells. Sialidase plays a role in processing antigen-presenting molecules on the cell surface. Sialidosis patients are prone to multiple infections.

In type 2 sialidosis, the phenotype more closely resembles that found in mucopolysaccharide storage disease. Patients show developmental regression and mental retardation. They may develop hepatosplenomegaly and frequently skeletal changes with characteristics of dysostosis multiplex. The *NEU1* mutations in these patients result in absence of enzyme activity (Seyrantepe et al. 2003 and Pattison et al. 2004).

A particularly severe form of sialidosis, galactosialidosis, may present in early infancy or even in fetal life with excess fluid accumulation and ascites. It is due to deficiency of cathepsin A. This protein forms a complex with sialidase and β-galactosidase and protects these enzymes from proteolytic degradation. Galactosialidosis is discussed further below

Free Sialic Acid Storage Diseases

In free sialic acid storage diseases, free sialic acid accumulates in the lysosomes as a result of a defect in the transport of sialic acid out of the lysosomes (Havelaar et al. 1998). Sialic acid (*N*-acetylneuraminic acid) is depicted in Figure 6–3. A form of free sialic acid storage disease known as Salla disease is relatively common in Finland. Early signs of the disorder are hypotonia and delayed motor development. Later, children develop spasticity, brisk reflexes, abnormal movements, and ataxia. Speech development is delayed, and growth is retarded. By adult life, patients are severely mentally retarded. In the late stages of the disease, facial coarsening may be marked. Death usually occurs in the third decade of life. Postmortem brain analysis has revealed severe reduction in cerebral white matter volume; on histology, stored material is observed in the perinuclear region of neurons (Sewell et al. 1996).

Infantile sialic acid storage disease is a more severe variant of Salla disease. Patients with this variant usually die in early childhood. This disorder occurs in individuals from different ethnic backgrounds. Infants with free sialic acid storage disease may present with significant swelling and ascites. The accumulation of fluids is similar to that seen in nephrotic syndrome.

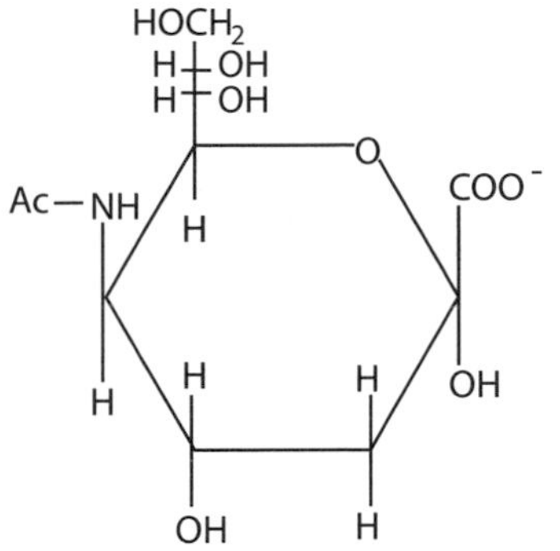

Figure 6.3. *N*-Acetylneuraminic acid accumulates in free sialic acid storage diseases.

Salla disease was mapped to chromosome 6q14-q15 through linkage studies. A common haplotype in this chromosomal region was found in 94% of Finnish patients. Infantile sialic acid storage disease was found through linkage studies to map to the same chromosomal region. To identify the gene defect in these disorders, Verheijen et al. (1999) used a positional cloning strategy. In the region where the disease gene maps, they searched for DNA sequence homologous to sequences that encode transporter proteins. The gene defect in sialic acid storage disease was found to be in a solute carrier gene, designated *SLC17A5*. The protein encoded by this gene is known as Sialin. Ninety-five percent of Finnish patients with sialic acid storage disease carry the same mutation, R39C. Salla disease has been found in other ethnic groups, primarily in Caucasians.

Preliminary diagnosis of sialic acid storage disease may be made by finding large quantities of free sialic acid in the urine and in medium in which a patient's cells are cultured. Specific diagnostic confirmation requires mutation analysis.

Defects in the Breakdown of Glycoproteins

Aspartylglucosaminuria

Aspartylglucosaminuria is due to deficiency of the enzyme aspartylglucosaminidase, which primarily cleaves asparagine coupled to *N*-acetylglucosamine (Savolainen 1976) (see Fig. 6–4). It has a worldwide distribution. In the Finnish population, it is most often due to a specific founder mutation.

Patients frequently present during the second or third year of life with developmental delay. Speech delay is particularly prominent. Cognitive skills are impaired; motor skills may be relatively unimpaired. Initially, development progresses, albeit slowly, until the mid-teens; it then ceases. During adult

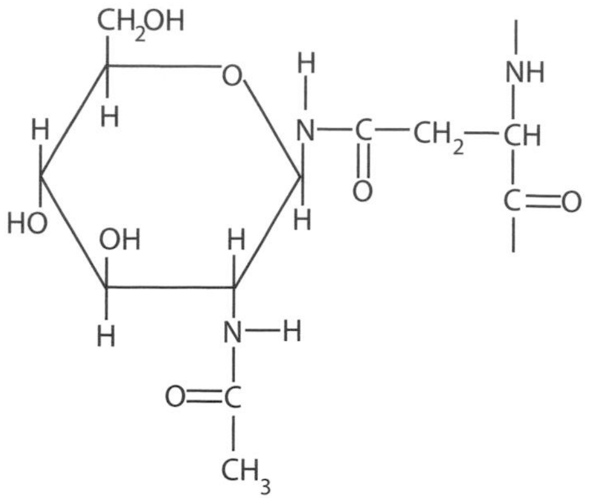

Figure 6.4. N-Acetylglucosylaminylasparagine accumulates in aspartylglucosaminuria.

life, patients may show significant deterioration and may develop seizures. Dysmorphism is subtle during childhood. In adults, dysmorphic features are more evident. They are primarily due to changes in connective tissue. These changes include sagging facial skin, thickened lips, and skin rash with dilated small blood vessels, similar to acne rosacea. Diagnosis may be made on the basis of finding increased urinary concentrations of aspartylglucosamine and other aspartylglycosamines (Aula et al. 2001).

Galactosialidosis (Schindler Disease)

In patients with Schindler disease, there is an abnormal accumulation of sialated and unsialated peptides, oligosaccharides, and glycosphingolipids that contain α-N-acetylgalactosamine residues. The enzyme N-acetylgalactosaminidase is one component of a lysosomal complex that contains α-neuraminidase, β-galactosidase, and the protective protein cathepsin A. In galactosialidosis, there is deficiency of β-galactosidase and neuraminidase that results from deficiency of cathepsin A.

Suzuki et al. (1981) and D'Azzo et al. (1982) reported that cultured fibroblasts from patients with this disorder were deficient in β-galactosidase and α-neuraminidase. They determined that activity of these two enzymes was restored in cultured cells treated with protease inhibitors. Subsequently, they determined that the patients' cells were deficient in a specific protein that prevents degradation of the β-galactosidase and neuraminidase enzymes in the lysosome.

In the severe infantile form of galactosialidosis, edema may be present; patients may present in infancy with ascites and inguinal hernias. Facial coarsening may also be noted.

In the later-onset infantile form of the disorder, patients may present with somatic features including facial coarsening, hepatosplenomegaly, and skeletal malformations. Neurological symptoms are usually present. These include myoclonus and ataxia. Psychomotor retardation is evident. Later, cortical blindness occurs, and children die within a few years. Storage of abnormal compounds is particularly prominent in axons. The stored compounds may be present as spheroidal bodies.

In some families, an intermediate form of galactosialidosis occurs. Patients may present with language delay and behavioral difficulties, including autistic behaviors. Later, moderate to severe psychomotor retardation occurs.

Galactosialidosis has been described in families from Europe, Japan, and Pakistan.

Glycosphingolipid Storage Diseases and Gangliosidoses

Sphingosine is synthesized from serine and palmitoyl CoA (see Fig. 6–5). Sphingosine then undergoes acetylation to form N-acylsphingosine (ceramide). Ceramide acts as a signaling molecule. The reaction of ceramide with phosphatidylcholine gives rise to sphingomyelin. Glycosphingolipids are synthesized in the Golgi apparatus by the progressive addition of monosaccharides to the core ceramide molecule. In these reactions, ceramide reacts with activated sugars, e.g., UDP-glucose or UDP-galactose, to give rise to glucosylceramide or galactosylceramide, respectively. Reaction of the latter compounds with active sulfate (adenosine-3-phosphate-5'-phosphosulfate) gives rise to sulfogalactosylceramide. Gangliosides are sphingolipids where sialic acid is present (see Fig. 6–6).

Glycosphingolipids are abundant in cell membranes in the outer layer of the lipid bilayer. Ceramide is embedded in the plasma membrane, and the

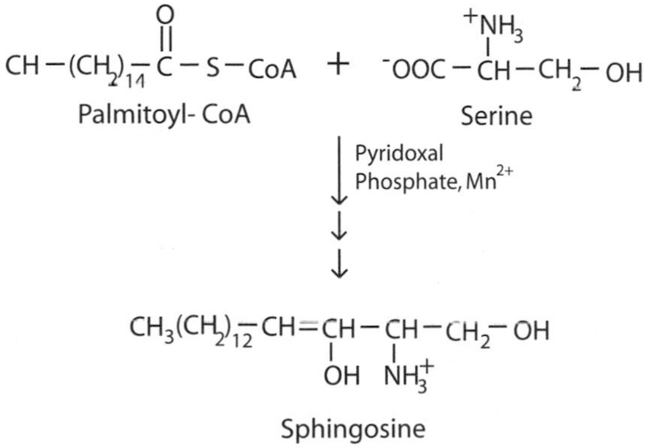

Figure 6.5. Synthesis of sphingosine. CoA, coenzyme A.

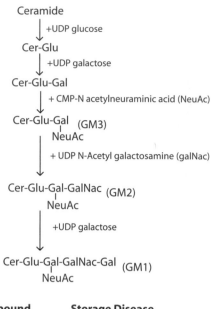

Figure 6.6. Synthesis of gangliosides. UDP, uridine diphosphate. CMP, cytidine 5′ monophosphate.

carbohydrate moieties of the glycosphingolipids extend out into the extra-cellular fluid. Glycosphingolipids are degraded in the lysosomes through the activity of hydrolases. Different types of glycosphingolipid storage disease occur; each type is due to deficiency of a specific hydrolase (see Fig. 6–7). Taken together, the frequency of the glycosphingolipidoses is 1 in 18,000 (Platt et al. 2003).

Gaucher Disease

In Gaucher disease, there is an accumulation of glucosylceramide and gluco-sylsphingosine due to decreased or absent activity of the enzyme β-glucosidase (Beutler and Grabowski 2001). This may be due to mutations in the gene that encodes β-glucosidase, which is located on chromosome 1q21. Decreased enzyme activity may be due to deficiency of the sphingolipid activator pro-teins saposin A and saposin C, which function as protein activators of β-glucosidase. Saposins A and C are derived through proteolytic processing from prosaposin (Sandhoff and Harzer 2001). A gene located on chromo-some 10q22.1 encodes prosaposin.

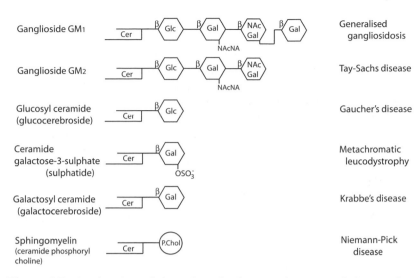

Figure 6.7. Gangliosides and glycosphingolipids accumulate in specific lysosomal storage diseases.

Gaucher disease type 1 is distinguished by absence of central nervous system symptoms. The most prominent symptoms arise as a result of involvement of bone, spleen, and liver. The degree to which each of these systems is involved and the age at onset of symptoms differ in different patients (Grabowski et al. 2004). The diagnosis may be made through the finding of unusual cells, Gaucher cells, in the bone marrow. These cells have a typical appearance on light microscopy. The cytoplasm of the cells has a wrinkled appearance, reminiscent of crumpled fabric or tissue paper.

The neuronal forms of Gaucher disease include type 2 and type 3. Glucosylceramide is stored in microglia in the brain and to some degree in neurons. Grabowski (2004) reported that the primary pathophysiology of brain symptoms is due to neuronal cell death. Key early signs of Gaucher disease are strabismus or oculomotor apraxia (impaired voluntary movements). Type 2 Gaucher disease, the acute neuronal form, is usually diagnosed in early infancy. Increased muscle tone and hepatosplenomegaly are often present. Children die within the first few years of life. Examination of the brain in these cases frequently reveals widespread neuronal loss and glial proliferation. Gaucher cells occur in perivascular tissue.

Type 3 Gaucher disease, the subacute neuronal form, leads initially to mild central nervous system manifestations, including developmental delay. Hepatosplenomegaly may be noted during the first few years of life. Neurological findings usually become evident during the first decade. These include limitation of eye movements, ataxia, abnormal movements (choreo-athetosis), and increasing cognitive impairment. Patients with type 3 Gaucher disease also experience bone crises and bone fractures, similar to those that commonly occur in type 1 Gaucher disease. Death usually occurs in the second to fourth decade of life. Neuronal loss may also be evident in this form of Gaucher disease. There is evidence that glucosylsphingosine, one of the compounds that accumulate in Gaucher disease, may have a toxic effect.

Diagnosis of Gaucher disease may be made through assay of β-glucosidase activity in leukocytes or fibroblasts. Diagnosis is sometimes made through detection of the typical Gaucher's cell in bone marrow. Enzyme activity assays are not useful for detecting heterozygotes. The β-glucosidase-encoding gene *GBA* maps to chromosome 1q21. A transcribed pseudogene of this gene maps 16 kb downstream. One group of mutations results from recombination between the *GBA* gene and the *GBA* pseudogene. Some mutations are due to gene conversion; exon 9 of *GBA* is replaced by exon 9 of the *GBA* pseudogene (Tayebi et al. 2003). The presence of the pseudogene may complicate mutation detection by DNA analysis.

A specific mutation, N370S, accounts for 80%–90% of cases of Gaucher disease type 1 in the Ashkenazi Jewish population. Homozygosity for this mutation is predictive of the absence of neurological symptoms. One of the more common mutations associated with neuronopathic Gaucher disease is the L444P mutation.

Patients with saposin C deficiency may present with symptoms of type 3 Gaucher disease. Recent breakthroughs in the treatment of lysosomal storage diseases, including Gaucher disease, will be discussed at the end of this chapter.

Niemann-Pick Disease: Types A and B

Niemann-Pick disease results from deficiency of the enzyme acid sphingomyelinase, which cleaves sphingomyelin to ceramide and phosphatidylcholine (Brady et al. 1966) (see fig. 6–7). A gene on chromosome 11.p15.1-p15.4 encodes this enzyme. Type A is the severe, infantile form of the disorder. Infants often present by 6 months of age with marked hepatosplenomegaly, enlarged lymph nodes, and anemia. Bone marrow microscopy reveals large foam cells that are typical of Niemann-Pick disease. Psychomotor retardation is apparent within the first year of life. This is followed by progressive loss of motor and cognitive abilities, and later, the infant loses contact with the surroundings. Death usually ensues within the first 2–3 years of life. Postmortem brain analysis reveals swelling of dendrites, deficiency of myelin, and lipid-laden foam cells (Schuchman and Desnick 2001).

Niemann-Pick disease type B patients may present during infancy or early childhood with hepatosplenomegaly; in some cases, diffuse infiltration of pulmonary tissue is found on chest X-ray. These patients do not usually have intellectual impairment. Neurological abnormalities may be absent, though some patients have cerebellar signs including ataxia (Schuchman and Desnick 2001).

Niemann-Pick Disease Type C

Niemann-Pick disease type C is due to deficiency in products of the genes *NPC1* and *NPC2*, which play a role in lipid trafficking (Patterson et al. 2001). The *NPC1* gene maps to chromosome 18; *NPC2* maps to 14q24.3. Neurological deterioration may begin in childhood, between 1 and 15 years of age. In some patients, symptoms begin only in adult life. Hypotonia and hepatosplenomegaly may be the earliest manifestations, followed by cognitive regression. Supranuclear or vertical gaze paralysis is often a characteristic sign of the disorder when it presents in adolescents and adults. These individuals may manifest dystonia, ataxia, epileptic seizures, and cognitive regression.

Patterson (2003) reported that Niemann-Pick disease type C is most often recognized in mid-childhood. Children may present with slowly increasing learning disabilities or behavioral difficulties. Sometimes they are diagnosed as having attention-deficit disorders. Cognitive impairments often become more marked over time, and children develop motor difficulties, including clumsiness, falling, and tripping. Later, ataxia becomes apparent. Patterson (2003) reported that approximately 20% of patients have episodes where they lose muscle tone (atonic episodes). Later, they may develop seizures.

Brain studies reveal widespread changes that involve cortical neurons. Fine granular inclusions are present that are visible on staining of tissue sections. These inclusions may also stain positively for cholesterol. Patterson (2003) emphasized that diagnosis should be considered in cases of unexplained cognitive impairment, especially when a movement disorder or ataxia is present. Vincent et al. (2003) emphasized that the effects of mutations in the *NPC1* and *NPC2* genes may differ in the brain and in other tissues. In the brain, there is an accumulation of cholesterol, glycolipids, glucosylceramide, and sialogangliosides. Accumulation of stored substances leads ultimately to neurodegeneration and brain atrophy. In fibroblasts, cholesterol is abnormally stored and may be detected with special staining (filipin staining). Cells fail to esterify cholesterol, and free unesterified cholesterol accumulates. The *NPC1* gene encodes a protein with 13 transmembrane spanning domains. Five of these domains form a sterol-sensing domain (Scott and Ioannou 2004).

Krabbe Disease, Also Known as Galactosylceramide Lipidosis or Globoid Cell Leukodystrophy

Krabbe disease occurs in two forms; the most common is the infantile form, which presents between 3 and 6 months of age. In the later-onset or childhood form, symptoms usually begin by the age of 3 years, although they may start later. The first signs in the infantile form may be irritability and hypersensitivity to light and sound. Infants rapidly develop spasticity and hyperactive reflexes; their vision and hearing deteriorate. In the later stages of the disease, they become hypotonic and atonic. On autopsy, the brain appears shrunken. Histology of the brain reveals the absence of myelin and presence of globoid cells. These are macrophages that are filled with the stored substance galactosylceramide, and they are abundant in white matter. The peripheral nervous system is often affected. Myelin is decreased in peripheral nerves, and there is an abnormal degree of fibrosis; macrophages filled with stored substance may also be present (Wenger et al. 2001).

In the late-onset form, there may be a history of developmental delay. By the age of 3 years, patients begin to lose previously attained cognitive and motor skills. Visual impairment occurs, and children become irritable. Later, spasticity develops and there are signs of central and peripheral neuropathy.

Krabbe disease is inherited as an autosomal recessive condition. It occurs in different populations, with a frequency of approximately 1 in 100,000. The frequency of this disease is higher in Sweden. It occurs with high frequency in the Druze population isolate in Israel.

This disorder is due to deficiency of the enzyme galactosylceramide β-galactosidase (GALC). In the absence of GALC, there is an accumulation of galactosylceramide and of sphingosine galactose, also known as psychosine. Svennerholm et al. (1980) reported that accumulation of these substances leads to rapid destruction of oligodendroglial cells. This in turn interferes with myelination.

The GALC-encoding gene maps to chromosome 14q24-q32. At least 60 different disease-causing mutations have been identified in this gene. One specific mutation is relatively common in affected individuals in Europe, the United States, and Mexico (Luzi et al. 1995). In this mutation, 30 kb of the genomic DNA sequence are deleted from the 3' end of the gene and there is a single nucleotide deletion at position 502 (502Tdel). It accounts for 50% of cases of Krabbe disease in the Dutch population and 75% of cases in the Swedish population (Kleijer et al. 1997).

Metachromatic Leukodystrophy

Metachromatic leukodystrophy is due to deficiency of the enzyme arylsulfatase A, which cleaves sulfogalactose-containing glycolipids (see Fig. 6–8). Sulfoglycolipids accumulate in lysosomes in the brain, nerves, liver, and kidney; and this accumulation leads to the presence in histological tissue sections of granules with an unusual staining pattern and unusual dye affinity (metachromatic granules).

The infantile form of this disorder usually presents in the first year of life. In other cases, signs of the disorder may first be detected in older children or in adults. The infantile form frequently manifests with reduced muscle tone in the limbs and with diminished tendon reflexes. Regression of development occurs. Later, optic atrophy may be detected. Peripheral neuropathy may develop; this leads to pain in the arms and legs and subsequently to spasticity. Later, feeding and respiratory difficulties become obvious. Seizures may occur, and patients may become blind. Children with this form of metachromatic leukodystrophy usually die before the age of 5 years (Von Figura et al. 2001).

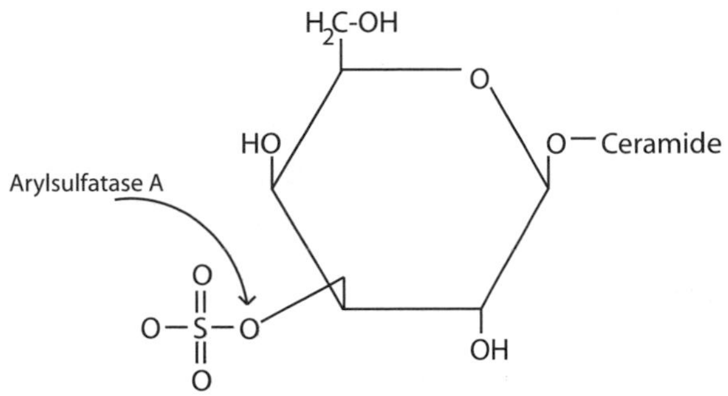

Figure 6.8. Arylsulfatase A cleaves sulfate from sulfogalactosylceramide. This enzyme is deficient in metachromatic leukodystrophy.

In juvenile metachromatic leukodystrophy, the earliest signs may be deterioration in abilities at school, clumsiness, and changes in speech. Children may also manifest behavioral problems. Later, children lose the ability to walk and become ataxic and spastic. Abdominal pain may be one of the symptoms due to involvement of the gallbladder and pancreas. Within a few years of onset of symptoms, children may develop feeding and respiratory difficulties.

Symptoms of metachromatic leukodystrophy may begin during adult life. The initial symptom is often a decline in intellectual performance.

In metachromatic leukodystrophy, deficiency of arylsulfatase A leads to accumulation of sulfated sphingolipids and sulfated glycolipids (Jatzkewitz and Mehl 1969). In brain, brain stem, and spinal cord, there is a reduction of white matter. Peripheral nerves are myelin-depleted. Metachromatic granules occur in macrophages, perivascular spaces, and oligodendrocytes. Occasionally, they may be present in neurons. The arylsulfatase A gene is relatively small, with eight exons. Metachromatic leukodystrophy is, however, due to a large number of different mutations.

Symptoms of metachromatic leukodystrophy may also occur in patients who have a deficiency of Saposin B (Gieselmann and von Figura 1990). Features of metachromatic leukodystrophy may also occur in cases of a very rare disorder, multiple sulfatase deficiency. In this disorder, there is a defect in the cysteine modification system that serves to modify the activity of a number of different sulfatases.

Gangliosidoses

Gangliosides are sphingolipids that contain neuraminic acid (sialic acid) (see Fig. 6–7). Deficiency of β-galactosidase, the enzyme that cleaves galactose from N-acetylgalactosamine in the GM_1 gangliosides, occurs in two different diseases, GM_1 gangliosidosis and Morquio syndrome type B.

GM$_1$ gangliosidosis is a neurodegenerative disorder in which other organs may also be affected. In Morquio syndrome, there is no involvement of the central nervous system and the disease primarily affects bone. Mutation analysis of the gene that encodes β-galactosidase has revealed that GM$_1$ gangliosidosis and Morquio syndrome are allelic disorders; i.e., they are due to different mutations in the same gene (Suzuki and Oshima 1993).

In the infantile form of GM$_1$ gangliosidosis, signs of the disease are usually evident by 6 months of age. Early signs include developmental delay and fluid accumulation in the abdomen (ascites) and in the extremities. Rapid neurological deterioration occurs, and infants develop an exaggerated startle response and brisk tendon reflexes; they may develop seizures. Patients develop hepatosplenomegaly, and corneal clouding may be present. Examination of the optic fundus reveals optic atrophy and a cherry red spot in the region of the macula. Skeletal dysplasia occurs; this includes frontal bossing (prominence of the forehead), kyphoscoliosis, and short, broad hands and feet. The tongue is often large and appears to be swollen.

In late-onset juvenile GM$_1$ gangliosidosis, signs develop early in childhood. There may be a history of developmental delay. Children lose previously attained skills. They develop stiffness of the limbs and have difficulty walking. Initially, hepatosplenomegaly may be absent. The disorder may progress slowly. Symptoms of GM$_1$ gangliosidosis may begin in adult life. The first symptoms may be difficulty in walking. Later, ataxia (poor muscle coordination) and dystonia (abnormal muscle tone) occur.

Neuroimaging studies in GM$_1$ gangliosidosis reveal cortical atrophy, enlarged ventricles, and reduced myelin. These findings are particularly prominent in cases of GM$_1$ gangliosidosis. This disorder is characterized by abnormal storage of galactosylceramide and lactosylceramide. Galactose-containing oligosaccharides and mucopolysaccharides, such as keratan sulfate, also accumulate.

The β-galactosidase gene is located on chromosome 3p21.3; it has 16 exons. A relatively large number of different mutations lead to GM$_1$ gangliosidosis. There is, however, a relatively good correlation between specific mutations and phenotypic manifestations (Suzuki et al. 2001).

Deficiency of other proteins may lead to GM$_1$ gangliosidosis manifestations. These include deficiency of protective protein, which associates with β-galactosidase, and deficiency of saposin B, an activator protein for β-galactosidase. Deficiency of protective protein leads to galactosialidosis, a disorder characterized by deficiency of both β-galactosidase and neuraminidase. Saposins facilitate substrate-enzyme interactions. Saposin B stimulates degradation of a number of substrates, including GM$_1$ gangliosides.

A precursor molecule, prosaposin, is encoded on chromosome 10q22.1. Prosaposin is transported from the cytoplasm to the cell surface and then to the lysosome. Within the lysosome, prosaposin is processed. Proteolytic processing of prosaposin by the protease cathepsin D gives rise to three saposins: A, B, and C.

GM₂ Gangliosidosis: Tay-Sachs Disease, Tay-Sachs Variants, and Sandhoff Disease

GM_2 gangliosidosis results from deficient activity of the enzyme hexosaminidase. Hexosaminidase A (HexA) is composed of two subunits, α and β. Hexosaminidase B (Hex B) is composed only of β subunits. A gene on chromosome 15q23 encodes the α subunit. A gene on chromosome 5q13 encodes the β subunit. In combination with the GM2A activator protein, HexA, cleaves GM_2 gangliosides. Activator protein, Hex A, and Hex B are synthesized in the endoplasmic reticulum and processed in the Golgi. They are then targeted to the endosomes and lysosome through the mannose-6-phosphate targeting system. The B form hydrolyzes a number of different substrates, including GM_2 gangliosides.

Tay-Sachs disease and Tay-Sachs variants result from deficiency of the α subunit of HexA. This deficiency leads to an elevation in the quantity of HexB. The term *Tay-Sachs disease* usually refers to the acute or infantile form of the disorder. Deficiency of HexA may, however, be associated with later-onset symptoms (Gravel et al. 2001).

Sandhoff disease is due to deficiency of HexB. The infantile form of Sandhoff disease and the late-onset forms are clinically indistinguishable from Tay-Sachs disease.

Deficiency of the GM_2 activator protein leads to a disorder that is clinically similar to infantile Tay-Sachs disease. However, the activities of HexA and HexB enzymes, as regularly assayed using artificial substrates, are normal. Also, the DNA sequences of the genes encoding α and β hexosaminidase subunits are normal. The GM_2 activator protein gene maps to chromosome 5q32-q33.

The infantile form of Tay-Sachs disease, Sandhoff disease, and GM_2 activator deficiency present the same clinical picture. Onset of symptoms occurs at 3–5 months. An exaggerated startle response to sound and light may be the first clinical sign. Development ceases to progress, and acquired developmental skills may be lost.

On examination, infants have poor muscle tone. They may develop seizures. They are not visually attentive, and they have abnormal eye movements. Eye examination reveals evidence of optic atrophy and the presence of a cherry red spot in the macula. Later, often by the second year of life, affected infants become progressively less responsive; they have difficulty swallowing and breathing, and decerebrate rigidity develops.

The earliest symptoms of subacute GM_2 gangliosidosis may be noticed in children between 2 and 10 years of age. Symptoms include poor coordination and loss of previously acquired cognitive and motor skills. This form of the disorder progresses more slowly than the infantile form. However, the same long-term complications occur. Children usually die between 10 and 15 years of age.

Chronic GM_2 gangliosidosis frequently has onset during childhood, and symptoms increase gradually. In some cases, the first symptoms present during adult life. Symptoms include ataxia, abnormal movements, abnormal muscle tone, and muscle wasting. Psychomotor regression may occur. Some patients manifest symptoms of psychosis.

Two common mutations in the HexA gene that encodes the α hexosaminidase subunit are encountered in Tay-Sachs disease patients of Ashkenazi Jewish origin. The most frequent mutant allele has a 4 bp insert in exon 11. This mutation leads to mRNA instability. The second common mutant allele is a point mutation at a splice junction in intron 11. This mutation leads to exon skipping. In Tay-Sachs disease patients of other ethnic groups, at least 92 different mutations in the HexA gene have been described. Sandhoff disease is associated with a number of different mutations.

Recent approaches toward therapy of Tay-Sachs disease and other lysosomal storage diseases will be described below.

Neuronal Ceroid Lipofuscinoses

Homozygous defects in any one of at least nine different genes give rise to a rare group of neurological diseases, the neuronal ceroid lipofuscinoses (NCL) (Mole 2004; Schulz et al. 2004). The disease name derives from the abnormal autofluorescent pigment that accumulates in the brain, other tissues, and leukocytes.

Linkage studies and positional cloning strategies have led to isolation of the diverse group of genes that cause these disorders. Deficiency of the lysosomal palmitoyl protein thioesterase leads to an infantile-onset form of NCL. This enzyme cleaves the thioester bond between cysteine groups and fatty acids.

The juvenile-onset form of NCL is known as Batten disease. In this disease, there is deficiency of a lysosomal membrane protein. Development is initially normal. In early or late childhood, cognitive and motor development slows or becomes static. Subsequently, acquired skills are lost. Children develop seizures; vision deteriorates and, later, children become blind. Detection of the abnormal staining pigment in cultured cells or leukocytes by electron microscopy may confirm the diagnosis (Hoffman and Peltonen 2001).

Advances in the Treatment of Lysosomal Storage Diseases

Enzyme Replacement Therapy

Since 1991 a number of investigators have treated Gaucher disease type 1 with purified and modified human acid β-glucosidase. The enzyme is modified to expose carbohydrate residues on its surface. The modification facilitates enzyme targeting to endosomes and lysosomes via the mannose-6-phosphate receptor.

Grabowski (2004) reviewed results of enzyme replacement therapy in non-neuronopathic Gaucher disease. He noted that in the majority of patients who received modified β-glucosidase there was a reduction in hepatosplenomegaly; anemia, thrombocytopenia, and leukopenia became less marked; and there were fewer bone lesions detectable on X-ray. Adverse effects included allergic reactions, which subsided on treatment with antihistamines. Five percent of the patients who were treated developed antibodies that neutralized β-glucosidase enzyme activity. This subgroup of patients required higher doses of enzyme. Grabowski (2004) noted that in neuronopathic Gaucher disease enzyme replacement therapy has not led to improvement of symptoms. For many families, the cost of treatment of Gaucher disease, US$140,000–$300,000, is prohibitive.

Enzyme replacement therapy has been developed for a few other lysosomal storage diseases. Laronidase, a form of α-L-iduronidase, is available for treatment of the milder forms of Hurler disease (Mucopolysaccharidosis type 1).

Bone Marrow Transplantation

Bone marrow transplantation has proven useful in the treatment of a number of lysosomal storage diseases (Krivit et al. 1999). It has proven effective even in disorders with neurological symptoms that arise as a result of abnormal storage of substrate in the brain. The mechanism for this finding has been elucidated. Monocytes that occur in bone marrow and circulate in blood give rise in tissues to macrophages. Monocytes in the circulation give rise to microglial cells in the brain. The monocytes that are present in transplanted bone marrow or that arise from hematopoietic stem cells give rise to macrophages and to microglial cells. The enzyme that is present in donor-derived macrophages and in microglial cells degrades stored substance in the tissues and brain of the recipient.

Bone marrow transplantation as a treatment for lysosomal storage diseases is limited by the difficulty in finding matched donors. In addition, the whole-body irradiation required in pre-transplantation preparation has a significant complication rate.

Cord Blood Transplants

Cord blood from unrelated donors is proving to be an excellent source of stem cells for transplantation. Staba et al. (2004) reported results of cord blood transplantation in patients with Hurler syndrome. Each patient in their study received a cord blood transfusion with cells from an unrelated donor; donor cells matched patient cells at three out of six human leukocyte antigen (HLA) loci. In 10 of the 20 patients they studied, ABO blood type of donor and patient blood did not match. Cord blood samples with the highest numbers of nucleated cells were used for transplantation. Prior to transplantation, patients were treated with busulfan, cyclophosphamide, and antithymocyte antibodies to reduce their B and T stem cells. Patients were monitored between 1995 and 2002. During the course of monitoring, three patients died.

Following transplantation, growth velocity was normal in most patients. In six patients, kyphosis of the spinal column partially resolved. After transplantation, neurocognitive function was stable in some patients; in others, it improved. Staba et al. (2004) noted that three of the four oldest children studied after transplantation had average to high intelligence quotient (IQ) scores. In these children, results of enzyme protein analysis, prior to transplantation, predicted severe disease.

Cord blood samples are of value since monocytes, derived from stem cells present in cord blood, give rise to circulating macrophages and microglia. These two cell types are transported in the circulation to tissues and brain, as described above.

In a number of lysosomal storage diseases, the stored substances in tissues, including the brain, induce an inflammatory response. As part of this response, macrophages and, in the case of the brain, microglia infiltrate the tissues. In this way, donor macrophages and microglia, which contain normally active enzyme, invade tissue and degrade stored substrate.

Hematopoietic Stem Cell Transplantation

Bone marrow, umbilical cord blood, or peripheral blood may be used as a source of hematopoietic stem cells. Hematopoietic stem cells have been used with promising results in the treatment of Hurler syndrome, mannosidosis, Krabbe disease, and X-linked leukodystrophy (discussed in the following section of this chapter). The primary goal of treatment is to optimize quality of life (Wenger et al. 2000; Peters and Steward 2003; Staba et al. 2004).

Emerging Treatments of Lysosomal Storage Diseases

The development of mouse models of a number of lysosomal storage diseases has enabled investigation of a number of different strategies for treatment.

Advances in Gene Therapy

Biffi et al. (2004) carried out studies on mice with metachromatic leukodystrophy. These investigators used lentiviral vectors that carried the normal arylsulfatase A gene to transduce hematopoietic cells from affected mice. Following transplantation of these stem cells into affected mice, they noted that mice improved in their motor coordination and learning abilities. They demonstrated that normal enzyme was present in macrophages and in endoneural macrophages. Biffi et al. (2004) concluded that transduction of patient hematopoietic stem cells with lentiviral vectors containing normal enzyme likely represents an effective treatment strategy for metachromatic leukodystrophy.

Lentiviral vectors are recombinant vectors based on human immunodeficiency virus-1 (HIV1). They have been used to target nondividing cells such as T lymphocytes, macrophages, and monocytes.

A mouse model of Gaucher disease has been developed. Kim et al. (2004) used this model to test the efficacy of HIV1 lentivirus-based vectors for vascular delivery of the glucocerebrosidase gene. Intravascular injection of the recombinant vector led to high concentrations of glucocerebrosidase in liver. Following treatment, they noted that there were no significant problems due to lentiviral vectors.

Chemical Chaperones

Mutations that lead to deficiency of a specific lysosomal enzyme frequently do not affect the active site of the enzyme. They lead instead to protein forms that are misfolded, unstable, or subject to incorrect trafficking within the cell. In a number of lysosomal storage diseases, the activity of the mutant enzyme is enhanced through the use of enzyme inhibitors. A number of investigators have postulated that small molecules that are inhibitors act to stabilize the mutant enzyme at neutral pH. This stabilization increases the quantity of enzyme that is transported to the lysosome. Within the lysosome, the inhibitor is likely displaced from the enzyme by the ambient low pH or by the high concentrations of the natural substrates for the enzyme.

Fan et al. (1999) reported the first example of the use of an inhibitor that chaperoned a lysosomal enzyme. These investigators demonstrated that a molecule known to inhibit the enzyme α-galactosidase, 1-deoxygalactonojirimycin, increased the activity of a mutant form of the enzyme present in Fabry disease.

The β-glucosidase mutation N370S occurs in 98% of Jewish patients with Gaucher disease and in 50% of non-Jewish patients with this disease. Sawkar et al. (2002) demonstrated that the activity of the enzyme present in patients with a homozygous N370S mutation increased twofold using the chemical chaperone N-(n-nonyl)deoxynojirimycin. These authors reported that a modest increase in β-glucosidase enzyme was sufficient to achieve a therapeutic clinical effect.

Lin et al. (2004) identified a β-glucosidase inhibitor, N-octyl-β-valienamine (NOV), that increased the activity of the F213I mutant β-glucosidase sixfold in cultured fibroblasts. Treatment with NOV also cleared ^{14}C-labeled glucosylceramide from cultured cells of patients who were homozygous for the F213I mutation. This mutation occurs in 15% of Japanese patients with Gaucher disease.

Matsuda et al. (2003) synthesized a galactose derivative, N-octyl-4-epi-β-valienamine (NOEV), that acts as a potent inhibitor of GALC. Activity of GALC is deficient in GM_1 gangliosidosis and in Morquio syndrome. They tested the effect of NOEV on human and mouse cells in which GALC activity was deficient. They also examined the effect of oral administration of

NOEV on GALC in mice that were GALC-deficient and had accumulated GM_1 gangliosides in their brain tissue. They demonstrated a marked increase in the catalytic activity of GALC in NOEV-treated mice. Following 1 week of treatment, they observed a marked decrease of GM_1 and GA_1 (asialoganglioside) in neuronal cells in the frontotemporal cortex and brain stem. Matsuda et al. (2003) noted that two of the advantages of inhibitor therapy, also known as chaperone therapy, are that these chemicals reach the brain and can be administered by mouth. They also demonstrated increased activity of GALC in cell lines with the R201C and R201H GALC mutations.

Tropak et al. (2004) reported results of studies in which cultured fibroblasts from patients with Tay-Sachs disease were grown in culture medium with HexA inhibitors. In the presence of inhibitors, HexA activity levels and protein levels were increased to approximately 10% of normal. These investigators noted that individuals with HEXA enzyme levels that are 10% of normal have been found to be free of symptoms. In the chronic or adult Tay-Sachs variant, patients have enzyme levels that are approximately 5% of normal. Tropak et al. (2004) concluded that chaperone therapy is an option in the treatment of patients who have residual enzyme activity.

Substrate Reduction Therapy of Glycosphingolipidoses

Platt et al. (2003) investigated the use of chemicals that inhibit the synthesis of glycosphingolipids in the treatment of glycosphingolipid storage diseases. The rationale of this treatment is that if accumulation of the substrate can be retarded, even in the presence of low levels of enzyme activity, severe disease may be converted to milder disease.

Platt et al. (2003) used imino sugar and alkylated derivatives of imino sugars to inhibit glycosphingolipid synthesis. The inhibitor that is most widely used is N-butyldeoxynojirimycin (NBDNJ). At concentrations of 2 mM, NBDNJ is nontoxic to tissue culture cells. Platt et al. studied mice deficient in HexA and mice deficient in HexB. The NBDNJ was well tolerated by mice at concentrations that will lead to 70% depletion in concentrations of stored glycosphingolipids. They demonstrated that NBDNJ crosses the blood–brain barrier. In Sandhoff disease mice, treatment extended life by 40%.

A specific advantage of decreasing concentrations of stored glycosphingolipids in the brain may be related to the fact that these compounds reduce the inflammatory response in the brain (Moyses 2003).

Peroxisomal Disorders

Peroxisomes are spherical organelles in the cytoplasm that are 0.1–1 μ in diameter. They have a single membrane. Within their matrix they contain at least 50 different enzymes that play a role in a number of different metabolic processes that include β-oxidation of very long and long chain fatty acids;

metabolism of plasmalogens, cholesterol, bile acids, leukotrienes, and pros-taglandins; synthesis of peroxide (H_2O_2); detoxification of peroxide by cata-lase; and oxidation of D-amino acids (Gould et al. 2001; Weller et al. 2003). Recently, peroxisomes have also been shown to play a role in the α-oxidation of phytanic acid.

Peroxisomal matrix proteins are synthesized on free ribosomes in the cytoplasm. They are then targeted to the peroxisomes through a specific pep-tide sequence, usually serine–lysine–leucine, at the C-terminal end of the protein. Less commonly, matrix proteins have an N-terminal target sequence.

Peroxisomal membranes are composed of phospholipids, sterols, fatty acids, and proteins. Specific protein molecules in the membrane include the receptor proteins PTS1 and PTS2, which recognize the targeting sequence on proteins destined for the peroxisomal matrix. Specific protein molecules play a role in the transport of proteins across the peroxisomal membrane.

Peroxin genes (*PEX* genes) encode proteins that play a role in the forma-tion of peroxisomes, proteins that constitute the peroxisomal membrane receptors, and proteins that transport molecules across the peroxisomal mem-branes (Gould et al. 2001). At least 19 *PEX* genes are known (Weller et al. 2003).

Peroxisomal disorders may be classified into two broad categories. In the first category are disorders that are due to defects in the formation of peroxi-somes, peroxisomal biogenesis disorders. In the second category are disorders that are due to defects in single peroxisomal enzymes.

Peroxisomal Biogenesis Disorders

Peroxisomal biogenesis defects occur in Zellweger syndrome and Zellweger variants, rhizomelic chondrodyplasia punctata (RCDP), neonatal adreno-leukodystrophy, and infantile Refsum disease. Zellweger syndrome, its vari-ants, and RCDP represent disorders where mental retardation is accompanied by dysmorphology (Baumgartner and Saudubray 2002). Two-thirds of pa-tients with Zellweger syndrome have *PEX1* gene mutations. Patients with RCDP most commonly have *PEX7* mutations. These disorders were also discussed in Chapter 4. *Infantile Refsum disease* is now considered to be an inappropriate name for a disorder that is genetically heterogeneous. The name *Refsum disease* was given to disorders where phytanic acid accumulates. It is now known that this compound accumulates in a number of different per-oxisomal disorders. Neonatal adrenoleukodystrophy is characterized by fa-cial dysmorphology, abnormal skin hyperpigmentation, evidence of cortisol deficiency, and adrenal atrophy. These symptoms may arise in infants with homozygous mutations in any one of at least six genes, including *PEX* genes and the *PTS1* receptor gene, which recognizes the targeting sequence on pro-teins destined for the peroxisomal matrix.

Patients with peroxisomal biogenesis disorders are deficient in multiple peroxisomal functions, including plasmalogen biosynthesis. Plasmalogens are phospholipids in which one of the two fatty acids is linked to the glycerol moiety in ether linkage. They may contain phosphatidylethanolamine, inositol serine, or choline. Plasmalogens comprise 10% of the phospholipids in the brain. Peroxisomal biosynthesis defects lead to inadequate α- and β-oxidation of fatty acids and reduced biosynthesis of polyunsaturated fatty acids and bile acids. In these disorders, abnormal storage occurs in lysosomes (Ferdinandusse et al. 2004). Layered inclusions occur in lysosomes; they are composed of very long chain fatty acids and cholesterol.

Diagnostic tests are based on quantitation of plasmalogen levels; this is frequently carried out using red blood cells. Analysis of serum levels of long chain fatty acids is also useful.

Peroxisomal Disorders That Present with Congenital Malformations, Dysmorphology, Neurological Problems, and Developmental Delay

The dysmorphic features associated with Zellweger syndrome and Zellweger variants include large fontanelle, high forehead, epicanthal folds, and malformations of the external ear. Other malformations include neuronal migration defects leading to neuronal heterotopias and gyral abnormalities. Cerebral myelination may also be abnormal. Stippled calcification of bone epiphyses may occur. Patients with Zellweger syndrome or its variants have hypotonia, seizures, and developmental delay. In classical Zellweger syndrome, death usually occurs during the first year of life. There is, however, variation in length of survival; children may survive for several years (Baumgartner and Saudubray 2002).

Rhizomelic Chondrodysplasia Punctata

Rhizomelia refers to the shortening of the proximal limbs that occurs in this disorder. Patients have facial dysmorphism including frontal bossing (prominence of the lateral regions of the forehead), flat nasal bridge, and small nose. Calcium stippling occurs not only in the bone epiphyses but also in other tissues. Compromised liver and renal function may also occur. Patients with this disorder manifest psychomotor retardation and visual problems.

Treatment of Peroxisomal Biogenesis Disorders

Dietary supplementation with the polyunsaturated fatty acid docosahexaenoic acid (DHA) has proven to be beneficial in some patients with Zellweger syndrome and its variants. This treatment has been particularly beneficial in patients with milder forms of the disease and in cases where treatment commenced before 6 months of age. Martinez (2001) reported that treatment improved muscle tone and liver functions. On brain magnetic resonance imaging (MRI), there was evidence of normalization of myelination. Plasma levels of very long chain fatty acids decreased. Docosahexanoic acid plays a role in building membranes. Zellweger syndrome patients have very low levels of DHA in brain, retina, and other tissues.

Another treatment strategy that is sometimes applied in peroxisomal biogenesis disorders is use of compounds that increase the number of peroxisomes. These compounds include the hormone dehydroepiandrosterone and 4-phenylbutyrate.

Deficiency of Single Peroxisomal Enzymes

D-Bifunctional Protein (Also Referred to as D-Bifunctional Enzyme)

D-Bifunctional enzyme plays a role in the β-oxidation of straight chain and branched chain fatty acids. Patients with deficiency of this enzyme accumulate very long chain fatty acids, including C26.0 and C24:0. They also accumulate abnormal quantities of branched chain fatty acids (including pristanic acid and phytanic acid) and bile acid intermediates (cholestanoic acid). Deficiency of D-bifunctional enzyme leads to severe developmental delay, hypotonia, and seizures. Neuropathology studies reveal severe reduction in neurons and impaired nerve myelination (Wanders et al. 2004).

Diagnosis may be made through demonstration of elevated plasma levels of very long chains fatty acids. The serum carnitine profile is abnormal due to the coupling of very long chain fatty acids to carnitine. Abnormal carnitine may be detected using tandem mass spectrometry. The latter serves as a rapid screening method for fatty acid oxidation defects (Rizzo et al. 2003).

X-Linked Adrenoleukodystrophy

X-Linked adrenoleukodystrophy occurs in all ethnic groups. The approximate frequency is 1 in 50,000. In approximately 40% of cases, male patients with this disorder develop normally and symptoms begin between 3 and 10 years of age. In approximately 35% of cases, symptom onset is between 11 and 21 years of age. Onset of symptoms in adult life is less common (Moser et al. 2001).

In childhood- and adolescent-onset adrenoleukodystrophy, the first symptoms may be difficulties in school due to behavioral problems and diminishing cognitive function. Patients may become progressively more withdrawn; they may manifest symptoms of attention-deficit hyperactivity disorder. Patients experience progressively greater difficulty understanding speech. They may also develop abnormal eye movements or strabismus (squint). Many patients develop seizures.

Brain MRI reveals symmetrical lesions in the parietooccipital regions. These lesions are due to loss of myelin, gliosis, and inflammatory response. Neurological signs and symptoms usually precede manifestations of adrenal insufficiency. However, patients with neurological symptoms frequently show abnormally low cortisol secretion in response to corticotropin administration. Patients later develop sphincter problems, with urinary and fecal incontinence.

Early symptoms of adult-onset X-linked adrenoleukodystrophy include stiffness, clumsiness, and urinary incontinence. Symptoms of corticosteroid deficiency develop, including weakness and weight loss. Depression and emotional disturbances also occur.

Female heterozygous carriers of the X-linked adrenoleukodystrophy gene defect may manifest symptoms. These may include declining school performance during adolescence.

Gene Defect in X-linked Adrenoleukodystrophy

The gene that is defective in X-linked adrenoleukodystrophy was identified through positional cloning, i.e., through genetic linkage studies and sequencing of genes in the region where adrenoleukodystrophy mapped. Sarde et al. (1994) characterized the genomic structure of adrenoleukodystrophy and determined the gene function. On the basis of sequence homology of the adrenoleukodystrophy gene with other known genes, they determined that adrenoleukodystrophy encodes an adenosine triphosphate binding cassette transporter, ABCD1. The X-linked *ABCD1* gene shows significant homology to the *ABCD2* gene on chromosome 12q11. It is interesting to note that the ABCD2-encoded protein can carry out some of the same functions as ABCD1.

The ABCD1 protein is targeted to peroxisomal membranes through a 14–amino acid motif. Landgraf et al. (2003) described deletions of amino acids in this targeting motif in patients with X-linked adrenoleukodystrophy.

In X-linked adrenoleukodystrophy, there is an accumulation of very long chain fatty acids (C26.0 and C24:0) in the brain, adrenal glands, and plasma. It is likely that ABCD1 transports very long chain fatty acids into peroxisomes for degradation. McGuiness et al. (2003) proposed that the ABCD1-encoded protein, also known as ALDP, facilitates interaction between peroxisomes and mitochondria and that this interaction plays a role in the β-oxidation of very long chain fatty acids. At the time of writing, debate continues regarding the degree to which β-oxidation of very long chain fatty acids occurs in the peroxisomes versus the mitochondria.

Treatment of X-Linked Adrenoleukodystrophy

In 2002, results were published of a 10-year study on 107 boys who were treated with Lorenzo's oil, the fatty acid erucic acid. A chemist, working in collaboration with a parent of a patient with X-linked adrenoleukodystrophy, developed Lorenzo's oil treatment (Senior 2002). Moser reported, "continuous treatment with Lorenzo's oil brought about significant reductions in the levels of very long chain fatty acids that correlated with a reduced risk of developing neurological abnormalities."

Bone marrow transplant has also been useful in the treatment of patients with X-linked adrenoleukodystrophy, particularly at an early stage of the disease (Shapiro et al. 2000). Hitomi et al. (2003) reported that bone marrow transplant significantly reduced neurological symptoms in patients with this disorder.

Borker and Yu et al. (2002) reported successful treatment of X-linked adrenoleukodystrophy with hematopoietic cell transplants enriched for CD34 stem cells.

Pharmacological substances that increase expression of the *ABCD2* gene have proven efficacious at reducing disease pathology in a mouse model of X-linked adrenoleukodystrophy. Such substances include thyroid hormone (Fourcade et al. 2003), dehydroepiandrosterone (Gueugnon et al. 2003), and cholesterol-lowering drugs (Rampler et al. 2002). Weinhoffer et al. (2002) reported that cholesterol regulates ABCD2 expression.

Menkes Syndrome and Occipital Horn Syndrome

Menkes and occipital horn syndromes are due to disorders of copper metabolism resulting in increased intracellular accumulation of copper. In classical Menkes syndrome, patients are normal for the first 2 months of life; thereafter, they manifest developmental delay and growth delay. They develop hypotonia, seizures, and hypothermia. Their hair is unusual, with a texture that resembles steel wool; it is lightly pigmented and often gray or dull blond. Patients have pale skin that does not tan on exposure to sun. Connective tissue abnormalities are a prominent feature. Joints are lax. Weakness of connective tissue leads to aneurysms of major blood vessels and smaller vessels and to the presence of diverticulosis of the intestine and bladder. Diverticula are prone to sepsis and rupture. Bones are poorly mineralized. Death usually occurs in early childhood. Milder forms of Menkes syndrome occur, and in these cases intellectual impairment may be the most striking feature (Kaler 1998 a,b; Culotta et al. 1999).

In patients with occipital horn syndrome, neurodegeneration is less prominent and the most striking abnormalities involve connective tissue and skeleton. Skeletal manifestations include prominences on the skull (occipital horns), short clavicles, and abnormalities of the long bones that include flaring at the bone ends. Blood vessel malformations, including aneurysms, and diverticulosis of the bowel and bladder are common. The skin is very lax and easily stretched. This condition is sometimes referred to as X-linked cutis laxa or Ehlers-Danlos syndrome type IX. Patients may be mildly retarded or may have normal intelligence (Kodama et al. 1999).

In both disorders, the plasma levels of copper and ceruloplasmin are abnormally low. Elevated levels of intracellular copper occur in cells of the gastrointestinal tract and in cultured cells, fibroblasts, and lymphoblasts.

Menkes syndrome and occipital horn syndrome are due to mutations in the *ATP7A* gene, which maps to chromosome Xq13.3-q21.1 (Vulpe et al. 1993;

Chelly et al. 1993). It encodes a protein that pumps copper from the cell into a secretory pathway. When *ATP7A* function is defective, intracellular copper levels are increased. The excess intracellular copper binds to metallothionein and is not available to act as a catalyst for copper-requiring enzymes. This results in reduced activity of a number of different copper-requiring enzymes, including cytochrome *c* oxidase and dopamine β-hydroxylase.

Large deletions in the *ATP7A* gene account for 15%–20% of cases of classical Menkes syndrome; the mutation spectrum is quite broad. Mutation analysis is the most efficient method to identify Menkes syndrome carriers; measurements of serum and intracellular copper are not reliable for carrier detection (Tumer et al. 2003).

A number of investigators have administered copper, usually as copper histidine, to treat Menkes syndrome. Treatment is apparently effective only if it is initiated early, prior to 2 months of age. Treatment may slow neurological deterioration but does not improve connective tissue laxity (Kodama et al. 1999).

Rett Syndrome

Rett syndrome occurs predominantly in female indvidiuals. In many cases, development is initially normal for the first year or more; thereafter, regressive changes begin. Since Rett syndrome has been molecularly defined as a chromatin modification disorder, it was briefly discussed, along with other chromatin modification disorders, in Chapters 4 and 8. Mutations in *MECP2* sometimes occur in association with nonsyndromic mental retardation (Gomot et al. 2003). We have therefore included a brief discussion of Rett syndrome in the context of nonsyndromic mental retardation in Chapter 6.

Mental retardation, behavioral changes, loss of speech, and loss of purposeful hand movements characterize this syndrome. It has onset in early childhood. In the majority of cases, Rett syndrome occurs sporadically, and affected female patients have unaffected parents. Rare familial cases of Rett syndrome have been described. In these families, more than one affected sibling occurs. Gonadal mosaicism may be present in a parent: one population of cells in the gonad has a normal X chromosome, while in another cell population a mutation in the Rett gene occurs on the other X chromosome. These rare familial cases facilitated mapping of the disorder to Xq27.3-Xqtcr (Van den Veyver and Zoghbi 2002).

In the period of regression, Rett syndrome patients may develop autistic behaviors (including social withdrawal and communication difficulties), hand flapping, seizures, and episodes of hyperventilation, ataxia, and hypotonia. Arrest of growth in height and head circumference also occurs. Patients may survive to adolescence or early childhood. Death is due to apnea, wasting, or cardiac arrhythmias.

Neuroimaging in the early stages of Rett syndrome may be normal. Later, MRI reveals progressive atrophy in a number of brain regions. There is reduction of gray and white matter in the basal ganglia, particularly in the caudate nucleus, midbrain, and cerebellum (Jellinger 2003).

Histopathological studies of the brain reveal reduction in neuronal size, loss of dendrites from pyramidal cells, and shortening of apical and basilar dendrite branching in cortical layers 3 and 4. Dendrites without branches occur in the frontal and temporal cortex. There is often a marked decrease of melanin in the striatal cortex. Cerebellar lobes exhibit atrophy and marked loss of Purkinje cells. In older patients, axonal degeneration of spinal tracts may occur.

Belichenko et al. (1997) related the autistic behaviors and cognitive deficits in Rett syndrome to cerebral architectural abnormalities and neuronal loss. Gait and motor dysfunction are likely related to cerebellar neuronal loss and to corticospinal tract degeneration. Movement disorders (e.g., abnormal hand movements) may be related to dysfunction of the dopaminergic system. Reduced levels of dopamine, serotonin, and 5-hydroxyl-indoleacetic acid occur in the substantia nigra.

Molecular Genetics of Rett Syndrome

The mapping of Rett syndrome to Xq27.3-Xqter led to analysis of candidate genes in this region, including the *MECP2* gene that had been mapped by Kriaucionis and Bird (2003). A breakthrough in defining the etiology of Rett syndrome occurred when Amir and coworkers (1999) discovered that *MECP2* mutations occur in this syndrome. The *MECP2* gene encodes a protein that binds to methylated cytosine in the CpG configuration. The *MECP2* protein localizes to chromatin during interphase and to chromosomes during metaphase (Nan and Bird 2001). This protein binds to methylated cytosine through an 80–amino acid domain near its amino terminal. It acts as a transcriptional repressor. There is evidence that repression of transcription requires that MECP2 bind to other proteins, such as the histone deacetylase complex Sin3A and HDAC1 and -2. The majority of missense mutations in MECP2 that lead to Rett syndrome occur in the methylcytosine binding domain or in the transcription repression domain. Rett syndrome is frequently due to deletion or insertion mutations in the *MECP2* gene; these occur throughout the gene. A number of mutations in Rett syndrome patients occur in the 3' gene region. This indicates that as yet undiscovered functional regions likely exist there (Kriaucionis and Bird 2003).

Laccone et al. (2004) reviewed reports of mutation analysis Rett syndrome patients. They noted that in 25% of cases of classical Rett syndrome detailed analysis of *MECP2* failed to reveal mutations. One possible explanation is that there is another as yet undiscovered gene responsible for the Rett phenotype. Another possibility is that mutation detection methods fail to detect

MECP2 mutations. They noted that in cases where large deletions occur in the *MECP2* gene in one X chromosome, polymerase chain reactions (PCR) primers might amplify fragments only from the normal X chromosome. They carried out dosage PCR studies on DNA from 151 girls with typical Rett syndrome manifestations where previous DNA analysis had failed to detect mutations or deletions. Using dosage-sensitive PCR, they identified 15 large *MECP2* deletions.

Laccone et al. (2004) noted that the *MECP2* gene sequence is highly enriched for repeat elements. Intron 2 is highly enriched for Alu repeat and Chi repeat sequence elements (gctggtgg). Breakpoints of deletions frequently occur in these repeats.

MECP2 Gene Expression

The *MECP2* gene is expressed to a variable extent in tissues throughout the body. In the brain, it is expressed in neurons but not in glia. Expression is higher in postnatal life than during fetal life. The gene exerts its effects primarily through modification of histone H3. The precise pathogenesis of disease manifestations caused by insufficient or abnormal MECP2 protein remains to be elucidated.

Environmental Causes of Late-Onset Cognitive Impairment

A number of environmental causes of late-onset impairment of cognition also contribute to impaired development of the brain and nervous system during fetal life.

Neurodevelopmental Effects of Malnutrition in Early Childhood

Animal studies have revealed that nutritional deficits in early life lead to poor cognitive ability (Pinero et al. 2001). There is also evidence that malnutrition in early life leads to poor cognitive ability in humans. Making the direct link between malnutrition and cognitive outcome is often confounded by the fact that poor nutrition is frequently accompanied by psychosocial deprivation.

Galler et al. (1984, 1990, 1998) followed a series of 204 children who required hospitalization for malnourishment at a specific time point. Following initial treatment of malnutrition, the children, who lived in Barbados, were followed over an extended period to ensure that they did not relapse into malnutrition. Each child was matched by socioeconomic levels, gender, and age with a control child. Galler et al. (1998) determined that children with previous malnutrition had IQ scores that were 10–12 points below those of matched controls. The IQ level was measured at different ages. Galler et al.

(1998) noted further that children with earlier severe malnutrition had shorter attention spans, and 60% were diagnosed with attention-deficit disorder. Previously malnourished children scored significantly lower on academic examinations at 11 years. Lower scores were particularly correlated with attention-deficit hyperactivity disorder.

Liu et al. (2003) carried out a study of 1559 children on the island of Mauritius, aged 3 and 11 years. They analyzed four indicators of malnutrition: hemoglobin concentration, evidence of protein malnutrition (kwashiorkor), angular stomatitis (cracking at the corners of the mouth), and sparse thin hair. Angular stomatitis is an indicator of vitamin deficiency. At 3 years of age, they assessed basic verbal, spatial, and cognitive ability using Boehm tests. At 11 years of age, they assessed verbal IQ, full-scale IQ, and scholastic ability based on standardized academic tests used in the local schools. In the statistical analyses, 14 measures of psychosocial adversity were entered as variables. They determined that malnutrition at 3 years was associated with poorer verbal and cognitive ability. Malnutrition at 11 years was associated with lower IQ, poorer reading ability, and poorer psychological performance. The differences between the malnourished group and the control group remained statistically significant even after controlling for the 14 measures of psychosocial adversity. Liu et al. (2003) also demonstrated a close relationship between the numbers of indicators of malnutrition and the extent of cognitive deficit.

Lozoff et al. (2000) reported poor long-term behavioral and developmental outcomes in children who had severe iron deficiency anemia during infancy. Severely iron-deficient children scored lower on measures of mental and motor function than controls. The differences remained statistically significant even after background factors were taken into account.

Pesticide Exposure in Children and Neurocognitive Deficits

Inner-city children are exposed to insecticides, often applied on a monthly basis, in apartment buildings. The most commonly used insecticides include organophosphates, carbamates, and pyrethroids.

Organophosphates and Carbamates

Organophosphates are esters, amides, or thiol derivatives of phosphoric acid. Carbamates are esters of carbamic acid. These compounds are widely used as pesticides. Neurotoxic agents including nerve gases such as sarin and soman are derived from organophosphates. Workers may contaminate their clothing and skin while using pesticides and then carry the pesticides into their homes. Contamination of runoff water with pesticides leads to water source and soil accumulation. In addition, effluents from manufacturing plants and waste sites may be a source of water and soil contamination.

Organophosphate esters inhibit serine-containing esterases. They phosphorylate serine residues at the active sites in these enzymes, thereby disrupting their activity. Many of the toxic effects of organophosphates depend on their ability to inhibit the enzyme acetylcholinesterase and other acetylcholine hydrolases. These enzymes play a role in detoxification reactions and in fatty acid metabolism. They are present in neuronal cells, hepatocytes, adipocytes, cells of the renal tubules, and cells of the reticuloendothelial system. Acetylcholine is released by cholinergic neurons, and this stimulates cholinergic receptors on postsynaptic neurons in the central nervous system and the autonomic nervous system. Acetylcholine receptors also occur at the myoneural junctions of skeletal muscle and smooth muscle. Following activation of the receptors, acetylcholine is released and then hydrolyzed by acetylcholinesterase.

Organophosphates and carbamates are absorbed through the mucosa of the gastrointestinal tract and the respiratory system. They are also absorbed through the skin. Acute poisoning leads to intestinal cramps, vomiting, laryngospasm, respiratory muscle paralysis, convulsions, and cardiac arrhythmias. Following the acute phase, peripheral neuropathy may develop. The effects of chronic exposure include impairment of memory and learning and altered behavior (Marrs 1993; Steenland et al. 2000).

Extensive studies on the genotoxic effects of organophosphates and carbamates have demonstrated that these compounds react with nucleic acids and lead to alkylation of nitrogen bases. Specific genotoxic effects that have been documented in human and animal cells include increased chromatid exchange (Lander and Romme 1995), increased frequency of chromosomal aberrations, impaired chromosomal segregation, and increased mutation rate (Desc et al. 1998).

Kilburn and Thornton (1995) studied control subjects and exposed subjects in an apartment complex where a subset of dwellers was exposed to high levels of organochloride pesticide. They demonstrated protracted impairment of neurophysiological function in adults and children.

Lu et al. (2001) reported results of an analysis of urine samples obtained from preschool children living in urban and suburban Seattle. They determined that metabolites of organophosphates were present in 99% of samples obtained in the spring and summer.

In rural areas, children are exposed to pesticides, especially organophosphates, that are present in dust and brought into homes on the clothes of parents who are engaged in agricultural activities (Curl et al. 2002). Guillette et al. (1998) studied two groups of 4- to 5-year-old Yaqui children in northwestern Mexico. The children had similar genetic and social backgrounds but differed with respect to their exposure to pesticides. In the Yaqui Valley, children were exposed to pesticides. Pesticides were also found at high levels in cord blood and in breast milk. In the foothill areas above the valley, pesticides were not used. Guillette et al. determined that pesticide-exposed children had decreased coordination of gross and fine movements, decreased drawing ability, and decreased 30-minute short-term memory.

Neuropathy Target Esterase and Response to Organophosphates

Winrow et al. (2003) studied the effects of reduced levels of a specific enzyme, neuropathy target esterase (Nte1), in mice. Activity of this enzyme is reduced by exposure to organophosphates. Winrow et al. (2003) developed strains of mice where Nte1 activity was reduced through genetic mutation. They demonstrated that genetic or chemical reduction of Nte1 led to hyperactive behavior in mice. This study raises the interesting possibility that genetic variation may influence the outcome following exposure to organophosphates. It also raises the possibility that organophosphate exposure in humans, particularly in individuals who carry *NTE1* mutations, may lead to hyperactivity disorders.

The neuronal membrane protein NTE1 is highly expressed in hippocampal neurons, Purkinje cells of the cerebellum, and the spinal cord. It is involved in neuronal development (Winrow et al. 2003). It is also expressed at high levels in the lens of the eye and in the testes.

Organophosphates lead to inhibition of NTE1 activity through phosphorylation of the serine residue at the active site of the enzyme. Detoxification of organophosphates depends on the activity of the enzyme paraoxonase. Berkowitz et al. (2004) demonstrated increased sensitivity of individuals with genetically determined low paraoxonase activity to chloropyrifos pesticide exposure.

Polychlorinated Biphenyls and Dioxin

Dioxins and polychlorinated biphenyls (PCBs) are both members of a family of halogenated aromatic hydrocarbons that are chemically and biologically resistant to degradation. The PCBs are synthetic compounds comprised of two benzene rings linked through a carbon bond. A chlorine group replaces each of the hydrogen atoms in the two rings. The PCBs are widely used in the making of adhesives and flame retardants. They are also present in electrical equipment and transformers and are acid-, alkali-, and heat-resistant. They are combustible at high temperatures. The products derived from burned PCBs may be more hazardous than the original substances. The PCBs accumulate in water and soil, and vapors containing these chemicals accumulate in air. They may be present in food such as fish, meat, and poultry. Breathing PCB-contaminated air may also lead to accumulation of these toxic substances in the body. These chemicals accumulate in fat-rich tissue. They also pass to breast milk and cross the placenta. Specific domains of neurodevelopment most vulnerable to the toxic effects of PCBs include attention, memory, and overall cognition (Dick et al. 2001).

A number of investigators have demonstrated that PCBs impair cognitive function in children in a dose-dependent manner (Darvill et al. 2000; Schantz and Widholm 2001). Vreugdenhil et al. (2002) carried out a study in the Netherlands and demonstrated subtle neurobehavioral deficits in children who were exposed to levels of dioxin and PCBs that are currently considered safe.

Exposure to Heavy Metals

There is an extensive body of knowledge on the consequences to the nervous system of exposure to lead. The neurocognitive and neurobehavioral consequences of lead exposure in children led in most Western countries to legislation that prohibited the addition of lead to household paint and to reduction of the quantity of lead in gasoline. The current "permissible" level of lead in the blood of children is 10 μg/dl. A number of investigators have proposed that the target level of lead in the blood of children under 1 year should be below 5 μg/dl.

In older housing, there is still a risk of lead poisoning. Between 1993 and 1997, in the city of Chicago, there was no decline over time in the number of children with blood lead levels between 15 and 45 μg/dl (Bernard and McGeehin 2003).

Specific neurocognitive and neurobehavioral effects of lead exposure include increased reaction time, impaired visual–motor integration, impaired fine motor skills, attention deficit, withdrawn behavior, impaired socialization, and lower IQ scores (Bellinger 2004).

The developing brain is particularly susceptible to damage by mercury. Organic mercury in fish is the principal source of mercury contamination in humans. Infants may also be exposed to mercury from breast milk in mothers who consume fish as a major part of their diet. Inorganic mercury may be released as vapor in industrial and mining operations. At the time of writing, the relationship of mercury exposure, due to addition of thimerosal (ethyl mercury) to vaccines, and the rising frequency of autism is being debated.

7

Nonsyndromic Mental Retardation, Autism, and Language Deficits

Mental retardation is categorized as syndromic if it is associated with clinically recognizable physical, neurological, or biochemical features. In nonsyndromic or nonspecific mental retardation, significant developmental delay and mental retardation represent key features and distinct dysmorphic features as well as neurological and metabolic abnormalities are absent. The distinction between syndromic mental retardation and nonsyndromic mental retardation is, however, not as clear-cut as it may seem. Following identification of genes for nonsyndromic forms of X-linked mental retardation, investigators who undertook detailed phenotypic analysis in patients with defects in a specific gene often found subtle but distinct clinical abnormalities. In some instances, patients with a specific gene defect had associated biochemical abnormalities or specific MRI findings. Furthermore, it has become clear that different mutations in a particular gene may have different consequences. Some may lead to syndromic mental retardation, while others lead to nonsyndromic mental retardation (Frints et al. 2002).

X-Linked Mental Retardation

Within all grades of mental retardation worldwide, there is an excess of affected male subjects. The ratio of affected male to affected female subjects is approximately 1.3:1. This observation indicates that many genes that determine mental function map to the X chromosome. Herbst and Miller (1980) reported that 1.8 per 1000 male individuals carry a gene for X-linked mental retardation. Ropers et al. (2003) estimated that approximately one-third of these cases have syndromic forms of X-linked mental retardation. Fragile X mental retardation may be considered in the category of syndromic mental retardation (see Chapter 4). However, the dysmorphology in this syndrome is very subtle, and the disorder is difficult to diagnose on the basis of clinical findings. Fragile X syndrome should therefore be considered in male children who present with mental retardation and who have no clear evidence of dysmorphology.

Since the discovery of the gene defect in fragile X mental retardation in 1991, there has been considerable progress in identifying X-linked genes that play a role in cognition (Barnes and Milgram 2002). Progress is in large part due to the efforts of investigators who established an international consortium to pool clinical resources. Their strategy includes collection of blood samples and clinical information from families that fulfill criteria for X-linked mental retardation. In these families, there are two or more affected male individuals related through female individuals who themselves are unaffected or mildly affected (Hamel et al. 2003). In all male patients affected with mental retardation, routine cytogenetic studies and analysis for fragile X mental retardation is performed. Deoxyribonucleic acid (DNA) samples from family members are prepared and used for analysis of polymorphic markers on the X chromosome to determine if mental retardation segregating in a specific family can be linked to a specific region of the X chromosome (Yntema et al. 1998, 2002, and X linked mental retardation database) (http://www.molgen.mpg.de/~abt_rop/mrwelcome.html).

A second strategy developed by the consortium is collection of blood and cultured cell samples (fibroblasts) from individuals with mental retardation who have a previously detected structural abnormality on the X chromosome. Molecular genetic studies are then carried out to identify genes interrupted as a result of translocation or inversion and to detect dosage changes in specific genes that occur in consequence of the microdeletion or duplication.

A third component of the consortium study is the extensive use of databases of gene maps and gene sequences to search for candidate genes for mental retardation in X-chromosome regions determined to be of interest on the basis of linkage studies or chromosomal analyses. Candidate genes are then examined in families linked to a specific chromosomal region or in families where the number of affected individuals is too small to undertake linkage. In carrying out mutation analysis, investigators make use of database information and analysis of DNA from control individuals in order to distinguish sequence changes that constitute polymorphisms (normal variation) from mutations that lead to changes that are deleterious to function of the gene product (des Portes et al. 1999; Chiurazzi et al. 2004).

At least 72 different forms of syndromic X-linked mental retardation have been described and mapped (Chiurazzi et al. 2004; Siderius et al. 1999; Frints et al. 2003) (see also Chapter 4). Twenty-two genes that play a role in nonsyndromic X-linked mental retardation have been characterized (Chiurazzi et al. 2004). These genes were usually isolated on the basis of analysis of chromosomal translocations and deletions in a specific patient or family. They were then analyzed for mutations in other families with nonsyndromic X-linked mental retardation. The genes thus far described turn out to be only rarely mutated in these families, with the exception of the *FMR1* gene and the *SLCA6* creatine transporter gene (Rosenberg et al. 2004). Genes involved in nonsyndromic mental retardation are listed in Table 7–1.

It is important to note that for a number of genes listed in Table 7–1 specific mutations give rise to nonsyndromic mental retardation, while other mutations or gene deletions give rise to syndromic mental retardation. This is true for *FGD1*, *OPHN1*, *ARX*, and *FACL4* (Chiurazzi et al. 2004).

Ropers et al. (2003) noted that in 30% of all families with X-linked mental retardation, linkage analysis reveals that the disorder maps to Xp11.2 to Xp11.3. The *ZNF41* gene, which maps in that region, was interrupted as a result of an X:7 chromosomal translocation. Subsequently, mutations were found in other patients with mental retardation, language problems, and aggressiveness. Jensen et al. (2005) undertook a systematic analysis of brain-expressed genes in the pericentromeric region of the X chromosome, including Xp11 to Xp11.3, in 210 families with X-linked mental retardation. They identified mutations in the gene *JARID1C* in affected members of seven of the families. The *JARID1C* gene maps in Xp11.2-p11.21 and encodes a protein that plays a role in transcriptional regulation and chromatin remodeling. Studies by Jensen et al. (2005) indicate that *JARID1C* plays an important role in cognition.

It is interesting to consider the possibility that non-protein-coding genes in Xp11.2-11.3 may play a role in X-linked mental retardation. Examination of the Sanger database of micro-ribonucleic acids (RNAs) reveals that a cluster of microRNAs maps in this region (http://www.sanger.ac.uk/Software/Rfam/mirna).

Rett Syndrome

In the classic form of Rett syndrome, development is normal before 1 year of age. In the period of regression, girls may exhibit behavioral changes, loss of speech, and loss of purposeful hand movements. Subsequently, patients become mentally retarded. In the majority of cases, Rett syndrome occurs sporadically; affected female patients have unaffected parents. Rare familial cases of Rett syndrome have been described.

Mutations in the *MECP2* gene, which maps to Xq28, (Vilain et al. 1996; Amir et al. 1999) are responsible for Rett syndrome. The classical form of this syndrome is discussed in Chapter 6 under the category of disorders of chromatin modification.

Variant Forms of Rett Syndrome

More comprehensive searches for *MECP2* mutations in subjects with mental retardation have led to the recognition that variant forms of Rett syndrome occur (Couvert et al. 2001). Gomot et al. (2003) reported results of *MECP2* mutation analysis in three families with nonsyndromic X-linked mental retardation. In each of these families, affected male patients occurred who were linked through unaffected female carriers. In one family, a *MECP2* deletion mutation occurred. This led to loss of 80 amino acids in the

Table 7-1
Gene Defects in Nonsyndromic Mental Retardation

Location	Gene	Function	Reference
Xp22.3	NLGN4	Neuronal cell surface protein, interacts with DLG2	Laumonnier et al. (2004)
Xp22.3-p21.1	IL1RAPL1 (interleukin-1 receptor accessory protein-like 1)	Interleukin receptor; signal transduction, learning and memory	Carrie et al. (1999)
Xp22.1-21.3	ARX (aristaless-related homeobox)	Expressed in central and peripheral nerves; involved in development	Kato et al. (2004)
Xp13.1	DLG3 (human homolog 3 of Drosophila Discs large, dlg)	Encodes synapse-associated protein SAP102, interacts with NMDA receptors	Tarpey et al. (2004)
Xp12	OPHN1 (oligophrenin-1)	Rho GTPase activation	Billuart et al. (2000)
Xp11.4	TM4SF2 (transmembrane 4 superfamily 2)	Cell surface glycoprotein, involved in neurite outgrowth	Maranduba et al. (2004)
Xp11.3	ZNF41 (zinc finger protein)	Transcriptional repressor	Shoichet et al. (2003)
Xp11.3	GDI1 (GDP dissociation inhibitor)	Regulates GDP–GTP exchange on Rab proteins in neuronal membranes	des Porte et al. (1999) Bienvenu et al. (1998)
Xp11.23	ZNF81 (zinc finger protein)	Plays a role in transcription	Kleefstra et al. (2004)
Xp11.23	PQBP1 (polyglutamine binding protein)	Nuclear protein binds to proteins with polyglutamine repeats	Lenski et al. (2004)
Xp11.23	FTSJ1 (Homolog of Escherichia coli Ftsj)	RNA methyltransferase, transcriptional regulation	Freude et al. (2004)
Xp11.2	FGD1 (Rho GEF)	Stimulates GDP–GTP exchange, binds to Rho GTPase	Lebel et al. (2002)

Locus	Gene	Function	Reference
Xp11.2	*JARID1C* (*SMCX*, Jumonji AT-rich domain)	Transcriptional regulation, chromatin modification	Jensen et al. (2005)
Xq22.1–q23	*FACL4* (*ACSL4*, long chain acyl CoA synthase 4)	Converts long chain fatty acid into acyl CoA esters, lipid biosynthesis	Meloni et al. (2002)
Xq23	*PAK3* (p21-activated kinase)	Links Rho GTPases to cytoskeleton reorganization; involved in synaptic plasticity	Allen et al. (1998)
Xq23	*NLGN3* (neuroligin 3)	Neuronal surface protein involved in remodeling of synapses	Jamain et al. (2003)
Xq26.3	*ARHGEF* (Rho GEF)	Links cytoskeleton to cell membrane, involved in synaptic plasticity	Kutsche et al. (2000) Rosenberger et al. (2003)
Xq27.3	*FMR1* (*FRX4*, fragile X mental retardation)	Transcriptional and translational control	Verkerk et al. (1991)
Xq28	*MECP2* (methyl CpG binding protein)	Transcriptional repressor binds to methylated DNA	Van den Veyver and Zoghbi (2002)
Xq28	*SLC6A8*	Creatine transporter	Rosenberg et al. (2004)
Xq28	*FMR2* (*FRXE*)	Fragile site E	Gecz et al. (1997)

GDP, guanosine disphsphate; GTP, guanosine triphosphate; CoA, coenzyme A; NMDA, *N*-methyl-D-aspartate; GEF, guanine nucleotide exchange factor.

C-terminal end of the MECP2 protein. In the other two families, missense mutations occurred.

Nonlethal Rett syndrome has also been reported in male subjects with exon 4 mutations. Male subjects who are somatic mosaics for MECP2 mutations have also been encountered. Huppke et al. (2002) reported that mutations that involve the nuclear localization signal domain in MECP2 lead to a more severe phenotype. They noted that truncating mutations in the C-terminal region led to a less severe phenotype. One common point mutation that leads to an amino acid substitution, R133C, is associated with a less severe phenotype in female individuals (Smeets et al. 2003).

The proportion of cells in which the X chromosome that carries the mutant form of MECP2 is inactivated may influence the effects of a specific mutation of MECP2 in female individuals.

Huppke et al. (2002) described patients with MECP2 mutations who had normal motor function and symptoms typical of autism, including social withdrawal, language delay, and stereotypical hand movements.

Other studies have reported a higher frequency of missense *MECP2* gene mutations in patients with mental retardation or autism (Shibayama et al. 2004). It is not clear whether or not some of these represent disease-causing mutations or polymorphisms. Further studies are required to determine the functional significance of specific missense mutations. Studies on the extent of *MECP2* polymorphisms in the general population are also required.

Forms of Nonsyndromic Mental Retardation That Manifest Autosomal Recessive Patterns of Inheritance

Identification of causative autosomal genes for nonsyndromic mental retardation is difficult because deficits in a large number of different genes likely lead to this disorder. Furthermore, there are few clinical criteria that enable recognition of different subgroups. Linkage studies in large multigeneration families or in consanguineous families with a number of cases of mental retardation have led to identification of at least three loci for autosomal recessively inherited forms of nonspecific mental retardation. Using such studies, Molinari et al. (2002) mapped a gene locus for autosomal recessively inherited mental retardation to chromosome 4q24. They carried out mutation analysis in genes that mapped in this region and concluded that the gene that encodes neurotrypsin was defective in this family. Higgins et al. (2000) mapped a gene locus for autosomal recessive mental retardation to 3p25–pter on the basis of linkage studies in a large family with multiple cases of mental retardation.

Basel-Vanagaite et al. (2003) carried out linkage studies in three large consanguineous Arab families with the same last name. Multiple individuals in the families manifested mild psychomotor delay in early childhood. Later in life, they manifested severe retardation and had only single words. Affected subjects had no physical abnormalities and their height, weight, and head circumference were normal. Basel-Vanagaite et al. analyzed 400 microsatellite markers spaced at 10 centimorgan intervals throughout the genome. In each family, the investigators examined marker data to determine if affected individuals were homozygous for specific alleles and if different affected individuals shared the same alleles. The four families had a common haplotype on chromosome 19p13.12-p13.2. These findings strongly support the conclusion that a gene mutation that leads to nonsyndromic mental retardation maps to this region.

Multifactorial or Complex Inheritance and Mental Retardation

It is highly likely that complex inheritance plays an important role in the etiology of mental retardation. In his monograph *The Biology of Mental Defect*, published in 1972, Lionel Penrose wrote "the type of inheritance most commonly observed in human genetical material is due to the combined actions of more than one gene. Indeed the number of genes involved can be very large" (Penrose 1972, p. 108).

The terms *multifactorial disease* and *genetically complex disorder* are used to describe conditions that exhibit familial clustering but do not exhibit clearcut mendelian inheritance. In multifactorial diseases both genetic and environmental factors may play a role. In genetically complex disorders, variation at specific gene loci leads to an increased risk of developing the disorders. Disease manifestations depend upon the interaction of mutations at a number of different gene loci. In multifactorial and genetically complex disorders the risk to siblings of an affected patient is higher than in the general population (Todd 2001).

The etiology of disorders such as mental retardation may be dependent upon the interaction of genes and environment. The term *heritability* is used to define the contribution of genetics to the phenotype.

Proof that a phenotypic character or disease is genetically determined usually requires that it exhibits some degree of familial clustering and that the risk to a relative of someone who has a specific disease is higher than the risk to an individual in the general population. Since families share environment and genetic factors, the two cannot always be clearly separated. Analysis of the co-occurrence of a specific trait in monozygotic versus dizygotic twins has been used to measure the genetic contribution to risk of a specific disease. Studies on twins separated at birth have been particularly useful in this regard (Gottesman 1997; Gottesman and Erlenmeyer-Kimling 2001). Twins separated at birth have, of course, shared the same intrauterine environment.

Identification of gene loci for genetically complex disorders may be accomplished more easily in populations that are more homogeneous, e.g., inbred populations.

Strategies to Identify Gene Loci That Contribute to Genetically Complex Disorders

The first problem in the analysis of genetically complex disorders has to do with classification of the phenotype. This is particularly a problem with behavioral disorders. A second problem involves the appropriate selection of specific parameters required for the statistical analysis of data. In parametric linkage analysis, it is necessary to include information on the population frequency of the disease, the mode of inheritance, and the penetrance of the gene. *Penetrance* is defined as the percentage of cases that have phenotypic manifestations when the disease mutation is present. In genetic linkage studies in complex disorders, nonparametric linkage analyses are usually applied. This form of analysis is model-free; for example, a specific mode of inheritance is not included in setting up the analysis. Evidence for linkage is based on the extent to which affected relatives, for example, sib pairs, share specific alleles at a particular locus.

Association Studies

To identify gene loci that play a role in the etiology of complex diseases in a specific population, investigators frequently carry out association studies. The goal of these studies is to determine if a specific allele at a particular locus occurs more frequently in affected individuals than in controls. A specific allele at a particular gene locus may be associated with a disease because there is a direct connection between that gene and the disease (Botstein and Risch 2003). The connection may, however, be secondary and due to the fact that individuals are descended from a common ancestor. Secondary association occurs in families and in populations. If association studies are carried out to determine association of a specific allele in subjects affected with a certain disorder, it is important that the frequency of that allele be determined in unaffected control individuals drawn from the same population.

Linkage Disequilibrium

The terms *linkage disequilibrium* and *allelic association* are applied when specific alleles at two or more loci occur together more frequently than would be predicted based on their population frequencies at each locus. Linkage disequilibrium studies may be used to map genetically complex disorders (Clark 2003; Botstein and Risch 2003). They may also be applied to the analysis of disorders that follow a simple mendelian pattern of inheritance.

In families where a genetically determined disease is transmitted through several generations, it may be possible to determine if there are regions of shared alleles that passed through the generations and are present in affected individuals and in individuals who transmitted the genetic disorder. Similarly, in nuclear families with more than one affected child, it is important to determine the degree to which affected siblings share specific alleles at a particular locus. Such regions are defined as regions that are in linkage disequilibrium with the disease. Genes that map within a genomic region that is in linkage disequilibrium with the disease gene are disease candidate genes. Definitive characterization of the disease gene requires a DNA sequence search for evidence of DNA mutations.

DNA Sequence Changes and Complex Diseases

The question that frequently arises is whether or not a specific DNA difference that occurs in an affected individual constitutes a significant change and whether or not the change plays a role in the pathogenesis of the disorder. In disorders that follow a simple mendelian pattern of inheritance, there are standard guidelines that may be applied to determine the significance of a particular mutation (Strachan and Read 1999). Examples of mutations that alter gene function include the following:

1. Small intragenic deletions or duplications that introduce a frameshift so that the transcript that is derived cannot be correctly translated. Frame-shift mutations may lead to absence of a protein or to the presence of a truncated protein.
2. Base substitution near the intron–exon splice site may lead to abnormal splicing of the primary transcript and generation of an abnormal mature messenger RNA transcript.
3. A base substitution may lead to an alteration in the amino acid present in the gene product. This may be a functionally silent mutation. However, if the usual amino acid is one that shows a high degree of evolutionary conservation across species, it is likely that its replacement will have functional consequences. Amino acid substitutions are more likely to have consequences if they occur in the active site of an enzyme or in locations that play a role in determining interactions with other proteins or with specific substrates. Base substitutions may convert the three-letter codon for an amino acid to a stop codon so that transcription is halted.

In complex genetic diseases, it is possible that the base changes associated with the disease phenotype represent changes that have a more subtle effect on the function of the gene product. It is also possible that the mutation in one specific gene is not sufficient to cause disease and that mutations in a number of different genes are required for the disease to manifest. Interactions between specific gene mutations and specific environmental factors may also be important. The question then arises whether certain combinations of alleles at different loci increase the likelihood of developing the disorder.

It is also important to consider whether or not the different loci that are shown to be in linkage disequilibrium with the disorder encode products that impact the same biochemical pathway or a specific physiological function.

In the case of nonsyndromic mental retardation, it seems unlikely that the linkage disequilibrium approach will help define specific disease genes except in inbred populations.

Autism

In 1943, Leo Kanner first described a behavioral disorder in children that he referred to as "autism." Patients with this disorder have difficulties with social interactions and social reciprocity. They have difficulties sharing experiences with other people and are frequently unable to correctly interpret the emotions that underlie specific facial expressions. Individuals with autism have language and communication deficits. These range from mute status to adequate speech with poor conversation skills. Approximately 50% of individuals with autism do not develop functional spoken language.

Speech quality is often abnormal, with atypical intonation. Subjects often exhibit difficulty with integration of language and gesture. They exhibit abnormally stereotyped interests and repetitive behaviors. They strongly resist changes in environment or routines. They frequently engage in repetitive actions or repetitive types of play. Their actions are often ritualized (Eigesti et al. 2003).

Lockyer and Rutter (1969) suggested that autism has an organic (biological) basis. They reported that 75% of cases of autism had mental retardation and that 40% of cases had epilepsy. Only a small percentage of cases have a history of pre- or postnatal infections or exposure to toxins. Autism may occur in patients with monogenic diseases such as tuberous sclerosis or fragile X mental retardation. Autistic symptoms have also been described in patients with chromosomal abnormalities, e.g., duplications of chromosome 15q11-q13 (Dykens et al. 2004) or deletions of chromosome 2q37.3 (Smith et al. 2001; Lukusa et al. 2004). Routine cytogenetic studies provide evidence for chromosomal abnormalities in a low percentage of cases with autism. The possibility that higher-resolution techniques, such as fluorescence in situ hybridization or microarray analysis, may detect chromosomal abnormalities in a higher percentage of subjects with autism cannot, however, be ruled out.

Cases of autism where there is no evidence of a single-gene disorder or of chromosomal abnormalities are sometimes referred to as "idiopathic autism." There is evidence that genetic factors play a role in the etiology of this condition. This evidence comes from twin studies and from studies in families. The concordance rate for autism in monozygotic twins is reported to be 60%–92%, while the concordance rate in dizygotic twins ranges 0%–10% in different reports. Autism rates in siblings also suggest that genetic factors play a role. The recurrence risk (3%) in families with one autistic child is higher than the population prevalence (5.2 per 10,000). Many investigators are of the opinion that autism is a complex genetic disorder where, in each affected patient, a series of different but interacting gene mutations occur and determine the clinical picture (Lamb et al. 2002; Risch et al. 1999). However, the fact that monozygotic twins are not always concordant for autism suggests that epigenetic and/or environmental factors underlie the development of autistic behaviors.

Epidemiology of Autism

Prior to 1996, the prevalence of autism was estimated as 5.2 per 10,000. If milder forms of autism (e.g., Asperger syndrome) are included in the calculations, the prevalence is 16–19 per 10,000. Later reports indicate a great increase in the frequency of autism. Other reports question whether this increase is real or whether it reflects changes in ascertainment. Psychometric tests used to establish a diagnosis of autism have changed in each decade since Kanner first recognized the condition in 1943. Initially, Kanner's diagnostic criteria were used. Later, Rutter's criteria were applied. Following this *Diagnostic and Statistical Manual* third edition (DSMIII), the DSMIII revised, and *International Classification of Diseases* tenth edition criteria were frequently used. More recently, additional psychometric testing instruments were developed to diagnose autism. These include standardized autism diagnostic interviews and observation schedules (Lord and Volkmar 2002). During the time period, when psychometric tests for autism were modified, the estimated prevalence increased from 6 per 10,000 to 60 per 10,000. Fombonne (2003) reported that a clear-cut conclusion regarding an increased incidence of autism could not be made.

A consistent feature in epidemiological studies is the fact that male individuals are more frequently affected than female individuals. The ratio of male to female subjects is 4 to 1. The ratio of male to female subjects is lower, 2 to 1, among the mentally retarded autistic.

Another consistent feature across different epidemiological studies is the 70% incidence of mental retardation in autistic subjects. Thirty percent of individuals are mildly to moderately retarded; 40% score in the severely retarded range. There is no clear-cut relationship between autism and ethnicity or autism and socioeconomic background (Fombonne 2003).

Neuropathology of Autism

Kanner (1943) noted that children with autism frequently had macrocephaly, i.e., head circumference above the 97th percentile. Later studies reported that macrocephaly is usually not present in autistic subjects during the first year of life; it develops after that time (Stevenson et al. 1997). Neuroimaging studies have confirmed larger head size in autistic children (Filipek 1996) and that there is an increase in cerebral white matter visible on MRI. Excessive white matter connection suggests a failure of the normal process of cortical pruning.

Neurohistology

Ritvo et al. (1986) reported cerebellar changes in autism; they noted a reduction in the number of Purkinje cells. Kemper and Bauman (2002) and Bauman and Kemper (2003) confirmed that Purkinje cell numbers are reduced in autism. In addition, they noted abnormalities in the hippocampus, amygdala, and mamillary bodies; in these structures, autism is characterized by the presence of small densely packed neurons.

Studies by Bailey et al. (1998) confirmed that the brains of autistic subjects are usually larger than those of controls. They presented evidence that increased neuronal cell numbers underlie this increase in brain size. They pointed out that the increased cell numbers in autistic brains could be due to increased cell replication or impaired cell death.

Neuropsychological Functioning in Autism

Minshew et al. (1997) administered a comprehensive battery of neuropsychological assessments to 33 high-functioning autistic subjects and matched controls. They determined that autistic subjects manifested deficits in complex motor movements and had difficulties in higher-order information processing. They had difficulties with interpretative aspects of language and concept formation. Minshew et al. (2002a,b) noted that mentally retarded subjects with autism had the same qualitative cognition profile as non-mentally retarded autistic subjects. Namely, higher-order skills were disproportionately affected. Minshew et al. (2002a,b) proposed that reduced connectivity between neural systems constitutes the neural basis of autism.

Eigsti et al. (2003) reported that individuals with autism have a jagged profile in cognitive performance. They exhibit strengths in some areas and weaknesses in others. They manifest difficulties in planning and in integrating practical knowledge. Their working memory is impaired. Approximately 10% of subjects exhibit savant status, e.g., with calculations or rote memory.

One of the most striking features of autism is language deficit. In addition, many children with autism have a hyperactive response to sensory input, particularly to sound (Casanova et al. 2002). Gage et al. (2003) used the noninvasive technique magnetoencephalography to analyze auditory cortical function in autistic children and controls. They determined that early cortical encoding of sounds and neural conduction of sound were slowed in autistic subjects. They postulated that abnormalities in early auditory processing lead to abnormal sound reactivity and to language dysfunction in autism.

Mapping of Genome Regions Related to Autism

Between 1998 and 2004, much effort was expended and some progress was made in identifying regions of the genome that play a role in autism. A number of investigators have carried out linkage studies in families where several members have autism (multiplex families). They used polymorphic markers located throughout the genome. Results of comprehensive genomewide linkage scans have been published by at least eight groups. No two groups have identified the same overall pattern of genomic regions that are linked to autism. No single chromosome has been associated with autism in all studies. However, there are a few regions that show linkage in several studies, e.g., regions in chromosomes 7q, 2q, and 19p13-q13 (International Molecular Genetic Study of Autism Consortium 1998, 2000; Buxbaum et al., 2001; Auranen et al. 2002; Shao et al. 2002). Thus far, sequencing analyses have failed to identify specific autism-determining genes on these chromosomes.

Association studies have been carried out by a number of different groups. Intragenic polymorphisms, especially single nucleotide polymorphisms, have been analyzed both in multiplex families and sibling pairs. One goal of association studies is to determine if a particular allele at a polymorphic locus occurs more frequently in affected individuals than in their non-affected siblings. Different association studies have usually highlighted different autism-associated genes; positive associations found by one group have frequently not been confirmed in later studies by others. However, a number of different groups have found positive associations on chromosome 7q and on chromosome 17q11.2. Bonora et al. (2005) reported evidence for association of autism with a missense mutation in the *LAMB1* gene (laminin-β1) on chromosome 7q24. They also reported association between autism and several polymorphisms in the promoter and untranslated regions of *NRCAM* (neuronal cell adhesion molecule) on 7q31.

As of 2004 there are no autism and marker polymorphism associations that examine whether or not any combination of alleles at two loci that map on different chromosomes occur more frequently in affected individuals.

Structural Chromosomal Abnormalities in Autism

Identification of chromosomal abnormalities in individuals with autism may serve to highlight specific genomic regions that play an important role in the pathogenesis of this disorder. In fact, many different chromosomal abnormalities are associated with autism. The most frequent chromosomal abnormality in autism involves chromosome 15q11-q13 (Bolton et al. 2004). There are reports of chromosome 2q32-2q34 abnormalities in autism (Gallagher et al. 2003; Pescucci et al. 2003). There are at least 10 reports of 2q37.3 region deletions associated with autism (Smith et al. 2001; Lukasa 2004). Chromosome 7q emerges as the region that shows linkage and association with autism, and chromosomal abnormalities of 7q have been reported in cases with autism (Bonora et al. 2005). The significant region for autism is large, 7q21-7q36. Chromosome 15q11-q13 also emerges as being significant in autism through association studies (Dykens et al. 2004). One of eight genome scan reports provides evidence for linkage autism to chromosone 15.

Are There Subtypes in Autism?

One question that is relevant to linkage studies in autism is whether or not there are groups of patients in whom particular autism spectrum features predominate. Are there specific features that show familial aggregation, that is, decreased variance, within families? There is some evidence that this may be the case. Evidence for linkage of autism to chromosome 7 was more striking when linkage studies were carried out in a subgroup of autism patients with severe language impairment (Lamb et al. 2002).

Evidence for linkage of autism to chromosome 15 became more striking when a subgroup of patients were studied who manifested many stereotypic behaviors and striking "insistence on sameness"; i.e., they were very intolerant of changes in their environment (Shao et al. 2003).

Gene Defects Associated with Autism

Autism and Genome Regions That Are Involved in DNA Methylation and Chromatin Modulation

Identification of the genetic defect in Rett syndrome by Amir and coworkers (1999) has important implications for autism. Rett syndrome and autism are both classified as pervasive developmental disorders. Rett syndrome and autism have many features in common, including loss of social, cognitive, and language skills and development of repetitive stereotypic behaviors (Zoghbi 2003). A number of investigators have reported results of *MECP2* analysis in autistic subjects. Results of these studies revealed that *MECP2* mutations occur in a low percentage of cases with autism.

We described a patient with autism who had a deletion on chromosome 15q22-q23 (Smith et al. 2000). The deletion in this patient leads to hemizygosity for the gene that encodes Sin3A. This protein interacts with MECP2 protein and histone deacetylases to regulate gene transcription.

Autism occurs in patients with chromosome 15q11-q13 abnormalities, such as duplication of this region (Bolton et al. 2004). Autistic features sometimes occur in Prader-Willi syndrome (Veltman et al. 2004) and in Angelman syndrome (S. U. Peters et al. 2004). Samaco et al. (2005) reported reduced expression of two genes in the 15q11-q13 region, *UBE3A* and *GABRB3*, in Rett syndrome, Angelman syndrome, and autism brains and in brains of *Mecp2*-deficient mouse strains compared to controls. They suggest that there is an overlapping pathway of dysregulation of 15q11-q13 genes in Angelman syndrome, Rett syndrome, and autism.

Fragile X Syndrome

Symptoms of autism frequently occur in patients with fragile X syndrome. However, a relatively low percentage of all cases of autism are due to fragile X mutations. Kaufman et al. (2004) reported that a range of autistic spectrum disorders occur in fragile X syndrome. Some patients manifest classical autism, while others manifest pervasive developmental disorder. They noted further that male subjects with fragile X particularly manifest defects in the social interaction domains.

Autism occurs in a significant percentage of cases of tuberous sclerosis.

Autism: Questions and Hypotheses

If we consider genome regions identified thus far as playing a role in autism, several key questions arise. First, do gene defects in these different regions lead to autism through different mechanisms, or do they interact in a common pathway? Second, do some of these gene regions harbor regulatory elements that influence gene expression? These elements may not be identified as being defective in autism if we consider only protein-encoding genes as candidates and confine mutation analysis to such genes.

Speech and Language Disorders and Developmental Delay

By the age of 4 years, many children have a vocabulary of several thousand words and are able to construct complex sentences. Impaired language development may be a manifestation of mental retardation, autism, hearing loss, cleft palate, or cerebral palsy. In many cases, language deficit occurs as an isolated developmental problem (Fisher et al. 2003).

Language impairment is classified into subtypes. It is not clear, however, that subtypes have different etiologies. DSMIV subtypes include the following:

1. Phonological disorders characterized by a failure to use speech sounds correctly
2. Deficits in expressive language with normal receptive language
3. Mixed expressive and receptive language disorder

For a diagnosis of isolated language disorder to be made, there must be a discrepancy between verbal intelligence quotient (IQ) and nonverbal IQ. There is, however, evidence that early language problems influence later development (Tomblin and Pandich 1999).

Speech and language difficulties tend to cluster in families, suggesting that genetic factors play a role in their etiology. Other evidence for genetic risk factors is that the concordance rate for language deficiencies is much higher in monozygotic twins (average 70%) than in dizygotic twins (average 46%).

Autosomal Dominant Speech and Language Deficit

Significant progress in the elucidation of a genetic factor in speech and language disorders began when Hurst et al. (1990) described a three-generation pedigree from the United Kingdom, where speech and language difficulties segregated as an autosomal dominant trait. The language problems in affected members of this family were initially defined as "developmental verbal dyspraxia." This condition is characterized by difficulty in controlling the complex mouth movements that are necessary for speech. Affected members showed no evidence for dyspraxia or apraxia in other parts of the body. Subsequent studies revealed that affected family members had deficits in receptive language and in written language.

The speech defect in this family was designated "SPCH1" and mapped to chromosome 7q31 by Lai et al. (2000). Four candidate genes were mapped in the region of linkage. A further breakthrough came when an individual from a different family was identified who had a translocation between chromosomes 7 and 5, receptive language deficits, and articulation difficulties. The translocation breakpoint in 7q31 interrupted a gene that encodes a transcription factor. This factor, Forkhead box P_2 (FOXP2), has a specific protein domain, a forkhead winged helix domain that binds to DNA (Lac et al. 2001).

All affected members in the large family with speech and language deficits described by Hurst et al. (1990) were shown to have a specific mutation in the *FOXP2* gene, a G-to-A substitution in exon 14 that leads to arginine being replaced by histidine in the FOXP2 protein. Arginine is highly conserved in different species and directly involved in the binding of the forkhead transcription factor to DNA. The *FOXP2* gene also encodes two adjacent polyglutamine tracts that may be susceptible to expansion.

Molecular Evolution of FOXP2 and Development of Articulated Speech

Enard et al. (2002a,b) studied the molecular evolution of FOXP2. These investigators noted "the ability to develop articulate speech relies on capabilities such as fine control of the larynx and mouth that are absent in chimpanzees and other great apes." (p. 869) Sequence analysis of the FOXP2 protein-coding regions revealed that chimpanzee, gorilla, rhesus monkey, and macaque monkey have an identical sequence. Furthermore, the sequence in these primates differs only by two amino acids from that in humans. These differences are encoded in exon 7 of *FOXP2*, where in humans threonine at position 303 is replaced by asparagine and at position 325 asparagine is replaced by serine. Enard et al. note that the human-specific change at position 325 is likely to have functional consequences since it creates a potential target site for phosphorylation by protein kinase. Phosphorylation of FOXP2 may potentially allow for a greater degree of transcriptional regulation. They propose that the FOXP2 amino acid changes were positively selected during human evolution. This led in turn to the capability for improved articulation of mouth movement and development of proficiency in spoken language.

The *FOXP2* gene maps in 7q31, a region that is linked to autism. Gauthier et al. (2004) and Newbury et al. (2002) carried out mutation screening analysis of *FOXP2* in autistic subjects. They concluded that coding variants of *FOXP2* do not segregate with autism. Interestingly, in 2004, Gong and coworkers reported significant association between autism and *FOXP2* single nucleotide polymorphisms in the Han Chinese population.

8

Genomics, Functional Genomics, and Epigenetics: Relevance to Mental Retardation

In this chapter, we will consider how information obtained through genomic analysis will continue to impact research into the etiology of developmental delay and mental retardation.

Genomes, Genetic Information, DNA, and Chromatin

A *genome* is defined as the total genetic information present in an organism. The human genome has been almost completely sequenced through research conducted as part of the Human Genome Project. The next phase of genomic analysis will involve research on functional genomics and analysis of factors that control gene expression. This will include identification of deoxyribonucleic acid (DNA) sequence elements that may be located at some distance from the genes they control. It will also include analysis of the complete array of messenger ribonucleic acid (mRNA) transcripts that are derived from a particular gene (The Transcriptome Project) and definition of the proteins that are translated from these transcripts (The Proteome Project). Other research efforts under way include in-depth analysis of the relationship between variations in expression of specific genes and the metabolic state of the cell or organism (Metabolomics).

The DNA is enclosed in chromatin. Chromatin remodeling plays a key role in gene expression since it determines accessibility of DNA to transcription factors. Chromatin modifications and their consequent effects on the readout of genetic information are sometimes referred to as "epigenetics." Analysis of regulation of gene expression requires that we examine not only DNA sequence but also chromatin structure.

Genomic sequencing has led to the identification of "new" genes, loci that have the sequence characteristics of genes and the potential to give rise to mRNA transcripts and to encode proteins. However, in many cases, the biological functions of these new gene products are unknown. Biological dissection of the functions of these genes and the consequences of mutations within their sequences will be facilitated through studies in model organisms and in cell culture systems (see also Chapter 1). Interference RNA methodologies will be applied to block RNA of a specific gene and to analyze the consequences to the cell or organism of the loss of gene expression (He and Hannon 2004).

It is possible that a substantial number of genes that are presently in the category of genes of unknown function play an important role in brain development and in cognition.

Freimer and Sabatti (2003) and Scriver (2004) have emphasized the need for a Phenome Project. Freimer and Sabatti wrote "the term phenotype can refer to any morphologic, biochemical, physiological or behavioral characteristic of an organism. Phenotypes, like genotypes can by definition, vary between individuals and it is this variation we wish to understand." (Freimer and Sabath 2003, pp. 15–16) Scriver wrote "Individuality in phenotypes is embedded in components of the phenome (transcriptome, metabolome, proteome, etc)." (Scriver 2004, p. 305)

As we analyze genes and regulatory factors involved in developmental delay and mental retardation, it will continue to be critically important to analyze the phenotype of patients. Detailed and accurate clinical descriptions are required to establish genotype–phenotype correlations. Assays of metabolites and proteins will continue to be an important part of phenotypic analysis. One goal will be to determine if there is a direct connection between gene expression, gene mutations, and changes in metabolic activity. Mass spectrometry and proton nuclear magnetic resonance spectroscopy are increasingly being used for metabolite and protein analysis. Application of these techniques enables more comprehensive analysis and reduces the cost of analysis (Griffin 2004).

Over the past few decades much of the research aimed at understanding the etiology and pathogenesis of mental retardation and developmental disabilities has been concentrated on the analysis of proteins and enzymes. It is now possible to examine the genome more comprehensively and to investigate factors that control gene expression. Such investigations are facilitated by the availability of cloned, mapped segments of DNA and the availability of reference DNA sequence information and techniques to investigate chromatin structure. More comprehensive analysis of gene expression is now possible through the application of array techniques.

Resources Made Available through the Genome Project

Improved Resources for Analysis of Genome Dosage Changes

The availability of sequenced and mapped segments of DNA provides a resource that may be used to search for chromosomal changes and dosage alterations. This may be achieved through direct hybridization of isolated, amplified segments of DNA to chromosomes as in fluorescence in situ hybridization (FISH). Dosage analysis may also be carried out using microarray analysis (Shaw-Smith et al. 2004). For microarray analysis, cloned DNA segments are bound to a solid matrix, such as a microscope slide or computer chip. Differentially, samples of test DNA and control DNA are sheared or cleaved to generate small segments of DNA. Control and test DNA specimens are differentially labeled, each with a different-colored fluorescent dye. They are mixed at equal concentrations and then hybridized to this slide or chip. The slide is then scanned at wavelengths corresponding to those emitted by each individual dye. The fluorescent signal obtained indicates whether or not labeled segments within the control and test DNA samples hybridize equally to the corresponding fragment of cloned DNA immobilized on the slide. If signal from the test DNA is less intense than signal from the control DNA at a particular location on the slide, this will indicate that there is likely a deletion in the test DNA in a region of the genome that corresponds to that cloned segment. Similarly, if signal from the test sample is more intense than that from the control sample, one may conclude that there is duplication of a DNA segment in the test sample (Schoumans et al. 2004).

Availability of DNA sequence information enables the design of polymerase chain reaction (PCR) primers to investigate loci and specific regions of the genome. Fine mapping of genome dosage changes may be carried out through application of quantitative PCR techniques.

Resources of DNA sequence information will enable analysis of sequences located near the site of structural chromosomal anomalies and provide insight into factors that predispose to breaks and rearrangements.

Resources of Genomic DNA Sequences and Expressed Gene Sequences

Advances in information technology have led to development of improved resources to analyze DNA sequence information and to identify new or previously unknown genes. Through the genome project, thousands of new genes of unknown function have been identified. Continued research to identify domains that may be homologous to protein domains of known function may shed light on the function of new genes. The Encyclopedia of DNA Elements (ENCODE) Project seeks to evaluate new computational methods of sequence analysis to identify functional elements.

Through availability of both genomic (chromosomal) sequence and expressed sequence information (mRNA or complementary DNA [cDNA]), it is possible to define gene structure, exon/intron structure, 5' regulatory sequences, promoter regions, transcription start sites, and 3' regulatory elements (Sogayar et al. 2004). Availability of this information facilitates design of assays of specific gene regions, e.g., by PCR amplification and sequencing, to search for gene mutations in affected individuals.

The availability of segments of cDNA corresponding to expressed sequence, arrayed and attached to a solid matrix, e.g., microscope slide, enables analysis of samples of cells and tissues to determine expression of multiple genes. In this way, networks of gene expression can be characterized. Furthermore, environmental and other effects on gene expression can be analyzed. Messenger RNA isolated from cells exposed to different environmental toxins or qualitatively or quantitatively different metabolites may be analyzed on arrays to search for alterations in gene expression. Array analysis will facilitate the search for changes in gene expression that distinguish pathological states from normal states.

Of continued importance in the identification of gene function is the profiling of genes that are expressed in different structures at different stages of development. Ultimately, it will be possible to consider screening individuals who have specific structural abnormalities for defects in genes that are expressed in that structure. The development of organ-specific libraries enables the identification of genes that encode products specific to the function of that organ. A number of genes that, when mutated, lead to, e.g., deafness have been identified using resources such as cDNA libraries developed from mRNA isolated from organs of the inner ear, i.e., cochlea and organ of Corti.

Methods for Comprehensive Gene Expression Analysis

High-throughput analysis of gene expression is facilitated through microarray analysis. In these analyses, oligonucleotide probes corresponding to thousands of genes are bound to solid matrices and may then be hybridized to mRNA isolated from cells of specific tissue at a defined stage of development. In this way, a comprehensive analysis of spatial and temporal gene expression may be obtained. Microarrays of DNA corresponding to genes and their 5' regulatory regions are used to analyze the interactions between genetic transcription factors and other DNA binding regulatory elements.

Expanded Resources for Gene Linkage and Association Analyses

Information on common sequence variants (polymorphisms) in mapped segments of DNA scattered throughout the genome provides a resource for linkage and association studies. If all affected members in a family with a specific disorder inherit the same alleles at a set of contiguous loci within a specific segment of DNA, i.e., have an identical haplotype in a specific region of the genome, database information on genes that lie within that segment can be analyzed to identify candidate genes for the disorder. These genes may then be examined to search for DNA sequence interruptions or mutations that may play a role in the pathogenesis of the disease. Figure 8–1 illustrates the use of polymorphic markers to identify a region of chromosome 9 that segregates with tuberous sclerosis.

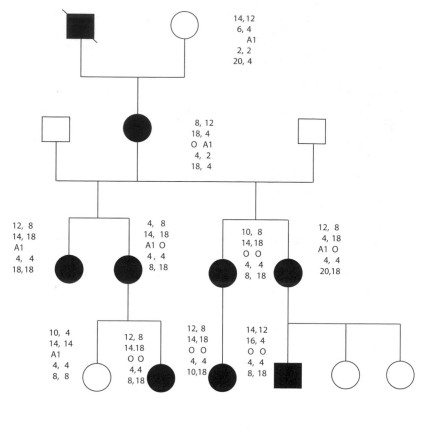

Figure 8–1. Use of polymorphic markers including DNA markers and ABO blood groups to identify a region of chromosome 9 that segregates with the dominantly inherited disorder tuberous sclerosis. Seven out of eight affected individuals inherited the same five-marker haplotype on chromosome 9q34. A recombination event in the male family member in the fourth generation resulted in inheritance of the same alleles as other affected family members at the three distal loci in the haplotype. The recombination event in this individual places the *TSC1* gene distal to the marker D9S125.

Improved Resources to Move from Gene Mapping to Analysis of Function

Mapping of a locus for mental retardation or developmental defect to a specific segment of the genome through genomic dosage studies or through linkage will be followed by an analysis of protein-coding candidate genes within that region. It will, however, also be important to analyze non-protein-coding DNA elements.

Processes involved in the production of a gene product include transcription of the gene, generation of mRNA, translation of the protein, protein folding, and compartmentalization or secretion. To date, most studies designed to investigate candidate genes in a specific gene region linked to or associated with chromosomal defects in mental retardation have focused on the exons of a gene. Core promoters at the 5' end of a gene determine the start of transcription. However, a gene may have several promoters. Specific DNA elements within the promoter region bind to factors that influence transcription. Promoters are influenced by regulatory elements, e.g., enhancers that may be located at some distance from the promoter.

Insights through Genomic Analysis: Long-Range Regulation of Gene Expression and Position Effect

There are now a number of examples of long-range regulation of gene expression. Kleinjan and Van Heyningen (2005) determined that deletions of DNA sequences located 125 kb beyond the final exon of the PAX6 gene led to defective expression of that gene and resulted in aniridia (absence of the iris) in heterozygotes. Homozygous deletion of the distant regulatory element of PAX6 led to neurodevelopmental abnormalities including polymicrogyria, subcortical heterotopias, and abnormalities of the cerebellar vermis, pineal gland, and corpus callosum. Another example of long-range effects on gene regulation is the Townes-Brocks syndrome, a condition characterized by skeletal, renal, and ear anomalies; deafness; and sometimes mental retardation. In some patients, this syndrome is due to mutations in the gene that encodes the transcription factor SALL1. In other families, it is due to a mutation in noncoding DNA that occurs approximately 180 kb telomeric of SALL1 (Marlin et al. 1999).

Chromosomal deletions or rearrangements may cause a gene to be removed from its upstream regulatory elements. Alternately, they may cause a gene to come under the control of a different set of regulatory elements or perhaps to be transcribed in an antisense direction. Tufarelli et al. (2003) described an individual who had thalassemia due to a chromosome 16 deletion that flanked the α-globin gene but did not interrupt it. They found that in this patient there was an RNA transcript that was antisense to the hemoglobin A2 (HBA2) gene. They determined that the deletion resulted in the juxtaposition of the 3' end of *HBA2* and the gene *LUC7L*, which is transcribed in the opposite direction from *HBA2*. In the deletion patient, *LUC7L* transcription continued into the *HBA2* gene in a direction that was anti-sense to the normal *HBA2* transcript. The deletion had removed the 3' transcription termination site in the *LUC7L* gene. Further investigation revealed that the 5' CpG island in the promoter region of *HBA2* was methylated, suggesting that the antisense transcript led to methylation in the 5' region of *HBA2*. Tufarelli et al. (2003) noted that their findings identified new mechanisms underlying human disease.

Chromosomal aberrations, translocations, e.g., may have phenotypic effects even though they do not interrupt a gene. It is likely that the phenotypic effects in such cases result from interruption of noncoding *cis*-regulatory elements.

As we search to identify the genes and DNA segments that lead to phenotypic changes, we will need to not only look within regions that are directly involved in chromosomal aberrations but also take upstream and downstream elements into consideration.

Evidence That Non-Protein-Coding DNA Elements Are Important

Evolutionarily Conserved DNA Elements

Availability of DNA sequence information of genomes of different organisms facilitates searches for conserved sequence elements through bioinformatics. Conserved sequence permits the identification of protein-coding genes and of non-protein-coding sequence elements. Dermitzakis et al. (2003) proposed that 0.3%–1% of the human genome corresponds to conserved non-protein-coding sequence elements. These elements are 100–200 nucleotides in length and are conserved in many different species. It is likely that elements that exhibit a high degree of sequence conservation through evolution have an important function. Such elements have, e.g., been found near genes that play an important role in embryonic development. Deletions, duplications, or mutations of such elements may have functional consequences.

Non-Protein-Coding RNA Transcripts in the Genome

Mattick (2003) noted that 97%–98% of the transcriptional output of the genome is noncoding since it is composed of intronic sequences. He reviewed the functions of noncoding RNA transcripts and reported that these transcripts control chromosomal architecture, mRNA turnover, and developmental timing of protein expression. Transcribed noncoding RNAs, e.g., microRNAs, are also derived from intergenic sequences. Antisense RNA transcripts are also non-protein-coding. A number of noncoding RNAs are specific to the nervous system. *DISC2* (disrupted in schizophrenia) is a locus that cosegregates with schizophrenia (Millar et al. 2000). A non-protein-coding RNA is derived from this locus. Scherer et al. (2003) determined that a 7q31.31 chromosomal translocation associated with autism led to disruption of a large non-coding RNA transcript.

Introns at a number of different loci produce small nucleolar RNAs (SNO RNAs) that are incorporated into nucleolar protein complexes. These RNAs play a role in RNA processing and in control of imprinting. Variation in mRNA processing may influence gene expression (Proudfoot et al. 2002).

MicroRNAs are a specific class of small RNAs that regulate mRNA translation. Noncoding RNAs are present in heterochromatin assemblies and are likely involved in alter chromatin structure (Krichevsky et al. 2003).

Mattick (2003) wrote:

> The prevailing orthodoxy has been that proteins not only constitute the primary structural and functional components of living cells but also constitute most of the regulatory control system in both simple and complex organisms. . . . This assumption must now be reassessed. (pp. 936–937)

Natural Antisense Transcripts

By February 2004 information was available on 2500 natural antisense transcripts (NATs). This suggests that NATs constitute a relatively common mechanism for control of gene transcription (Lavorgna et al. 2004). Antisense RNA may be identified through sequence searches in mRNA databases or from direct experimental evidence that reverse transcripts of specific genes exist.

Antisense RNA to a specific gene may be transcribed in *cis*, i.e., on the same chromosome as the coding sequence but starting from the 3' end of the gene rather than at the 5' end, the usual transcription start site. *Trans* antisense transcripts are derived from reverse transcription of the corresponding locus on the homologous chromosome (Kleinjan and von Heyningen 2003).

Lavorgna et al. (2004) reviewed mechanisms by which antisense transcripts modulate expression of coding sequence. There is evidence that when transcription of two strands occurs, starting at opposite ends of a gene, RNA polymerases collide and stall. Presence of an antisense transcript leads to interference of intron–exon splicing on the coding sequence. Sense and antisense transcripts may form duplexes. In mammalian cells, there are mechanisms that degrade double-stranded RNA molecules greater than 200 nucleotides in length. This degradation thus removes antisense and sense RNA. Sense mRNA is therefore not available for translation. There is also evidence that when antisense transcripts overlap sense transcripts, methylation of the 5' CpG region occurs and this shuts off further transcription of the sense strand.

Disease Relevance

Antisense transcripts play an important role in the imprinted region, e.g., in the Prader-Willi/Angelman syndrome region on chromosome 15q12-q13 and in the Beckwith-Wiedemann region on chromosome 11p15.5. Antisense transcripts also play an important role in gene expression in the insulin growth factor II/mannose-6-phosphate receptor region on chromosome 6q24.

Transcriptional Regulation

A large percentage of the genome of many organisms is dedicated to encoding products that determine spatial and temporal transcription of genes (Freiman and Tjian 2003). Transcription factors bind to DNA, and changes in transcription factors may lead to activation or repression of a large number of genes. Transcription factors are associated with the chromatin remodeling complexes.

Transcription factors are subject to secondary modification. They may be activated or de-activated by ubiquitination or deubiquitination. Ubiquitin is a 76–amino acid protein that becomes linked to lysine in target proteins. This linkage requires an enzymatic cascade that will be described below. There is evidence that monoubiquitination may enhance transcription factor activity, whereas polyubiquitination of a transcription factor may lead to its destruction.

Transcription factors are also modified through the activity of histone acetyltransferases and histone deacetylases. Removal of acetyl groups from the p53 protein stimulates its activity. Histone methyltransferases (HMTs) may also target nonhistone regulatory proteins. Arginine is targeted for methylation by HMT.

Freiman and Tjian (2003) concluded that the relatively limited differences in gene numbers between worms (*Caenorhabditis elegans*, 19,000 genes) and humans (30,000 genes) could not explain the vast differences in complexity of cell type, signal transduction, and behavior. They proposed that the complexity of regulation likely explains these differences. They noted that organisms have developed multiple mechanisms to modify their transcription factors. This permits the use of the same regulatory factor in different ways and allows for a more diverse expression profile.

Are Morphological and Behavioral Differences Largely Due to Quantitative Differences in Gene Expression?

King and Wilson (1975) demonstrated that DNA sequence in the coding regions of many genes in human and chimpanzees, the closest human primate relative, showed very few differences. They proposed that morphological and behavioral differences between humans are largely dependent on differences in gene expression rather than on differences in gene sequence.

Enard et al. (2002a) studied the transcriptome, i.e., protein-encoding transcripts, in several species including human, chimpanzee, macaque, and orangutan. They used membrane-bound cDNA clones to analyze mRNA from a number of different tissues including blood leukocytes, liver, and brain. They noted that the level of RNA expression in leukocytes and liver was similar in humans and chimpanzees. In human liver, the level of RNA expression was 1.3 times that in chimpanzees. However, the level of RNA expression in brain cortex is 5.5-fold higher in humans than in chimpanzees. Macaques and chimpanzees have similar levels of brain mRNA expression. These results demonstrate that there are evolutionary changes in levels of mRNA expression that are particularly striking in the brain.

Enard et al. (2002a) then undertook studies in protein expression. They used two-dimensional electrophoresis to study qualitative and quantitative changes in protein expression. Their studies revealed a large number of quantitative changes in expression of specific proteins between humans and chimpanzees. Qualitative changes in gene expression between humans and chimpanzees may be related to gene duplication, promoter changes, changes in transcription factors, and/or changes in cellular composition of specific tissues (Enard et al. 2002a; Pennisi 2002).

Human Genetic Variants (Polymorphisms) That Affect Levels of Gene Transcription

Yan et al. (2002) compared the relative expression of two alleles at the same gene locus through sequence analysis of mRNA from a specific cell type in heterozygous individuals. They examined single nucleotide polymorphisms (SNPs) in 13 genes in 96 individuals. In individuals who were heterozygous for polymorphisms, they examined mRNA from family members for SNP. In heterozygous individuals and their family members, they analyzed adjacent polymorphic microsatellite DNA markers. They demonstrated that altered levels of expression of the SNP alleles were consistently inherited together with a haplotype that contained at least two adjacent markers.

These findings indicate that inherited *cis*-acting factors play a role in determining inherited variation in gene expression. These results have relevance not only for physiological variations but also for pathological states. Yan et al. (2002) concluded that in some cases disease susceptibility might be based on changes in levels of gene expression and not on changes in encoded proteins.

Chromatin Insulators: Another Example of DNA–Protein Interactions That Influence Gene Expression

Chromatin insulators are stretches of DNA sequence that act as a barrier so that a particular gene is not influenced by enhancer elements in adjacent genes. Insulators may also serve to separate blocks of chromatin that are differently condensed. A specific regulatory protein, CTCF, binds to DNA in insulator elements and blocks enhancer activity. Its targets include loci involved in cell metabolism, neurogenesis, growth, and signaling.

Ohlsson and coworkers (2001) reported the occurrence of a network of CTCF binding sites within the genome. The CTCF binding sites are located in heterochromatin, intergenic regions, introns, intron–exon boundaries, and exons. The CTCF binding sites located in 11p15.5 protect against spreading of methylation from H19.

Alternative Splicing of RNA and Posttranscriptional Regulation

A particular gene may give rise to many different RNA transcripts. Different transcripts may arise through the use of different transcription start sites. Frequently, different combinations of exons of one gene are spliced together to give different mRNA isoforms. These may encode structurally and functionally distinct proteins. There is evidence that alternate splicing plays a major role in determining functional complexity. In specific tissues, different splice forms of the mRNA derived from a particular gene occur.

A further source of variation is the fact that mRNA transcripts derived from a specific gene may terminate at different sites in the 3' end of the gene. As a result, the different transcripts may have different polyadenylation sites. Polyadenylation differences result in differences in mRNA stability (Proudfoot et al. 2002; Dreyfus and Regnier 2002).

It is clear that temporal and spatial differences in the expression of a protein that is encoded by a specific gene are dependent not only on the DNA sequence of the gene but also on transcriptional differences and posttranscriptional modification of mRNA. These processes further enhance protein diversity.

The Epigenome, Epigenetics, and Epigenetic Diseases

Mendel's gene is not just DNA.
    —A. Petronis (2004)

Epigenetic diseases may be defined as disorders of gene expression where the specific genes that manifest altered expression do not manifest sequence changes. Epigenetic factors lead to differences in the readout of genetic information.

Genomes of a number of different species have now been sequenced. The estimated number of genes for the worm *C. elegans* is 19,000 and that for humans is 30,000. Several investigators have drawn attention to the fact that the great differences between species such as worms and humans cannot easily be explained by differences in gene number. It is likely that complexities in gene regulation are important contributing factors (Pastinen et al. 2004).

The DNA is enclosed in chromatin (see also Chapter 4). The basic unit of chromatin is the nucleosome. Strands of DNA are wound around the outside of bead-like structures, nucleosomes, which are composed of histone proteins. A helix comprised of approximately 165 bp of DNA is wound around a bead composed of eight subunits of histone, H3–H4 tetramers and H2A–H2B dimers. Histone H1 binds to the nucleosome and to linker strands of DNA that lie between the nucleosomes (Felsenfeld and Groudine 2003).

Weintraub and Groudine (1976) demonstrated that nucleosomes associated with active genes have a more open, less condensed structure than those associated with inactive genes. A striking example of highly condensed chromatin is the Barr body that is visible in interphase nuclei. The highly condensed DNA of one X chromosome is present in the Barr body, and it is not transcribed.

Chromatin remodeling plays a key role in determining accessibility of DNA to transcription factors. In the process of chromatin remodeling, histone complexes (octamers) move a short distance along the DNA strand so that different DNA sequences lie in the open regions between beads. Histone modification plays a key role in chromatin remodeling. Altered chromatin structure leads to differences in accessibility of transcription factors to DNA. This in turn influences gene expression, which is controlled by the binding of transcription factors to DNA, particularly to promoter regions of genes and to control elements.

Histone proteins are composed of a globular region and a tail. It is the tail region in particular that undergoes modification by acetylation, methylation, phosphorylation, and ubiquitination. Specific enzymes induce modifications at specific amino acids within histones.

Jenuwein and Allis (2001) proposed that histone modifications have three major consequences:

1. Specific modifications of the histone tails would influence their interaction with other chromatin-associated proteins.
2. Histone modifications may be interdependent; one type of modification may lead to another.
3. The properties of chromatin and the generation of higher-order structure, including the generation of euchromatin (lightly stained regions) and heterochromatin (darkly stained regions), are dependent on modification of histones and nucleosomes.

Jenuwein and Allis (2001) noted that the modification of histones extends the information content of the genome past the genetic code. The state of chromatin is dependent upon the concentration and combination of differentially modified histones, which leads to different epigenetic states in which there is a different readout of genetic information. They referred to this as the "nucleosome code."

They noted that chromatin is sensitive to the metabolic state of the cell and to concentration of substances such as coenzymes. The concentration of the coenzyme nicotinamide adenine dinucleotide (NAD) influences histone deacetylases activity.

They proposed that chromatin-based epigenetics impacts X inactivation, stem cell plasticity, imprinting, and developmental programming of differentiation as well as DNA replication and cell cycle progression. The chromatin-related epigenetic marking system serves as a regulatory mechanism that impacts cell fate decisions and development. They further proposed that significant phenotypic differences between organisms is in part due to epigenetic factors imposed at the level of DNA packaging and histones. An extension of this concept is that perturbations of this process may lead to specific pathologies.

Jiang et al. (2004) defined *epigenetic regulation* as a form of regulation that involves changes in chromatin structure and modification of DNA. They noted that the clearest impact of epigenetics on disease manifestation is to be found in disorders that are due to uniparental disomy. In this condition, both members of a chromosome pair are derived from the same parent. In a subgroup of patients, Prader-Willi syndrome is due to maternal uniparental disomy of chromosome 15. In these patients, the Prader-Willi gene region shows no evidence of DNA sequence alterations, yet genes in this region are not expressed because the maternal genes in the critical region are imprinted.

DNA Methylation and Histone Modification

Methylation and histone modification of DNA are closely associated processes. Following methylation of DNA at carbon 5 of cytosine in specific CpG dinucleotide sites, proteins bind to DNA at those sites. Approximately 50% of genes have CpG islands in their promoter regions or first exons. These are stretches of DNA sequence rich in cytosine and guanine residues that are frequently located upstream of transcription start sites. Methylation of these islands inhibits gene expression (Tucker 2001). Bound proteins recruit histone deacetylases. Enzymes responsible for histone deacetylation occur in the vicinity of repressed genes. Following deacetylation, DNA is silenced. Conversely, actively expressed genes are surrounded by acetylated histones.

The DNA methyltransferases DNMT1, DNMT2,DNMT3a, and DNMT3b catalyze methylation; DNMT3L acts by binding to other DNMT proteins and altering their DNA methylation activity (Okano et al. 1998). Several proteins have affinity for methylated DNA through their methyl binding domains; these include MBD1, MBD2, MBD3, and MECP2 (Nakao et al. 2001).

Following binding to methylated DNA, through its methyl binding domain, MECP2 recruits a complex that includes SIN3A and histone deacetylases (see Fig. 8–2). MBD2 and MBD3 also recruit histone deacetylases following their binding to methylated DNA. In addition, the MBD proteins recruit adenosine triphosphate (ATP)–dependent helicase, which alters chromatin structure and impacts the activity of RNA polymerase that is involved

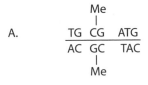

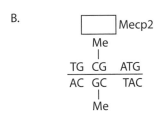

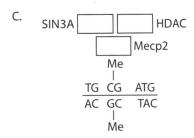

Figure 8–2. The Mecp2 protein binds to methylated DNA at CpG sites. It then recruits transcriptional repressors, including SIN3A and histone deacetylase (HDAC).

in DNA transcription. Acetylation of histones H3 and H4 leads to an open chromatin configuration. Deacetylation of histones via histone deacetylases leads to a closed structure that is not accessible to transcription factors.

The SIN3 proteins SIN3A and SIN3B are transcriptional corepressors that interact not only with MECP2 but also with other corepressors, including ALIEN.

The effect of histone methylation on gene transcription varies, depending on which lysine is methylated. Methylation of lysine 4 of histone H3 leads to active transcription. Methylation of lysine 9 is associated with nonexpressing genes. Khalil et al. (2004) reported that trimethylation of lysine 4 of histone H3 is a marker of the X chromosome that escapes inactivation. They noted that RNA polymerase II is present at the sites of trimethylated histone H3, indicating that these sites represent transcriptionally active chromatin. They observed that trimethylation of histone H4 also occurs in discrete regions of other metaphase chromosomes. It is not yet clear whether DNA methylation impacts histone methylation or vice versa.

The importance of methylation in determining chromosomal architecture and function is illustrated by the finding that deficiency of the DNA methyltransferase DNMT3B results in a syndrome characterized by immunodeficiency centromeric instability, and facial anomalies (ICF syndrome). Geiman et al. (2004) reported that DNMT3B normally localizes with the protein condensin on mitotic chromosomes and that there is a direct link between DNA methylation and mitotic chromosome condensation in mammalian cells.

Ubiquitin Modification of Chromatin-Associated Proteins

Ubiquitin is a 76–amino acid protein that becomes linked to lysine groups in target proteins. This linkage requires an enzymatic cascade that includes ubiquitin-activating enzymes (E1), ubiquitin-conjugating enzymes (E2), and ubiquitin ligase enzyme (E3). This is described in more detail below (see Proteomics).

Briggs et al. (2002) reported that ubiquination of histone H2B is necessary for the methylation of lysine 79 in histone H3. Lysine 79 is the only amino acid outside the histone tail that undergoes methylation. The ubiquitin-conjugating enzyme UBC2 mediates ubiquitination of histone H2B. Briggs et al. (2002) proposed that ubiquitination plays a role as a switch responsible for gene silencing. Dover et al. (2002) and Sun and Allis (2002) reported that ubiquitination of histone H2B on lysine 123 is the signal for methylation of histone H3. This leads to silencing of genes near telomeres.

Role of RNA in DNA Methylation and Chromatin Modification

Jeffery and Nakielny (2004) reported that DNMTs and MBD proteins form complexes with RNA. The formation of these RNA complexes inhibits binding on DNMTs and MBDs to DNA.

It is interesting to note that Mbd1 deficiency in the mouse leads to defective neurogenesis and aberrant hippocampal function (Zhao et al. 2003).

Stochastic Events and Epigenetic Variation

Temporal and spatial changes in DNA methylation and chromatin state within an individual result in modification of gene expression. These changes may arise in response to metabolic or environmental factors. The processes that modify DNA and/or chromatin structure occur in a random or stochastic manner.

Stochastic epigenetic variations are thought to be responsible for phenotypic differences between the two members of a monozygotic twin pair. Examples of such differences are the discordant expression of the antisense RNA KCNQ10T1 in monozygotic twins with Beckwith-Wiedemann syndrome as described by Weksberg et al. in 2002 (see below). Imprinting is one form of epigenetic variation. Parent-of-origin effects on disease occurrence indicate a role for imprinting. In Angelman syndrome, e.g., mutation in the *UBE3A* gene has a pathological effect only if it is maternally inherited and not when it is paternally inherited. This indicates that *UBE3A* undergoes imprinting and parent-specific expression.

Epigenetic Modification and Complex Traits

Bjornsson et al. (2004) proposed that epigenetic variation may explain the variation in quantitative traits and that this variation may be influenced by environmental factors. They noted also the late onset and progressive nature of complex traits may result from the combined impact of epigenetic and environmental factors.

In considering environmental factors that impact epigenetic status, it is important to consider metabolism of methionine, homocysteine, and folate (see also Chapter 3).

5,10-Methylene tetrahydrofolate is reduced by methylene tetrahydrofolate reductase (MTHFR) to 5-methyl tetrahydrofolate. This is then converted to methionine through the action of methionine synthase. The production of methyl groups for methylation of DNA is directly related to production of 5-methyl tetrahydrofolate and the subsequent production of methionine. Decreased MTHFR activity is also correlated with decreased conversion of homocysteine and decreased production of *S*-adenosylmethionine (Relton et al. 2004a,b).

In individuals who are homozygous for a mutation at position 677 in the MTHFR gene, 677 T/T, the degree of DNA methylation is directly correlated with folate status. Individuals with the *TT* genotype and low folate levels have DNA hypomethylation (Christensen et al. 1999).

Tools for investigation of the epigenome will include methods to analyze genomic methylation, including methylation of DNA and histones and analysis of specific gene expression.

Epigenetics, Imprinting, and Twins

One of the most powerful arguments for the importance of imprinting has to do with the fact that monozygotic twins who are genotypically identical vary with respect to specific traits. This has, e.g., been demonstrated in Beckwith-Wiedemann syndrome (BWS). This syndrome is characterized by somatic overgrowth, visceromegaly, enlarged tongue, abdominal wall defects, and a tendency to develop embryonal tumors including Wilms' tumor (nephroblastoma) and rhadosarcoma. Asymmetry and *hemihypertrophy* (a condition in which structures on one side of the body are larger than structures on the other side) occur in some patients with BWS. Reports indicate that developmental delay occurs in 4%–15% of patients with this syndrome. The syndrome occurs with a frequency of 1 in 10,000 live births. A number of investigators have described monozygotic twins who are discordant for BWS. These twins are predominantly female.

Beckwith-Wiedemann syndrome is due to genetic and epigenetic factors that impact expression of genes located in the 11p15.5 region on one member of the chromosome 11 pair. Diaz-Meyer et al. (2003) and Bestor (2003) reviewed genetic and epigenetic etiologies of BWS. Genetic factors include uniparental disomy, translocations, and deletions. Twenty percent of cases are due to paternal uniparental disomy: both members of the chromosome 11p15.5 region are derived from the father. Imprinting defects account for approximately 50% of cases. There are two adjacent autonomously imprinted subdomains on 11p15.5. One domain contains the *H19* (imprinted RNA), *IGF2* (insulin-like growth factor 2), and *INS* (insulin) genes. The second domain contains nine genes, including *KCNQ1* (potassium voltage-gated channel Q1 subtype), its antisense transcript *KCNQ1OT* (KCNQT overlapping transcript), and *CDKNIC* (cyclin-dependent kinase 1C). Each imprinted domain has its own imprint control region. One imprint control region is located 2.4 kb upstream of the *H19* gene. The second imprint control region lies within the promoter of the *KCNQ1OT1* gene. Loss of imprinting in either of the two domains can result in BWS. The phenotype of individuals with *KCNQ1OT1* defects is most often identical to that in individuals with imprint control defects in the *H19*, *IGF2*, and *INS* region. Wilms' tumor may be more common in individuals with imprint defects in the latter region. The *H19* gene is expressed only from the maternal allele, and *IgF2* is expressed only from the paternal allele.

The promoter region of the *KCNQ1OT1* transcript lies in an intron of the *KCNQ1* gene. It normally undergoes methylation on the maternally derived allele, and that allele is then silenced. It is expressed from the paternal allele, where it is unmethylated. Transcription of the antisense transcript leads to silencing on the paternally derived allele of *KCNQ1*, *CDKNIC*, and other genes in this imprinted region. The *IGF2* gene that lies in the second imprinted domain is also expressed from the paternal allele (Diaz-Meyer et al. 2003) (see Fig. 8–3).

Bestor (2003) proposed that the occurrence of BWS in twins and the twinning process might be related to methylation during early embryogenesis. Bestor noted that imprints are erased during early meiosis. Maternal imprints are subsequently established in oocytes that are arrested in the prophase of meiosis1 until fertilization. Paternal imprints are established in prospermatozoa, which then undergo multiple cell divisions. Establishment of imprints is dependent in part on DNMT1 (mouse Dnmt1), which acts as a de novo methyltransferase and transfers methyl groups to hemimethylated DNA during the S phase of the cell cycle. Different transcripts of DNMT1 occur, and these transcripts use different 5' promoters and different first exons. Sex-specific differences occur in transcript formation (Howell et al. 2001).

In sperm, DNMT1 transcripts include multiple short upstream exons. These transcripts are apparently inefficiently translated. In oocytes, DNMT1 transcripts are derived from downstream promoters; these transcripts, referred to as DNMT1o transcripts, are translated to shorter proteins that are more

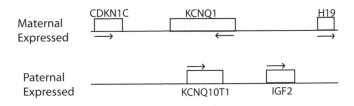

Figure 8–3. Two adjacent imprinted domains are present in the Beckwith-Wiedemann region on chromosome 11p15. The *H19* and *IGF2* genes are present in one domain, and the *KCNQ1* and *CDKN1C* genes are present in the second domain. *KCNQ1OT1* is an antisense transcript of *KCNQ1*; it is not expressed from the chromosome of maternal derivation.

stable. Following implantation, the zygote and early embryo produce full-length stable DNMT1 transcripts. Bestor (2003) noted that failure of DNMT1o to maintain methylation during S phase may lead to one chromatid that is methylated and one that is unmethylated. On cell division, the methylated chromatid may segregate to one blastomere (undifferentiated cell produced by early cleavage of the fertilized egg) and the unmethylated chromatid may segregate to another blastomere. This may lead to twinning or to hemihypertrophy.

Howell et al. (2001) demonstrated that removal of the Dnmt1o-specific allele in mice led to demethylation of half of normally imprinted alleles and reactivation of normally silenced alleles.

Bestor (2003) proposed that methylation of *KCNQ1OT1* is normally less efficient than that at other methylated regions and that BWS results when maintenance methylation of *KCNQ1OT1* is impaired. Since DNMT1 is also required for X-chromosome inactivation in females, it is likely that in women less DNMT1 is available for maintenance methylation. Females would then be more sensitive to relative deficiencies of DNMT1. Therefore, BWS is more likely to occur in female twins. Bestor noted that it is possible that other gene products derived from sperm impact maintenance methylation.

Twins and Autism: Do Epigenetic Factors Play a Role?

Greenberg et al. (2001) reported a striking increase in the incidence of twins among autistic sib pairs. Their data analysis revealed that the incidence of monozygotic twins was particularly increased in autistic sib pairs over that of the general population. Hallmayer et al. (2002) proposed that the observation published by Greenberg et al. (2001) was possibly due to ascertainment bias. Betancur et al. (2002) recruited families with two children with autism from eight different countries. Among 79 sib pairs, there were two sets of dizygotic twins and nine sets of monozygotic twins. This is a striking increase in the incidence of monozygotic twins over the expected rate for the population.

It is interesting to consider the possibility that monozygotic twinning and occurrence of autism may be related to the same biological factor. One possible factor is methylation and mechanisms such as Bestor (2003) described for the origin of twinning in BWS.

Proteomics: Insights into Variation in Functional Activity Due to Posttranslational Modification

Different forms of posttranslational modification may give rise to proteins and enzymes with different functional activity. The net effect of proteins and enzymes is dependent not only on rate of synthesis but also on rate of degradation.

The major extralysosomal mechanism for intracellular proteolysis in eukaryotic cells is the ubiquitin–proteosome system (Glickman and Ciechanover 2002; Pickart and Eddins 2004). This system is responsible for the degradation of abnormal or misfolded proteins but also for the degradation of regulatory proteins such as transcription factors, cell cycle-specific factors, and proteins whose levels are rapidly modulated during differentiation or development or in response to various physiological or metabolic effectors (Doskeland et al. 2001). In 2004, the Nobel Prize for chemistry was awarded to A. Hershko, A. Ciechanover, and I. Rose, who discovered and characterized the ubiquitin pathway of protein degradation.

Degradation is initiated by the "marking" of the protein substitute with a poly- (or multi-) ubiquitin chain. Ubiquitin is a 76–amino acid peptide, the primary sequence of which is highly conserved from yeast to mammals. Following polyubiquitination, the protein is degraded to the level of free amino acids and small peptides in the proteosome, while the multiubiquitin chain is recycled (as free ubiquitin monomers) by the action of ubiquitinases.

The formation of polyubiquitin chains on substrate proteins requires three enzymatic steps (see Fig. 8–4). The ubiquitin-activating enzyme, E1, catalyzes the formation of a high-energy ubiquitin–E1 thioester through the α-carboxyl group of the C-terminal glycine of ubiquitin. This step requires ATP and proceeds via an enzyme-bound ubiquitin adenylate intermediate.

Transfer of ubiquitin to one of a number of ubiquitin-carrier or -conjugating proteins (E2s, UBCs) occurs by transesterification to give a ubiquitin–E2 thioester. Multiple E2s have been identified in humans. They share a conserved region of substantial identity of approximately 130 amino acids, containing the active-site cysteine residue required for thioester formation. Some E2s contain extensions at their N-terminal, C-terminal, or both ends.

While some E2s are capable of transferring ubiquitin to an appropriate protein acceptor in vitro to form monoubiquitinated products, it remains largely unknown whether similar reactions occur in vivo. In most cases, specific E2s associate with specific E3s (ubiquitin–protein ligases) to transfer ubiquitin to substrates. The E3 or E2–E3 complex transfers a monoubiquitin

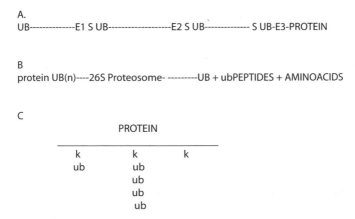

A.
UB-------------E1 S UB------------------E2 S UB------------- S UB-E3-PROTEIN

B
protein UB(n)----26S Proteosome- ---------UB + ubPEPTIDES + AMINOACIDS

C

PROTEIN

k	k	k
ub	ub	
	ub	
	ub	
	ub	

Figure 8–4. *A*: Three enzymatic steps, involving the enzymes E1, E2, and E3 and the thioester groups in ubiquitin are required for the linkage of ubiquitin to the lysine residues of protein. *B*: Ubiquitinated proteins are degraded in the proteosome to peptides and amino acids. *C*: Specific lysine residues may be monoubiquitinated, while others are polyubiquitinated.

moiety to a specific lysine residue of the acceptor protein, forming an isopeptide bond. The multiubiquitin chain arises by attachment of a second ubiquitin residue, in isopeptide linkage, to lysine 48 of the first ubiquitin, followed by additional such reactions to produce a "herringbone" structure.

The basis for the variability in protein stability, i.e., why some proteins are very short-lived while others are extremely stable, and the timing of protein degradation are of critical importance. Some proteins carry constitutive degradation signals within their primary structure that are recognized by specific E3s. In other cases, the signals on the proteins are "unmasked" by covalent modifications, such as phosphorylation or interaction with other proteins. In still other cases, specific protein targets are not recognized until E3s are activated by covalent modification or by association with other cellular proteins or viral proteins.

Degradation of polyubiquitinated proteins occurs in the proteosome, a large multicatalytic proteinase complex found in most eukaryotic species. The proteosome exits predominantly in two forms: a 20S complex with a mass of about 700 kDa and a larger 26S entity with a mass of about 1500 kDa. The 26S entity is formed by association of the 20S proteosome and a 19S regulatory complex.

The 20S proteasome is a cylindrical chamber formed by the stacking of four rings, two identical outer rings and two identical inner rings. Several different proteolytic activities have been identified in the 20S proteosome. These appear to be confined to the inner rings and face the inside of the chamber. The 20S proteasome is capable of degrading at least some nonubiquitinated proteins but degradation of multiubiquitinated proteins requires the 26S proteosome.

Role of Ubiquitin in Chromatin Structure and Remodeling

It is interesting to note that ubiquitin was first identified as a component of chromatin, where it is bound in isopeptide linkage to 10%–20% of histone H2A and H2B molecules. Studies in yeast have established that this monoubiquitination of H2B promotes the methylation of several lysine residues in histone H3, eventually leading to regulation of gene transcription. There is also a growing body of evidence that attachment of ubiquitin and other ubiquitin-like proteins (UBLs, see below) play other roles in modifying chromatin structure and in regulating the activities of transcriptional activators and RNA polymerase.

Genetics of the Ubiquitin–Proteasome System

E1

The *UBE1* gene mapping to chromosome Xp11.23 encodes the major human ubiquitin-protein ligase. Two genes, *UBE1C* and *UBE1L*, located on human chromosome 3 encode structurally related proteins.

E2

More than 20 E2s have been characterized in humans, and examination of the human genome database suggests that there may be twice that number of genes based on the presence of the conserved UBC domain. Studies in yeast and other lower eukaryotes in which individual E2 genes have been deleted suggests a certain amount of functional redundancy among the E2 genes.

E3

A limited number of E3s have been biochemically characterized, but based on homology to structural motifs found in these characterized E3s, analysis of the human genome suggests that many more E3s exist. This is consistent with the large number of proteins degraded by the ubiquitin–proteosome system and the relatively narrow substrate specificities of E3s.

Deubiquitinases

Deubiquitinases (DUBs) include enzymes which cleave monoubiquitin–lysine–isopeptide linkages, polyubiquitin–lysine–isopeptide linkages, and the isopeptide linkages that connect ubiquitin monomers to each other in multiubiquitin chains. Several families of DUBs have been identified, and human genome analysis suggests that more than 50 genes may encode DUBs.

The Ubiquitin Pathway and Genetic Disorders

A small number of genetic disorders have been directly associated with malfunctions in the ubiquitin–proteosome pathway. This number will almost certainly grow as functions for the large numbers of genes suggested to encode additional components of the system are identified. Mutations affecting recognition of degradation signals in protein substrates of the system leading to inappropriate stabilization or destabilization will probably also prove to be significant.

Angelman syndrome is characterized by mental retardation, poor speech, ataxia, and epilepsy. It is caused by loss of function of the maternal allele of UBE3A, a ubiquitin–protein ligase, located on chromosome 15q11-q13 (Kishino et al. 1997) (see also Chapter 4). The paternal allele is subject to silencing by genomic imprinting in neurons but not glia or nonneural tissues. Mutations leading to loss of UBE3A function include point mutations, large deletions, and uniparental paternal disomy. It is unknown which substrates of the UBE3A ubiquitin–protein ligase are impacted in Angelman syndrome.

Autosomal recessive Parkinson disease with juvenile onset is one of the most common familial forms of Parkinson disease (the great majority of Parkinson disease cases are sporadic and of late onset). Parkin, the gene product responsible for the disorder, has been shown to be a component of a ubiquitin–protein ligase (Kitada et al. 1998; Imai and Takahashi 2004). Although a number of proteins that are ubiquitinated by Parkin have been identified, it is not yet clear if the inappropriate accumulation of one or more of these (or as yet unidentified proteins) underlies the pathogenesis of the disease.

Ubiquitin-Like Proteins

A number of small proteins related to ubiquitin by sequence homology and/or structural similarity have been identified (Schwartz and Hochstrasser 2003). The most prominent members of this group are SUMO-1, -2, and -3 and NEDD8 (Rub1). Modification of target proteins by these UBLs requires E1, E2, and E3 activities that are distinct from those of the ubiquitin system itself. In general, only a single UBL molecule is attached to the target substrate. These modifications do not lead to degradation of the modified protein but to a variety of other effects, including protection from ubiquitination, activation, inhibition or recruitment of transcription factors, modulation of signaling pathways, chromatin remodeling, and nucleocytoplasmic transport. These modifications are reversible via the action of specific isopeptides that cleave the UBL–ligase bond. Although there is as yet no clear evidence that malfunctions in any of the UBL ligation systems result in disease, it seems only a matter of time before some are associated with the broad roles played by these systems in cellular physiology.

9

Establishing a Diagnosis and Determining Etiology in Developmental Delay and Mental Retardation

It can be argued that clinical acumen (the state of expert reasoning) is a skill which rests on an ability to combine research based knowledge (objective or propositional knowledge), professional knowledge (craft or non-propositional knowledge) and personal knowledge (experiential and reflective knowledge) with deductive reasoning and clinical thinking skills

—N. K. Poplawski (2003)

Developmental disabilities occur in 5%–10% of the pediatric population (Shevell et al. 2000). Deficits may exist in a single domain or across several domains. Included within the spectrum of developmental disabilities are global developmental delay, isolated speech and language delay, motor delay, cerebral palsy, pervasive developmental disabilities, and profound primary and sensory impairments such as deafness and blindness. Determining specific etiology in childhood developmental delay has implications for management. These include medical follow-up, prognosis prediction, and recurrence risk estimation. An important goal of the diagnostic evaluation is to ensure that appropriate rehabilitative services are arranged.

Implications of an Etiological Diagnosis

Specific etiological diagnoses have therapeutic implications. Success in establishing a diagnosis is in part dependent upon the design and thoroughness of the evaluation. Schaefer and Bodensteiner (1992) defined a specific etiological diagnosis as one that can be translated into useful clinical information for the family, such as information about prognosis, recurrence risk and preferred modes of available therapy.

Recommendations from Physicians
in Different Subspecialties

Physicians in different medical subspecialties and in different health-care systems frequently have somewhat different recommendations for the evaluation of children with developmental disabilities and mental retardation. In this chapter, we will review recommendations for these evaluations published by physicians in different specialties and from different countries: the United States, Italy, Canada, and Australia.

In Table 9–1, we list developmental milestones for children younger than 5 years. In Table 9–2, routinely used formal tests of development and cognition are listed.

Battaglia et al. (1999) reported a diagnostic algorithm that they established for evaluation of patients who were referred because of developmental delay. History and clinical evaluation data were used to design further evaluation. Prenatal, perinatal, and postnatal histories were documented; and family history was obtained to construct a three-generation pedigree. Physical examination included a search for congenital anomalies, including minor anomalies, and a neurological examination. Patients with major and minor anomalies were further evaluated for features of relevant multiple congenital anomaly syndromes, and cytogenetic studies were performed. In cases of developmental delay where no congenital anomalies were found, cytogenetic studies were also undertaken. Patients were evaluated clinically for signs of metabolic diseases, e.g., storage disease. In cases where physical examination revealed microcephaly or macrocephaly, electroencephalography (EEG) and neuroimaging were performed. Where neuromuscular defects were present, electromyography and nerve conduction studies were performed.

In the report published by Battaglia et al. (1999), 59% of cases were diagnosed with multiple congenital anomaly mental retardation syndromes. Cytogenetic studies were helpful in making a diagnosis in 15% of cases. These investigators noted that among the 120 patients they studied, six cases who were thought to have nonsyndromic mental retardation were found to have chromosomal anomalies. These included 7q+, inverted duplication of proximal 15q, deletion of 9p, XXY, and fragile X. They emphasized that cytogenetic studies are useful even in cases where multiple congenital anomalies are absent.

Battaglia et al. (1999) and Battaglia (2003) reported that the diagnostic yield of neuroimaging was low, 7.5% in their study. They emphasized that EEG studies had a diagnostic yield of 8.3% but that the finding of EEG anomalies may be helpful in designing therapy.

Shevell et al. (2000) reported results of a prospective study to determine etiological yield of diagnostic assessment of children less than 5 years of age with global developmental delay, developmental language disorder, autism spectrum disorder, and motor delay. The goal of their study was to determine

Table 9–1
Developmental Milestones

First month
  Motor activity: sucks well, has jerky movements of limbs, hands are held clenched

  Sensory activity: hearing is mature, may turn toward sounds, eyes wander and may sometimes cross, recognizes smell of milk, is soothed by smooth objects and gentle touch

1–3 months
  Motor activity: stretches and kicks legs, takes swipes at dangling objects, opens and closes hands, raises head while lying on stomach

  Sensory activity: turns head in direction of sound, smiles at voice sounds, makes sounds, watches faces, begins to track moving objects with eyes, begins to make more coordinated hand movements

  Social and emotional development: develops social smile, enjoys being played with, may be expressive with face and body

4–7 months
  Motor activity: rolls front to back and back to front; holds head in position when pulled to sit; sits with support at first then, by 7 months, without support; when held, supports weight on legs

  Sensory activity: tracking of moving objects improves, focuses on objects, responds to name

  Social and emotional development: distinguishes emotions and tones of voice, babbles in consonants, enjoys play

8–12 months
  Motor activity: crawls, stands when supported, reaches for objects, bangs objects together, places objects in container, pokes using index finger

  Sensory activity: explores objects by shaking, banging, and dropping; finds hidden objects

  Cognitive and emotional development: recognizes images in pictures when named; responds to verbal requests; uses gestures, shakes head for no; says "mama," "dada"; exclaims "Oh!"; is shy with strangers and anxious when parents or familiar caretaker leaves; imitates play; reaches for, handles, and eats finger foods; helps with dressing by extending arms

12 months to 2 years
  Motor activity: walks, pulls toys while walking, begins to run and climb; reaches by standing on tiptoe

  Sensory and cognitive development: sorts objects by shape or color; begins make-believe play; scribbles; pours objects from container; builds tower of four or more blocks; points to objects when named; by 15–18 months, says 15–18 words, repeats words; by 2 years, speaks in two- to four-word sentences

2–3 years
  Motor activity: climbs and runs well, walks up and down stairs, maintains balance while bending over, pedals tricycle

Table 9-1

Cognitive and emotional development: Follows commands with two or three components; recognizes common objects in pictures; says name and age; turns pages of book one at a time; holds pencil in writing position; uses crayon to make vertical, horizontal, and circular strokes; turns handles; screws lids; completes simple puzzles of three or four pieces; plays make-believe; expresses affection; separates more easily from parents or familiar caretaker; shows affection for playmates; understands "mine," "his/hers"; learns to take turns

3–5 years

Motor activity: hops on one foot, kicks balls, throws ball overhand, moves backward and forward

Cognitive and emotional development: cooperates in play, engages in fantasy, plays mom or dad, draws circles and squares, draws a person with two to four body parts, begins to copy letters, speaks in five- or six-word sentences, has a basic understanding of grammar rules, tells stories

By 5 years

Speaks in sentences of more than five words, says name and address, copies triangles, dresses and undresses without help, uses fork and spoon, cares for own toilet needs, washes and dries hands

Adapted from Shelov (1991).

variables that were likely to lead to successful determination of etiology. These investigators defined severity of delay by comparing functional age as a percentage of chronological age. Children with a functional age of 67%–100% of chronological age were designated mildly delayed; those with a functional age of 33%–66% of chronological age were designated moderately affected; those with a functional age of 33% or less of chronological age were defined as severely delayed. For each patient, at least two independent assessments of delay were made.

In their study, etiological determination was established in 44 of 80 cases with global developmental delay. In this category, the best predictors of defining etiology were aspects of family history, including consanguinity, history of intrapartum or neonatal complications, and history of developmental regression. The best predictors of etiological diagnosis in the category of physical findings were macrocephaly, microcephaly, dysmorphology, and congenital anomalies. Etiological diagnosis was established in 59.5% of cases with mild delay, in 44.1% of cases with moderate delay, and in all cases (four out of four) with severe delay.

The diagnostic yield of cytogenetic studies was not significantly different for cases with global developmental delay with dysmorphology than for cases with global developmental delay without dysmorphology. Shevell et al. (2001) reported that neuroimaging was twice as likely to contribute to diagnosis if

Table 9–2
Formal Tests of Development and Cognition

Children younger than 5 years
    Bayley Scales of Infant Development
    Denver Development Screening Test

Children older than 5 years
    Stanford-Binet
    Wechsler Intelligence Scale for Children, 3rd edition (WISC III)
    Vineland Adaptive Behavior Test
    Tests for autistic behavior
    Checklist for Autism in Toddlers (CHAT) autism screening questionnaire
    Childhood Autism Rating Scale (CARS)

there was a definite indication for this on clinical examination. Diagnostic information was obtained in 28% of cases where neuroimaging was carried out as a screening procedure in the absence of specific clinical indication. In cases of motor delay, evidence of cerebral palsy was most important in defining diagnosis.

Shevell et al. (2001) reported that 21 of their 44 cases with global developmental delay had a potentially preventable etiology. These included perinatal hypoxia, antenatal toxin exposure (e.g., alcohol exposure), and psychosocial neglect. In cases where developmental delay was confined to autistic disorder or developmental language disorder, etiology was determined in only 2%–4% of cases. Metabolic testing had a low yield in establishing diagnosis in their study. They noted, however, that there are significant genetic and therapeutic implications when metabolic abnormalities are found. Tests for such abnormalities should be considered. Important indicators for detailed metabolic studies include parental consanguinity, a family history of metabolic abnormalities or mental retardation, a history of developmental regression, or a history of episodes of acute illness and decompensation.

In 2003, the American Academy of Neurology (AAN) established practice parameters for the evaluation of children with global developmental delay (Shevell et al. 2003). They defined *global developmental delay* as "significant delay in two or more of the following developmental domains: gross/fine motor, speech/language, cognition, social–personal and activities in daily living." They noted that the term *global developmental delay* is applied to children less than 5 years of age, whereas the term *mental retardation* is applied to older children when intelligence quotient (IQ) testing is more valid and reliable. Thus according to the AAN, a diagnosis of mental retardation requires accurate IQ assessment, which they consider is not available for young children. They stress too that a child with developmental delay does not necessarily become mentally retarded. The importance of identifying a child with developmental delay is to enable the affected child to have the benefit of early intervention and rehabilitation services and to assess the family's needs. The importance of defining an underlying etiology is to improve outcome wherever possible.

Based on a literature review and data on diagnostic yield, the AAN published consensus-based recommendations for diagnostic testing. They recommended a staged approach to evaluation of the child with global developmental delay. Detailed history and physical, auditory, and visual examination are recommended in all cases. The AAN recommendation regarding special investigations is that a stepwise procedure be followed. They concluded that neuroimaging should be carried out since the diagnostic yield in their study was 55.3% for magnetic resonance imaging (MRI). The AAN reported that the diagnostic yield for cytogenetic studies is 3.5%–10%. They recommended that cytogenetic studies be carried out even in the absence of dysmorphology. They also recommended molecular genetic studies for fragile X. The AAN recommendations do not include routine metabolic screening since the diagnostic yield in their study was about 1%. They did not recommend lead studies unless there were identifiable risk factors. Thyroid studies were also not recommended unless the child had not had newborn screening. The AAN practice parameters recommended that specific aspects of the history and physical examination should be taken into account in the determination of special studies, to improve the diagnostic yield.

Poplawski (2003) published a genetic perspective on investigating intellectual disability. He reported that approximately 8.3 per 1000 schoolchildren in Australia have some degree of intellectual disability. Poplawski noted that a thorough history and clinical examination serve as the "cornerstone" of assessment of the child with intellectual disability. He tabulated details to be included in the history: maternal history, including obstetric history, previous pregnancies, miscarriages, stillbirths and neonatal deaths, as well as medical history. History of the current pregnancy should include details of any complications, maternal illnesses, possible teratogen exposure, and timing of fetal movements. The family history should include a three-generation pedigree with specific details on consanguinity, other family members with developmental delay, learning difficulties/congenital anomalies, and medical diagnoses. The child's early history should include information about mode of delivery; birth weight, length, and head circumference; resuscitation requirements; neonatal complications; and early feeding history. The child's subsequent history should include information on developmental progress or details of regression, eating habits, sleep patterns, physical problems, and medical conditions and behaviors.

Poplawski (2003) documented details of the physical examination that should be undertaken in the evaluation of the child with intellectual disability. These include defining growth parameters (height, weight, and head circumference) and searching for evidence of dysmorphology and abnormal skin manifestation that may indicate neurocutaneous symptoms. Skin evaluation requires the use of Wood's light to search for hypomelanotic macules that are typical of tuberous sclerosis. The examination should include a search for manifestations of storage disease, such as coarse facial features, corneal clouding, skeletal anomalies, hepato-splenomegaly, and cardiac murmurs. Poplawski also proposed evaluation of speech and hearing.

It is perhaps useful at this point to consider the neurological and dysmorphological examination of the child with developmental delay in greater detail.

Neurological Examination

A number of clinicians have emphasized that observation of the child interacting with a parent and at play constitutes an important aspect of the neurological examination (Diadori and Carmant 2002). Through such observation it may be possible to gauge whether development is age-appropriate, obtain insight into cognitive function, and determine whether or not motor deficits or abnormal movements are present.

General assessment includes evaluation of head size and shape, proportion of head circumference relative to height and weight, and the cranial to facial ratio. In infants, the size, shape, and tension of the fontanelle must be examined. In infants, it is important to determine if developmental reflexes are present and whether those that are present are appropriate for age. Developmental reflexes include rooting reflex, palmar grasp, tonic neck reflex, and Moro's reflex. In older infants, it is important to establish if pincer finger movements have developed. Muscle tone, strength of individual muscle groups, and stretch and plantar reflexes must be examined.

Sensory nerve function may be assessed through response to light touch and slight temperature change. Preliminary assessments of vision, hearing, and language should also be undertaken in older (8–12 months) infants and in children. More detailed evaluation of these functions and more detailed assessment of cognitive skills are important when developmental delay is clinically diagnosed.

Aspects of Dysmorphological Examination

Examination should include assessment of height, weight, and head circumference, including skull shape and size and shape of fontanelle. Hair examination should include assessment of sparseness or abundance and texture. Examine length of eyelashes, shape and length of eyebrows, presence or absence of synophrys (determine whether eyebrows meet in the middle). Examine the shape of the eyes and distance between the outer and inner canthi of the eyes; determine whether or not epicanthal folds are present and if pupils react normally to light. Note iris coloration and patterning; determine if cataracts are present. Determine if nose and lips are normal, whether the philtrum is of normal size, and whether the lengths of the upper and lower lips match; note the shape of the upper lip. Examine the palate and teeth;

note the position and spacing of teeth. Examine the position of the ears relative to the angle of the jaw; note the size and shape of helices. Examine the neck; note length and determine if webbing or excessive nuchal skinfolds are present. Examine the shape of the chest and the spacing of nipples; evaluate heart sounds and breathing. The abdomen should be palpated to rule out the presence of masses and enlargement of liver and spleen. Examine external genitalia.

Skeletal examination should include evaluation of body proportion (upper versus lower segments) and spine, including a search for abnormal curvature and bone defects. The upper and lower limbs must be evaluated to determine if the proportions of upper and lower arms and upper and lower legs are normal; range of motion of joints must be checked. Examine hands and feet; determine if the ratio of metacarpal/metatarsal length to phalangeal length is within normal limits. Examine fingers, toes, and nails to assess shape, length, and position. Examine palmar creases.

Skin examination should include a search for abnormal pigmentation, café-au-lait spots, skin tags, vascular lesions, and angiofibroma. The texture of the skin should be evaluated. Wood's lamp evaluation of skin should be undertaken to search for hypomelanotic macules.

It is often useful to examine photographs of the child at different ages to search for striking changes. Progressive facial coarsening may be indicative of lysosomal storage disease.

Features of the physical examination should be compiled. Measurement of height, weight, head circumference, intercanthal distances, hand size, and ear length should be plotted relative to age-appropriate control measurements. If anomalies are present, databases (e.g. Winter-Baraitser Dysmorphology Database) and references e.g. Smith's recognizable patterns of human malformations (Jones 1997) must be consulted to determine if the constellation of manifestations corresponds to a known chromosomal or dysmorphological syndrome.

Laboratory Tests

Poplawski (2003) recommended routine tests such as blood count and iron levels to search for anemia, measurement of creatine and creatinine to search for creatine deficiency disorders, liver function tests, and determination of lead levels to test for exposure. He noted that these tests might detect abnormalities that contribute to general "unwellness" of the patient. Poplawski wrote that thyroid-stimulating hormone (TSH) and thyroid hormone (thyroxine, T4) levels should be measured since signs of hypothyroidism may be subtle and because there is evidence that 5%–10% of neonates are not screened. Furthermore, when newborn screening is based solely on determination of TSH levels, infants with hypothalamic pituitary hypothyroidism or congenital hypothyroidism with delayed TSH elevations may be missed. He noted that in South Australia 2.25% of infants were not screened for phenylketonuria

(PKU) in 1999. It is important to take this into account and to screen for PKU where there is no definitive documentation of screening results. Furthermore, it is important to determine if the mother was screened for high levels of phenylalanine since this may result in fetal brain damage and microcephaly.

Poplawski (2003) reported that the diagnostic yield of chromosome studies in patients with disabilities is 4%–12%. He proposed that chromosome studies include high-resolution banding and full karyotype analysis to rule out autosomal and sex chromosomal anomalies. Fragile X studies through molecular testing should be routinely performed. Poplawski et al. (2001) and Poplawski (2003) acknowledged that there is controversy regarding routine testing of subjects with intellectual disability for inborn errors of metabolism but noted "diagnostic yield is not the sole parameter on which decisions should be made." They reported that in a study of 1447 individuals with intellectual disability, 1.1% were found to have metabolic disorders; however, specific therapies were available for 69% of those cases. They therefore proposed urine metabolic screen of amino acids and organic acids and suggested that other metabolic testing should be guided by clinical evaluation.

Biancalana et al. (2004) stressed that fragile X mental retardation (FMR) frequently occurs in individuals who have no family history of mental retardation. An affected male child with a clinically significant FMR CGG expansion may have a mother who is clinically asymptomatic but who has an FMR CGG expansion that is in the premutation range (54–60 repeats). They advocated that all patients who have significant developmental delay and language delay be tested for FMR through analysis of CGG repeat expansion in DNA.

Future Directions in Diagnosis of the Etiology of Global Developmental Delay

Microarray analysis will likely be used increasingly to search for chromosomal anomalies that lead to dosage changes (Schoumans et al. 2004). Dosage differences resulting from microdeletions or micro-duplications larger than 500 kb can be detected in genomic DNA from patients using microarray analysis. This enables comprehensive analysis of the genome at price that is close to that now charged for high-resolution chromosome banding. With the latter, the minimum size of deletion or duplication that can be detected is 3–5 Mb.

It is likely that tandem mass spectrometry will increasingly be used to examine metabolites in biological fluids. The cost of analysis of organic acids and amino acids will be greatly reduced from present levels. Furthermore, a comprehensive analysis of metabolites will become available, either through tandem mass spectrometry or through use of proton nuclear magnetic resonance spectroscopy (Chace et al. 2003; Filippi et al. 2002).

Proton nuclear magnetic spectroscopy (^{1}H NMR) was introduced for analysis of body fluids in 1985. This methodology facilitates simultaneous analysis of many types of component. Samples to be analyzed do not require prior chemical extraction or derivatization. The sample volume required is 1 μl. Samples are placed inside a static external magnetic field. A specific proton (^{1}H)–containing compound gives rise to a specific spin pattern and spectral shift so that a characteristic pattern, or fingerprint, is obtained. The signal intensity of the spin pattern and spectral shift are determined by the quantity of the specific compound. Proton NMR detects metabolites that are routinely detected in mass spectrometry (Engelke et al. 2004). In addition, metabolites are detected that are not usually found using other methodologies. Two examples of "new" inborn errors of metabolism that were only detected following introduction of ^{1}H NMR are dimethylglycine dehydrogenase deficiency and ureidopropionase deficiency. In dimethylglycine dehydrogenase deficiency, abnormal quantities of a normal metabolite are present. In ureidopropionase deficiency, abnormal metabolites arise because of a defect in pyrimidine metabolism. Moolenaar et al. (2003) reported two clinical indications for NMR spectroscopy: the presence in a family of two children with unexplained similar clinical signs and symptoms and finding that a patient has a peculiar body odor.

Proton magnetic resonance spectroscopy has also been applied to analysis of brain defects in inborn errors of metabolism (Kahler and Fahey 2003). Bianchi et al. (2000) reported studies on female siblings with developmental delay and severe language delay. Their metabolic workup was normal. Blood creatine levels were normal. Brain ^{1}H NMR studies revealed depletion of creatine. Oral creatine therapy led to dramatic improvement in their symptoms. Decreased levels of brain creatine were subsequently shown to occur in several different metabolic defects of creatine metabolism. In the following chapter, we will discuss how analysis of brain phenylalanine has provided new insight into genotype–phenotype correlations in PKU (Pietz et al. 2003).

The technique ^{13}C NMR spectroscopy is used to quantify cerebral metabolites such as glutamate, glutamine, *myo*-inositol, and *N*-acetylaspartate (Bluml 1999). The *N*-acetylaspartate:creatine ratio may be used as a marker of neuronal density. Neuronal loss leads to lower than normal ratios (Weisskopf et al. 2004).

Additional Routine Molecular Tests

It is likely that in addition to fragile X (FMR1) testing, other DNA tests may be introduced particularly for male subjects. Testing for mutations in the *SLC6A8* gene that predispose to one type of inborn error of creatine metabolism and for *ARX* mutations (aristaless homeobox gene) have been proposed.

Rosenberg et al. (2004) reported that in families with X-linked mental retardation the prevalence of *SLC6A8* mutation was 2.2%. Mandel and Biancalana (2004) reported that in families with evidence of X-linked mental retardation the incidence of fragile X abnormalities is 27% and the incidence of *ARX* gene mutations is 6.6%. There is a mutation hot spot in the *ARX* gene that is readily detected through DNA analysis.

10

Epilogue: The Value of Genetic Diagnosis—Applying Knowledge about Etiology to Prevention and Treatment

In this chapter, we will consider why a genetic diagnosis is useful. Much of the research in human genetics has been motivated primarily by the perception that certain genetic disorders cause suffering and severely impact life quality. Research activities are stimulated by the perception that it may be possible to prevent this suffering through an understanding of the cause and natural history of the disorder. It is clear this understanding evolves through research on individuals with disabilities and their families.

Presymptomatic Diagnosis and Disease Prevention: The Phenylketonuria Paradigm

Phenylketonuria (PKU) is a condition that, if left untreated, leads to mental retardation. The biochemical basis of this condition was discovered 70 years ago. Research led to an understanding of the basis of mental retardation in PKU. It also led to development and implementation of therapies. If instituted in a timely manner, these therapies prevent the deleterious consequences associated with inheritance of defective gene alleles. Analysis of the medical management of PKU also illustrates how our understanding continues to evolve over time. It is the investigation of the unusual patient and the unexpected biochemical findings that enhances our knowledge and points the way to more efficacious therapies.

Developing Treatment

As described in Chapter 1, Asborn Folling discovered in 1934 that excessive quantities of phenylpyruvic acid were present in the urine of two siblings who were mentally retarded. He went on to examine urine from several hundred individuals with mental retardation and discovered eight more cases. He postulated that excess phenylpyruvic acid resulted from a defect in phenylalanine metabolism.

Folling named this condition *imbecillitas phenylpyruvica*. Penrose and Quastel (1937) suggested that the disorder be named *phenylketonuria*. Penrose (1946) described the clinical features of untreated PKU. He noted that the majority of patients had moderate mental retardation; in one-third of patients, mental retardation was severe. Hyperkinetic digital mannerisms were often present. Head circumference was frequently reduced. Reflexes were brisk, and spasticity was present in some patients. The incidence of epilepsy was higher in PKU patients than in the general population. Patients were often short in stature and had lordosis of the spinal column. They were prone to dermatitis. Their hair color and eye color were diluted compared with those of family members.

In 1953, Jervis reported that PKU is caused by deficiency in the enzyme phenylalanine hydroxylase. In that same year, Bickel and associates demonstrated the efficacy of a phenylalanine-reduced diet in the treatment of PKU:

> We decided to keep a girl, aged 2 years with phenylketonuria on a diet low in phenylalanine. She was an idiot unable to stand, walk, or talk. She showed no interest in her food or in her surroundings and spent her time groaning crying and banging her head.
>
> The diet had to be specially prepared . . .
>
> The child was first treated in hospital so that careful observation could be made . . .
>
> The characteristic musty smell disappeared, the levels of phenylalanine fell to normal, excretion of phenylpyruvic acid ceased and the ferric chloride reaction became negative.
>
> During continued outpatient treatment a gradual improvement in the child's mental state took place within the next few months; she learnt to crawl, to stand and to climb on chairs; her eyes became brighter, her hair grew darker, and she no longer banged her head or cried continuously.
>
> In view of the importance of phenylketonuria as a cause of mental deficiency, further controlled trials are being made, special attention being paid to very young children who are likely to benefit most. (Bickel et al. 1953, pp. 812–813)

Screening for Phenylketonuria

In 1963, Guthrie and Susi developed a rapid test for analysis of blood phenylalanine in small samples of blood collected on filter paper. Subsequently, Guthrie and the National Association for Retarded Citizens persuaded governments to undertake newborn screening. Pass et al. (2000) noted that Guthrie was fortunate to have been advocating newborn screening during the early 1960s when John F. Kennedy was president. The president was interested in mental retardation, and he had the support of Congress. This led to generous support of programs to reduce mental retardation. Early detection and dietary treatment of infants with high levels of phenylalanine was shown to be effective at preventing mental retardation (Abadie et al. 2001).

Unusual Patients and New Discoveries I

In 1974, Smith and Lloyd described siblings with apparent PKU who, despite early detection and careful dietary management, developed neurological symptoms.

In 1978, Danks reported apparent cases of severe PKU that did not respond to treatment with a low-phenylalanine diet. This disorder was subsequently shown to be due to deficiency of the biopterin cofactor that is required for phenylalanine hydroxylase (PAH) activity and the activity of other hydroxylases. It is now known that approximately 2% of PKU cases are due to defects in biopterin synthesis or biopterin recycling. Danks demonstrated that intravenous administration of tetrahydrobiopterin (BH_4) in patients with atypical PKU led to reduction in plasma phenylalanine levels. Levodopa (L-Dopa) and 5-hydroxytryptophan were used in some cases along with biopterin.

Clinical features in biopterin deficiency patients include trunk hypotonia, hypertonia of the extremities, and myoclonic seizures. In some patients, head growth may be affected. Tetrahydrobiopterin is a cofactor for PAH, tyrosine hydroxylase, tryptophan hydroxylase, and nitric oxidase. Deficiency of BH_4 usually presents with hyperphenylalaninemia and deficiency of the neurotransmitter precursors L-dopa and 5-hydroxytryptophan. Deficiency of BH_4 impacts phenylalanine metabolism and synthesis of catecholamines and serotonins.

Tetrahydrobiopterin is a pterin that is synthesized from guanosine triphosphate (GTP) in a reaction that is catalyzed by three different enzymes (Fig. 10–1). There are known defects in the first two reactions in the pathway. In the first step in BH_4 synthesis, GTP is converted to 7,8-dihydroneopterin triphosphate by the enzyme GTP cyclohydrolase. The second step involves conversion of 7,8-dihydroneopterin triphosphate to 6-pyruvoyl-tetrahydrobiopterin through the activity of the enzyme 6-pyruvoyl tetrahydrobiopterin synthase (PTPS). In the third step, 6-pyruvoyl-tetrahydrobiopterin is converted to 5,6,7,8-tetrahydrobiopterin in a two-part reaction catalyzed by the enzyme sepiapterin reductase.

Following its oxidation, tetrahydrobiopterin is regenerated. Regeneration requires two enzymes, pterin-4-α-carbinolamine-dehydratase (PCD) and dihydropteridine reductase (DHPR).

Mutation in GTP cyclohydrolase does not usually give rise to hyperphenylalaninemia, but it leads to a form of dystonia that is responsive to L-dopa. Mutations in PTPS lead to hyperphenylalaninemia. Mutations in PCD may give rise to transient hyperphenylalaninemia. Deficiency of DHPR leads to a PKU phenotype and is the most common defect in biopterin metabolism.

Since biopterin deficiency is a severe but treatable disorder it is important to screen for it in all neonates with persistent hyperphenylalaninemia (Scriver and Kaufman 2001; Blau 2001). Screening tests include analysis of pterins in urine and measurement of DHPR in blood. Catecholamine levels should also be measured. A biopterin loading test may confirm diagnosis.

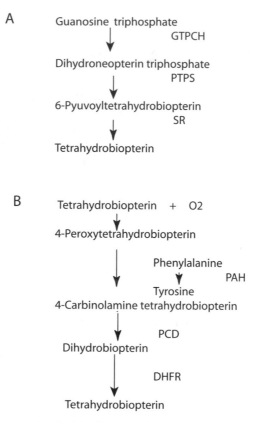

Figure 10.1. Enzymes involved in the metabolism of tetrahydrobiopterin and generation of cofactor for phenylalanine hydroxylase (PAH): GTPCH, guanosine triphosphate cyclohydrolase; PTPS, 6-pyruvolyltetrahydrobiopterin synthase; SR, sepiapterin reductase; PCD, pterin-4α-carbinolamine dehydratase; DHFR, dihydrofolate reductase.

Maternal Phenylketonuria

Mabry et al. (1963) and Frankenburg et al. (1968) recognized that high levels of maternal phenylalanine led to fetal brain damage. Further studies demonstrated that high levels of phenylalanine in the mother during pregnancy led to a number of different congenital anomalies, including microcephaly, congenital heart disease, and growth retardation (Lenke and Levy, 1980). The risk for congenital anomalies is a function of the maternal blood phenylalanine level. Levels above 15 mg% are associated with an 85% risk for microcephaly (Rouse and Azen 2004). To avoid fetal damage, blood phenylalanine levels must be maintained between 2 mg% and 6 mg%.

Phenylalanine Hydroxylase Gene Identification and Analysis

In 1982 Robson et al. isolated PAH encoding messenger ribonucleic acid (mRNA) from rat liver and developed complementary deoxyribonucleic acid (cDNA) clones from this. Woo et al. (1983) cloned the human PAH cDNA. Determination of the gene sequence opened the way for mutation analysis and for investigation of genotype–phenotype correlations.

Population Incidence of Phenylketonuria

Previously, PKU was considered to be a disorder that affected individuals of northern European origin. In Scotland, the incidence is 190 per million. It is interesting to note that the highest incidence of PKU occurs in Turkey, 385 per million. The disease occurs in Asian populations; in China, the incidence is 60 per million. The incidence in Arabic populations is 165 per million (Scriver and Kaufman 2001).

Hyperphenylalaninemia and Phenylketonuria

As more information was obtained, through screening of phenylalanine levels in newborns and follow-up of these patients, it became clear that different degrees of elevation of phenylalanine occur and that patients differ in their tolerance of dietary phenylalanine. Patients with hyperphenylalaninemia who maintain a blood phenylalanine level below 10 mg% (600 μM/l) on a normal diet may not require treatment (Weglage et al. 2001a).

In PKU the blood phenylalanine levels in untreated patients are above 15 mg% (1000 μM/l). The disease is subclassified into categories based on the amount of dietary phenylalanine that can be tolerated. In classic PKU, individuals tolerate less than 250–350 mg of phenylalanine per day and their diet must be severely restricted in its phenylalanine content to maintain safe plasma phenylalanine levels below 5 mg%.

Phenylalanine Hydroxylase Genotype and Patient Phenotype

Although genotype does not always predict clinical outcome, it is correlated with metabolic phenotype; and there is now consensus that the patient's genotype should be determined to predict the level of dietary control that will be required.

Gjetting et al. (2001) described features of mutant forms of PAH. They noted that approximately 60% are missense mutations that do not affect critical residues related to catalytic function. These mutations likely cause altered protein folding and altered subunit interaction. Misfolded proteins undergo accelerated degradation. More than 400 different mutations of the PAH gene lead to PKU (Erlandsen et al. 2003). Deletion mutations that lead to absence of phenylalanine protein are associated with the most severe phenotype. These mutations constitute 14% of mutations. The most common mutation in northern European populations is the missense mutation R408W, which occurs in 31% of the population. The splice mutation allele IVS12nt-1 occurs in 11%; the IVS10nt-11 splice allele occurs in 10%. In Asian populations, a broad range of different alleles occurs; R243Q and R413P each account for 13% of alleles.

Prognosis of Treated Phenylketonuria

Scriver and Ryan (2000) noted that the newborn screening test to identify infants with PKU has become routine in many countries because of evidence that the prognosis for individuals who have PAH deficiency is excellent if they are treated early. Untreated individuals with this deficiency are at risk for irreversible brain damage.

How long should treatment be continued? Initially, physicians proposed that treatment be continued from infancy until the age of 6 years. Later recommendations were for treatment to continue until the teenage years. Currently, life-long treatment is recommended. There is a general acknowledgment of the difficulties in sustaining treatment through adolescence (National Institutes of Health Consensus Development Panel 2001). It is particularly important that women be made aware of the importance of dietary control of phenylalanine levels prior to conception and during pregnancy.

Unusual Patients and New Discoveries II

Surprising differences in the phenotype of siblings with the same blood phenylalanine levels and the same PAH genotype support the conclusion that there are other genes that influence the final phenotype in PKU. Proton nuclear magnetic resonance (NMR) spectroscopy studies of brain provided evidence that siblings with the same elevated levels of blood phenylalanine differed with respect to their levels of brain phenylalanine. Weglage et al. (2001b) proposed that this variation results from genetic differences in an amino acid transporter. Koch et al. (2000) reported that 20 individuals who had high intelligence quotient (IQ) scores despite high levels of blood phenylalanine exhibited significantly low brain levels of phenylalanine.

Transport of Phenylalanine across the Blood–Brain Barrier

The passage of large neutral amino acids (LNAs) such as phenylalanine, tyrosine, tryptophan, valine, leucine, isoleucine, methionine, and histidine into the brain from the bloodstream is determined by an amino acid transport system, the L carrier system (Matalon et al. 2003). The degree of transfer of each of these amino acids is influenced by the concentrations of each of the other LNAs. Bidirectional transport occurs through this system. The L carrier system constitutes the rate-limiting step in regulation of the brain concentration of amino acids (Pardridge 1998).

Pietz et al. (1999) demonstrated using proton NMR that in the presence of high blood levels of phenylalanine the levels of brain phenylalanine were raised. When patients with elevated blood phenylalanine levels were given high levels of LNAs, their brain levels of phenylalanine dropped. These results indicate that by increasing blood levels of the other LNAs it may be possible to slow transfer of phenylalanine across the blood–brain barrier. Pietz et al. (1999) proposed that high levels of blood phenylalanine might impair transfer of other LNAs across this barrier, resulting in their deficiency in brain tissue and in pathology.

Biopterin in the Treatment of Phenylketonuria Due to Phenylalanine Hydroxylase Mutations

A major breakthrough in the treatment of PKU emerged when Kure et al. (2004) demonstrated that individuals with specific PAH mutations responded favorably to treatment with a stereoisomer of BH_4. Initial studies indicated that patients with the missense mutations I65T or Y414C responded to treatment. Waters et al. (1999) proposed that BH_4 acts as a chemical chaperone that prevents misfolding of mutant PAH, thereby delaying ubiquitin-mediated proteolytic degradation.

Trefz et al. (2001) recommended that in infants found through newborn screening to have high phenylalanine levels, a BH_4 loading test be performed. Lassker et al. (2002) reported that BH_4 responsiveness might not necessarily be demonstrated in the newborn period but that it may be present later. Muntau et al. (2002) noted that long-term administration of pharmacological doses of BH_4 improved dietary tolerance of phenylalanine in PKU patients with a variety of different PAH missense mutations. Kure et al. (2004) reported that normally suboptimal concentrations of BH_4 are present in liver and that activity of normal (wild-type) PAH can be enhanced through BH_4 administration. The only mutations that do not respond are null mutations that result in an absence of transcription and or translation.

All indications are that BH_4 therapy is useful in all PKU patients except those who have null mutations (Lucke et al. 2003; Matalon et al. 2004). Unfortunately, the cost of this compound is still high, and treatment for a child would likely cost several hundred dollars per day (Werner-Felmayer et al. 2002).

Newborn Screening and Presymptomatic Diagnosis

Implementation of screening programs and designation of resources to mitigate deleterious effects of underlying genes are dependent not on researchers and physicians but on societal attitudes and economic forces (Pandor et al. 2004).

There is consensus among different advocates of newborn screening that the following criteria should be applied.

1. Screen for conditions that are identifiable in a phase in which they would not be recognized clinically.
2. The available tests must have appropriate sensitivity and specificity.
3. There are benefits of timely identification and early intervention.
4. Newborn screening should report to the physician any findings of significance.
5. Newborn screening must be followed up with appropriate professional and family education.

The first newborn screening test was for phenylalanine levels in blood, as described above. In the 1970s, screening for congenital hypothyroidism was added following the demonstration by Dussault and Laberge (1973) that thyroxine (T4) and thyroid-stimulating hormone (TSH) could be adequately measured on dried blood samples collected on filter paper. Congenital hypothyroidism is the most frequent abnormality detected in newborn screening programs.

Newborn Screening Test for Hypothyroidism

Sporadic hypothyroidism occurs today in approximately 1 in 4000 infants in the United States. Fortunately, through newborn screening programs, this condition is detected early and can be vigorously treated (Dussault and Laberge 1973). Most commonly, it is due to abnormal development of the thyroid gland. In some cases, congenital hypothyroidism is an inborn error of metabolism (McGirr et al. 1959; Hutchison 1961; Madeiros-Neto and Stanbury 1994). In chapter 1, we outlined aspects of the history of goitrous cretinism and hypothyroidism.

Screening for Hemoglobinopathies

Screening for hemoglobinopathies was added to newborn screening programs in the United States in 1987. This addition was not implemented in all states, despite the clear rationale supporting its introduction. Early detection of sickle cell disease and thalassemia identifies the infant who should be included in a comprehensive health-care program. In sickle cell disease, prophylactic penicillin therapy and parental education regarding fever and hydration reduce the complications of vascular occlusion, including cerebral vascular occlusion and strokes.

Additional Newborn Screening Tests

Other tests that were subsequently added to newborn screening by some U.S. states include DNA testing for congenital adrenal hyperplasia and biotinidase assays. The introduction of tandem mass spectrometry to newborn screening programs in some states led to expanded testing that included screening for many aminoacidurias, organic acidemias, fatty acid dehydrogenase defects, and defects of carnitine metabolism. In Massachusetts, in one year, 160,000 newborns were screened using mass spectroscopy. Abnormal amino acid metabolism was detected in 22 infants, and abnormal organic acid metabolism was detected in 20.

Medium chain acyl-coenzyme A dehydrogenase deficiency and glutaricacidemia are readily detected by tandem mass spectrometry. These disorders respond well to treatment, particularly if it is initiated prior to the first episode of illness. In glutaricaciduria type I, carnitine treatment is particularly important. (For screening recommendations, see American College of Medical Genetics/American Society of Human Genetics Test and Technology Transfer Committee Working Group, 2000.)

Recommendation for Testing of Newborns for Deafness

Recently, screening of newborns for deafness has been added to the program in most U.S. states. The frequency of hearing loss in newborns far exceeds that of metabolic disorders. The incidence of deafness in newborns is 2 per 1000. Without screening, deafness is most commonly detected at 24–36 months of age. Motivations for testing include strategies to avoid the language and social difficulties that occur in deaf children. Early screening, identification, and early intervention may enable deaf children to enter school within the normal range of language development (DesGeorges 2003).

Tests for deafness are noninvasive. They include the otoacoustic emissions test, which is based on the fact that the inner ear generates sound of low intensity, and the auditory brain stem response test, which measures the registration of sounds in the brain. If a hearing deficit is diagnosed, it is imperative that rehabilitation procedures be instituted. Intervention most often requires assistive listening devices, including hearing aids, and, later possibly, cochlear implants.

Attitudes of Deaf People to Newborn Screening for Deafness

Taneja et al. (2004) reported that there are differences in attitudes of deaf individuals who associate with the deaf community and deaf individuals who have equal involvement with both deaf and hearing communities. More members of the latter group are accepting of newborn screening for deafness. It is important to note that many more deaf children are born to hearing parents than to deaf parents.

Causes of Hearing Loss in Infants Worldwide

It is estimated that 50% of cases of deafness in infants are genetic in etiology. Of these, 30% represent syndromic deafness and 20% are nonsyndromic.

Many genes have been found to be involved in hearing. However, more than half of the cases of nonsyndromic deafness have mutations in the Connexin 26 gene, which maps to chromosome 13q12.

Gene and environment interactions also play a role in deafness. For example, specific mitochondrial DNA mutations predispose to antibiotic (aminoglycosides) toxicity, leading to deafness.

In developing countries, rubella infections of mothers during pregnancy are an important cause of deafness and blindness in infants. Concerns about the safety of the measles, mumps, and rubella (MMR) vaccine have decreased its use in the United States and United Kingdom. It is possible that rubella infection rates in the population, including in pregnant women, may rise during the next few years. Cytomegalovirus infections during pregnancy are also an important cause of deafness. The recommendations of the American College of Medical Genetics /American Society of Human Genetics Test and Technology Transfer Committee Working Group (2000) are that newborns be screened for PKU, galactosemia, hypothyroidism, and biotinidase deficiency. Organic acidemias, amino acid metabolic defects, and carnitine metabolic defects should be screened using mass spectroscopy. Screening for abnormal hemoglobins should include HbS (sickle hemoglobin) and thalassemia testing. Newborns should be screened for deafness.

Universal newborn screening is the standard recommendation. A recent survey has revealed increasing disparity between the U.S. states in newborn screening. Newborn screening is not universal and not fair. While most states screen for three or four disorders (PKU, galactosemia, congenital hypothyroidism, congenital adrenal hyperplasia), selected populations receive more comprehensive screening. Screening for 20 different disorders occurs in 27% of infants in the United States. The extent of screening is often left to consumer initiative.

Galactosemia: Problems Despite Early Detection

Galactosemia due to deficiency of galactose-1-phosphate uridyltransferase may lead to severe jaundice, sepsis, and liver failure in young infants. It also leads to failure to thrive, hypotonia, and cataracts. Withdrawal of milk and formula that contains galactose leads to resolution of these problems. Early treatment of galactosemia may therefore be life-saving. Long-term follow-up of patients treated for galactosemia has revealed that they are at risk for cognitive and language difficulties and that female patients are at risk for hypogonadism.

Bosch et al. (2004) carried out a survey of treated galactosemia patients and their families. They reported that in the 6–11 year group, 44% of children attended special schools. In the general Dutch population, 3% of children attend special schools. Individuals in the patient group who were 16 years of age or older had significantly lower scores in the cognitive domain (memory, concentration, and attention) and in the social function domain. In the patient group older than 18 years, the percentage that had completed only basic school requirements and low vocational training was 61%. In the general Dutch population, 27.2 % complete only these requirements. In surveys, 91% of patients responded that they were able to have a good life. Bosch et al. (2004) concluded that additional research is required to understand the effects of galactosemia.

Prevention of Congenital Malformations and Perinatal Complications That May Predispose to Developmental Delay

In Chapter 3, we discussed the importance of pre- and periconceptual folic acid intake in the prevention of neural tube defects. Of growing concern is the increase in the incidence of diabetes in the population. The incidence of Type 2 diabetes is increasing, especially in patients who are obese. Maternal obesity and diabetes often lead to fetal overgrowth. This may lead to obstetrical complications (Hampton et al. 2004). There is also evidence that neural tube defects, including caudal regression syndrome, occur much more frequently in fetuses of diabetic mothers, especially those with insulin-dependent diabetes, than in the general population (Stroastrup Smith et al. 2004). The incidence of congenital malformation is 11 times higher in the infants of mothers with Type 2 diabetes. Congenital malformations that are more common include neural tube defects, congenital heart disease, urogenital anomalies, and vertebral defects.

Control of blood sugar levels and folic acid supplementation before conception and during pregnancy can reduce the incidence of fetal congenital malformation (Andreasen et al. 2004).

Preconceptual, Prenatal Genetic Testing and Carrier Testing of Individuals at Risk for Specific Genetic Diseases That Predispose to Severe Cognitive Impairment

One of the first applications of genetic carrier testing was the hexosaminidase assay in individuals of Ashkenazi Jewish origin to determine carrier status for Tay-Sachs disease. Community-based Tay-Sachs carrier screening, counseling, and prenatal diagnosis programs were implemented in the United States in 1970. In 2000, Kaback reported that these programs resulted in a 90% decline in the incidence of individuals with Tay-Sachs disease in the United States.

Carrier testing for Canavan's disease in the Ashkenazi Jewish population is also being considered in view of the fact that a specific mutation occurs in over 90% of cases of this disorder in that population.

Advances in DNA analysis have facilitated carrier testing for many genetic diseases, including fragile X mental retardation. There is a general consensus that carrier testing should be carried out on adults, not on minors. Carrier testing should be preceded by discussions of the goals and implications of the test. Posttest counseling is also important.

Advances in the Treatment of Inborn Errors of Metabolism That May Lead to Developmental Delay and Mental Retardation

During the 20-year period prior to 2004, improved treatments were developed for a number of inborn errors of metabolism. Clinical outcomes have been particularly improved for disorders that are responsive to dietary therapy and/or pharmacological doses of vitamins and cofactors. A number of new therapeutic strategies are improving outcomes in patients with lysosomal storage diseases. We will briefly review a number of the successful treatment strategies in specific diseases. This topic is addressed in part elsewhere in this book in sections that deal with specific biochemical disorders, e.g., in Chapters 5 and 6.

Treatment of Organic Acidemias

Organic acidemias include maple syrup urine disease, isovaleric acidemia, propionicaciduria, and methylmalonicaciduria. Ogier de Baulny and Saudubray (2002) reviewed treatment strategies for these disorders. Early detection through newborn screening would permit detection of at least some affected infants before they suffer an acute metabolic crisis.

In cases where infants undergo metabolic crises due to the accumulation of high levels of damaging organic acids, toxic compounds may be removed by dialysis or exchange transfusion. Carnitine supplements are available for treatment of patients with organic acidemias who have high levels of plasma acylcarnitine and reduced levels of free carnitine. Dietary management appropriate to the specific disorder involves the use of special formulas. For the treatment of maple syrup urine disease, isovalericaciduria, and propionicaciduria, special formulas with low content of branched chain amino acids have been developed. Special formulas depleted in branched chain amino acids and methionine are available for treatment of methylmalonicacidemia. Some cases of methylmalonicacidemia are vitamin B_{12}-responsive, and these generally have a better prognosis.

Marriage et al. (2004) reviewed metabolic therapies that are beneficial to treatment in mitochondrial oxidative phosphorylation defects. These include the specific cofactor coenzyme Q (ubiquinone) and antioxidants such as vitamins C, E, and K, and riboflavin. Thiamin, niacin and carnitine are also often recommended.

Kyllerman et al. (2004) reviewed results of treatment of glutaricaciduria type I. Treatment of this disorder includes protein restriction, in particular restriction of lysine and tryptophan, with riboflavin and carnitine supplementation. In infants who had already developed neurological symptoms, including dystonia, the treatment did not reverse neurological deficits; however, the deficits did not become more marked in treated infants. Kyllerman et al. (2004) noted that it is possible that neurological deficits may be averted if glutaricaciduria is detected early in life, e.g., through newborn screening, before the onset of symptoms.

Treatment of Fatty Acid Oxidation Defects

Key to the treatment of fatty acid oxidation defects is accurate diagnosis; it is critical to determine if the defect lies in the metabolism of long chain fatty acids, medium chain fatty acids, or short chain fatty acids. Treatment involves diets that are low in fats but supplemented with specific fats that are tolerated in a particular condition (Schuler et al. 2004). Thus, in patients with defects in metabolism of long chain fatty acid dehydrogenase, medium chain triglycerides may be used in therapy. In patients with short chain fatty acid dehydrogenase defects, treatment with long chain triglycerides may be beneficial. Roe et al. (2002) reported that treatment with odd chain fatty acids might be beneficial in patients with very long chain fatty acid dehydrogenase defects.

Supplementation with carnitine, avoidance of fasting, and adequate carbohydrate intake have improved outlook in fatty acid oxidation defects. These measures may also improve outcome in patients with defects in transport of long chain fatty acids across mitochondrial membranes due to carnitine:acylcarnitine translocase mutations (Iacobazzi et al. 2004).

Treatment of Biotin Synthesis and Recycling Defects

Weber et al. (2004) carried out a study of two groups of children with biotinidase deficiency. In the first group, treatment with biotin commenced after the development of symptoms. In the second group, biotinidase deficiency was detected on newborn screening, and treatment commenced soon thereafter. In both groups, biotinidase activity was absent.

Treatment after onset of symptoms did not reverse symptoms. Impairments in children treated late included delayed motor and speech development, impaired hearing, and visual impairment associated with optic atrophy. In contrast, 25 patients who were detected as being biotinidase-deficient on newborn screening and then treated demonstrated appropriate speech, language, and motor development. They had no auditory or visual deficits.

Therapy in Lysosomal Storage Diseases

Prognoses in a number of different lysosomal storage diseases have improved due to implementation of stem cell transplantation. In Gaucher's disease, improved prognosis is due to enzyme replacement therapy.

There are a number of reports on successful treatment of lysosomal storage diseases with hematopoietic stem cells derived from cord blood. Staba et al. (2004) reported results of studies on patients with Hurler's syndrome. Twenty consecutive patients were recruited for cord blood transplants from unrelated donors. The transplants were carried out following chemical myeloablation. Seventeen patients survived more than 905 days after transplantation. They had normal α-iduronidase levels, and the enzyme was donor-derived. Staba et al. reported that in transplanted patients neurocognitive performance improved and somatic manifestations of storage disease decreased.

Malm et al. (2004) reported the results of a 5-year follow-up study of two siblings with the lysosomal storage disease aspartylglucosaminuria who were treated with allogeneic bone marrow transplant. The donor cells were identical to these of the patients at the human leukocyte antigen (HLA) A and B and DR loci. Five years after transplant, the children had normal levels of aspartylglucosaminidase that was donor-derived. They had no evidence of neuropsychological and clinical features that are characteristic of the disease. Malm et al. concluded that the regression that is characteristic of aspartylglucosaminuria was averted by therapy.

Interesting new approaches to therapy of storage diseases are emerging. These include the use of cofactors and other chemicals that act as chaperones and the application of substrate reduction therapy. Derivatives of galactose act as chemical chaperones that enhance the activity of mutant forms of β-galactosidase that lead to GM_1-gangliosidosis. Matsuda et al. (2003) studied the effects of one such derivative, N-acetyl-4-epi-β-valienamine, in a mouse model of juvenile GM_1 gangliosidosis. They demonstrated that short-term oral administration of this compound enhanced β-galactosidase activity in the brain and in other tissues. Immunochemical staining revealed that treatment resulted in a decrease in compounds characteristic of GM_1 gangliosidosis in the frontal cortex (see also Chapter 6).

Substrate reduction therapy has been applied to the treatment of genetic diseases characterized by accumulation of glycosphingolipids. Andersson et al. (2004) used a galactose analog, N-butyldeoxygalactonojirimycin to inhibit the first step of glycosphingolipid synthesis in a mouse model of Sandhoff's disease. They demonstrated that this compound extended life expectancy and delayed symptom onset.

Lachmann et al. (2004) used miglustat, an inhibitor of glycosphingolipid biosynthesis, for in vitro substrate reduction therapy of Niemann-Pick disease type C. They demonstrated, using peripheral blood lymphocytes, that this compound normalized lipid trafficking in the lymphocytes. Their results have implications for therapy and provide further insight into the cause of the disease. Lachmann et al. concluded that glycosphingolipid accumulation is the primary pathogenetic event in Niemann-Pick type C.

Prognosis in X-linked adrenoleukodystrophy has greatly improved through introduction of Lorenzo's oil treatment prior to the onset of neurological symptoms (Moser et al. 2004a,b). C. Peters et al. (2004) reported that boys with early-stage disease benefit from the use of hematopoietic stem cell therapy.

In this work, we have sought to review the progress in understanding the etiology of specific forms of developmental delay and mental retardation. We have also reviewed examples of progress in the application of knowledge about etiology to presymptomatic disease detection and to therapy. Though much has been achieved, much remains to be done.

References

Abadie V, Berthelot J, Feillet F, Maurin N, Mercier A, de Baulny HO, de Parscau L. 2001. Neonatal screening and long-term follow-up of phenylketonuria: the French database. Early Hum Dev 65(2):149–58.

Abramsky L, Chapple J. 1997. 47,XXY (Klinefelter syndrome) and 47,XYY: estimated rates of and indication for postnatal diagnosis with implications for prenatal counselling. Prenat Diagn 17(4):363–8.

Adato A, Vreugde S, Joensuu T, Avidan N, Hamalainen R, Belenkiy O, Olender T, Bonne-Tamir B, Ben-Asher E, Espinos C, et al. 2002. USH3A transcripts encode clarin-1, a four-transmembrane-domain protein with a possible role in sensory synapses. Eur J Hum Genet 10(6):339–50.

Ahmed ZM, Riazuddin S, Wilcox ER. 2003. The molecular genetics of Usher syndrome. Clin Genet 63(6):431–44.

Akasaka-Manya K, Manya H, Kobayashi K, Toda T, Endo T. 2004. Structure-function analysis of human protein O-linked mannose beta1, 2-N-acetylglucosaminyltransferase 1, POMGnT1. Biochem Biophys Res Commun. 320(1):39–44.

Akefeldt A, Anvret M, Grandell U, Nordlinder R, Gillberg C. 1995. Parental exposure to hydrocarbons in Prader-Willi syndrome. Dev Med Child Neurol 37(12):1101–9.

Albrecht U, Sutcliffe JS, Cattanach BM, Beechey CV, Armstrong D, Eichele G, Beaudet AL. 1997. Imprinted expression of the murine Angelman syndrome gene, *Ube3a*, in hippocampal and Purkinje neurons. Nat Genet 17(1):75–8.

Allanson JE, Graham, G.E. 2002. Sex chromosome abnormalities. In: Rimoin DL, Connor JM, Pyeritz RE, Korf BR, eds. Emery and Rimoin's Principles and Practice of Medical Genetics. New York: Churchill Livingstone.

Allen KM, Gleeson JG, Bagrodia S, Partington MW, MacMillan JC, Cerione RA, Mulley JC, Walsh CA. 1998. PAK3 mutation in nonsyndromic X-linked mental retardation. Nat Genet 20(1):25–30.

American College of Medical Genetics/American Society of Human Genetics Test and Technology Transfer Committee Working Group. 2000. Tandem mass spectrometry in newborn screening. Genet Med 2(4):267–9.

American Breeders Association Eugenics Section 1912 Committee on sterilization and other means of eliminating defective germ-plasm. Preliminary report of the Committee of the Eugenic section of the American Breeders association to study and report on the best practical means for cutting off the defective germ-plasm

247

in the human population. Pamphlet 20 pages Wellcome Library London QZ50 1912.

Amir RE, Van den Veyver IB, Wan M, Tran CQ, Francke U, Zoghbi HY. 1999. Rett syndrome is caused by mutations in X-linked MECP2, encoding methyl-CpG-binding protein 2. Nat Genet 23(2):185–8.

Amos-Landgraf JM, Ji Y, Gottlieb W, Depinet T, Wandstrat AE, Cassidy SB, Driscoll DJ, Rogan PK, Schwartz S, Nicholls RD. 1999. Chromosome breakage in the Prader-Willi and Angelman syndromes involves recombination between large, transcribed repeats at proximal and distal breakpoints. Am J Hum Genet 65(2):370–86.

Anderson S, Bankier AT, Barrell BG, de Bruijn MH, Coulson AR, Drouin J, Eperon IC, Nierlich DP, Roe BA, Sanger F, et al. 1981. Sequence and organization of the human mitochondrial genome. Nature 290(5806):457–65.

Andersson U, Smith D, Jeyakumar M, Butters TD, Borja MC, Dwek RA, Platt FM. 2004. Improved outcome of N-butyldeoxygalactonojirimycin-mediated substrate reduction therapy in a mouse model of Sandhoff disease. Neurobiol Dis 16(3):506–15.

Andreasen KR, Andersen ML, Schantz AL. 2004. Obesity and pregnancy. Acta Obstet Gynecol Scand 83(11):1022–9.

Angelman H. 1965. Puppet children: a report of three cases. Dev Med Child Neurol 7:681–8.

Anton ES, Marchionni MA, Lee KF, Rakic P. 1997. Role of GGF/neuregulin signaling in interactions between migrating neurons and radial glia in the developing cerebral cortex. Development 124(18):3501–10.

Applegarth DA, Toone JR. 2001. Nonketotic hyperglycinemia (glycine encephalopathy): laboratory diagnosis. Mol Genet Metab 74(1–2):139–46.

Arai Y, Ijuin T, Takenawa T, Becker LE, Takashima S. 2002. Excessive expression of synaptojanin in brains with Down syndrome. Brain Dev 24(2):67–72.

Arnold PD, Siegel-Bartelt J, Cytrynbaum C, Teshima I, Schachar R. 2001. Velo-cardio-facial syndrome: implications of microdeletion 22q11 for schizophrenia and mood disorders. Am J Med Genet 105(4):354–62.

Assadi AH, Zhang G, Beffert U, McNeil RS, Renfro AL, Niu S, Quattrocchi CC, Antalffy BA, Sheldon M, Armstrong DD, et al. 2003. Interaction of reelin signaling and Lis1 in brain development. Nat Genet 35(3):270–6.

Association AB. 1913. A History of Mental Retardation. Baltimore: Brookes Publishing.

Augustine GJ, Santamaria F, Tanaka K. 2003. Local calcium signaling in neurons. Neuron 40(2):331–46.

Aula P, Jalanka A, Peltonen L. 2001. Asparty/glucosaminuria. In: Scriver CR, Beaudet AL, Sly W, Valle D, eds. The Metabolic and Molecular Bases of Inherited Diseases. New York: McGraw-Hill.

Ausio J, Levin DB, De Amorim GV, Bakker S, Macleod PM. 2003. Syndromes of disordered chromatin remodeling. Clin Genet 64(2):83–95.

Auranen M, Vanhala R, Varilo T, Ayers K, Kempas E, Ylisaukko-Oja T, Sinsheimer JS, Peltonen L, Jarvela I. 2002. A genomewide screen for autism-spectrum disorders: evidence for a major susceptibility locus on chromosome 3q25-27. Am J Hum Genet 71(4):777–90.

Avery OT, MacLeod CM, McCarty M. 1944. Studies on the chemical nature of the substance inducing transformation of pneumococcal types. Inductions of transformation by a desoxyribonucleic acid fraction isolated from pneumococcus type III. J Exp Med 79:137–58.

Avner P, Heard E. 2001. X-Chromosome inactivation: counting, choice and initiation. Nat Rev Genet 2(1):59–67.

Bachman KE, Rountree MR, Baylin SB. 2001. Dnmt3a and Dnmt3b are transcriptional repressors that exhibit unique localization properties to heterochromatin. J Biol Chem 276(34):32282–7.

Bailey A, Luthert P, Dean A, Harding B, Janota I, Montgomery M, Rutter M, Lantos P. 1998. A clinicopathological study of autism. Brain 121(Pt 5):889–905.

Bally-Cuif L, Hammerschmidt M. 2003. Induction and patterning of neuronal development, and its connection to cell cycle control. Curr Opin Neurobiol 13(1):16–25.

Bar I, Tissir F, Lambert de Rouvroit C, De Backer O, Goffinet AM. 2003. The gene encoding disabled-1 (DAB1), the intracellular adaptor of the Reelin pathway, reveals unusual complexity in human and mouse. J Biol Chem 278(8):5802–12.

Barlow GM, Chen XN, Shi ZY, Lyons GE, Kurnit DM, Celle L, Spinner NB, Zackai E, Pettenati MJ, Van Riper AJ, et al. 2001a. Down syndrome congenital heart disease: a narrowed region and a candidate gene. Genet Med 3(2):91–101.

Barlow GM, Micales B, Lyons GE, Korenberg JR. 2001b. Down syndrome cell adhesion molecule is conserved in mouse and highly expressed in the adult mouse brain. Cytogenet Cell Genet 94(3–4):155–62.

Barnes AP, Milgram SL. 2002. Signals from the X: signal transduction and X-linked mental retardation. Int J Dev Neurosci 20(3–5):397–406.

Barnes ND, Hull D, Balgobin L, Gompertz D. 1970. Biotin responsive propionic acidemia Lancet ii:244.

Bartsch O, Locher K, Meinecke P, Kress W, Seemanova E, Wagner A, Ostermann K, Rodel G. 2002. Molecular studies in 10 cases of Rubinstein-Taybi syndrome, including a mild variant showing a missense mutation in codon 1175 of CREBBP. J Med Genet 39(7):496–501.

Basel-Vanagaite L, Alkelai A, Straussberg R, Magal N, Inbar D, Mahajna M, Shohat M. 2003. Mapping of a new locus for autosomal recessive non-syndromic mental retardation in the chromosomal region 19p13.12-p13.2: further genetic heterogeneity. J Med Genet 40(10):729–32.

Bassez G, Camand OJ, Cacheux V, Kobetz A, Dastot-Le Moal F, Marchant D, Catala M, Abitbol M, Goossens M. 2004. Pleiotropic and diverse expression of ZFHX1B gene transcripts during mouse and human development supports the various clinical manifestations of the "Mowat-Wilson" syndrome. Neurobiol Dis 15(2):240–50.

Bateson W. 1902. Mendel's Principles of Heredity: A Defense. Cambridge: Cambridge University Press.

Bateson W. 1909. Mendel's Principles of Heredity. Cambridge: Cambridge University Press.

Battaglia A. 2003. Neuroimaging studies in the evaluation of developmental delay/mental retardation. Am J Med Genet 117C(1):25–30.

Battaglia A, Bianchini E, Carey JC. 1999. Diagnostic yield of the comprehensive assessment of developmental delay/mental retardation in an institute of child neuropsychiatry. Am J Med Genet 82(1):60–6.

Baulac S, Huberfeld G, Gourfinkel-An I, Mitropoulou G, Beranger A, Prud'homme JF, Baulac M, Brice A, Bruzzone R, LeGuern E. 2001. First genetic evidence of

GABA(A) receptor dysfunction in epilepsy: a mutation in the gamma2-subunit gene. Nat Genet 28(1):46–8.

Bauman E. 1895. Uber das normale vorkommen van Jod im Thierkorper. Z Physiol Chem 21(319).

Bauman ML, Kemper TL. 2003. The neuropathology of the autism spectrum disorders: what have we learned? Novartis Found Symp 251:112–22; discussion 122–8, 281–97.

Baumgartner MR, Saudubray JM. 2002. Peroxisomal disorders. Semin Neonatol 7(1):85–94.

Baumgartner MR, Dantas MF, Suormala T, Almashanu S, Giunta C, Friebel D, Gebhardt B, Fowler B, Hoffmann GF, Baumgartner ER, et al. 2004. Isolated 3-methylcrotonyl-CoA carboxylase deficiency: evidence for an allele-specific dominant negative effect and responsiveness to biotin therapy. Am J Hum Genet 75(5):790–800.

Bayes M, Magano LF, Rivera N, Flores R, Perez Jurado LA. 2003. Mutational mechanisms of Williams-Beuren syndrome deletions. Am J Hum Genet 73(1):131–51.

Beadle G, Tatum E. 1941. Genetic control of biochemical reactions in *Neurospora*. Proc Natl Acad Sci USA 27:499–506.

Bear MF, Abraham WC. 1996. Long-term depression in hippocampus. Annu Rev Neurosci 19:437–62.

Beck M. 2000. Mucopolysaccharidoses and oligosaccharidoses. In: J Fernandes JM Saudubray, G. van den Berghe, eds. Inborn Metabolic Diseases. Berlin, Heidelberg, New York: Springer Verlag.

Beique JC, Chapin-Penick EM, Mladenovic L, Andrade R. 2004. Serotonergic facilitation of synaptic activity in the developing rat prefrontal cortex. J Physiol 556(Pt 3):739–54.

Belichenko PV, Hagberg B, Dahlstrom A. 1997. Morphological study of neocortical areas in Rett syndrome. Acta Neuropathol (Berl) 93(1):50–61.

Bellinger DC. 2004. Lead. Pediatrics 113(4 Suppl):1016–22.

Beltran-Valero de Bernabe D, Currier S, Steinbrecher A, Celli J, van Beusekom E, van der Zwaag B, Kayserili H, Merlini L, Chitayat D, Dobyns WB, et al. 2002. Mutations in the *O*-mannosyltransferase gene *POMT1* give rise to the severe neuronal migration disorder Walker-Warburg syndrome. Am J Hum Genet 71(5):1033–43.

Berbel PJ, Escobar del Rey F, Morreale de Escobar G, Ruiz-Marcos A. 1985. Effect of hypothyroidism on the size of spines of pyramidal neurons of the cerebral cortex. Brain Res 337(2):217–23.

Berger W, van de Pol D, Warburg M, Gal A, Bleeker-Wagemakers L, de Silva H, Meindl A, Meitinger T, Cremers F, Ropers HH. 1992. Mutations in the candidate gene for Norrie disease. Hum Mol Genet 1(7):461–5.

Berkowitz GS, Wetmur JG, Birman-Deych E, Obel J, Lapinski RH, Godbold JH, Holzman IR, Wolff MS. 2004. In utero pesticide exposure, maternal paraoxonase activity, and head circumference. Environ Health Perspect 112(3):388–91.

Bernard C. 1853. Nouvelle Fonction du Foie Considere comme Organe Producteur de Matiere Sucree chez l'Homme et les Animaux. Paris: Bailliere.

Bernard SM, McGeehin MA. 2003. Prevalence of blood lead levels ≥ 5 µg/dL among US children 1 to 5 years of age and socioeconomic and demographic factors associated with blood of lead levels 5 to 10 μg/dL. Third National Health and Nutrition Examination Survey, 1988–1994. Pediatrics 112(6 Pt 1):1308–13.

Bestor TH. 2003. Imprinting errors and developmental asymmetry. Philos Trans R Soc Lond B Biol Sci 358(1436):1411–5.

Betancur C, Leboyer M, Gillberg C. 2002. Increased rate of twins among affected sibling pairs with autism. Am J Hum Genet 70(5):1381–3.

Beutler E, Grabowski G. 2001. Gaucher disease. In: Scriver CR, Beaudet AL, Sly W, Valle D, eds. The Metabolic and Molecular Bases of Inherited Disease. New York: McGraw-Hill.

Biancalana V, Beldjord C, Taillandier A, Szpiro-Tapia S, Cusin V, Gerson F, Philippe C, Mandel JL. 2004. Five years of molecular diagnosis of fragile X syndrome (1997–2001): a collaborative study reporting 95% of the activity in France. Am J Med Genet 129A(3):218–24.

Bianchi MC, Tosetti M, Fornai F, Alessandri MG, Cipriani P, De Vito G, Canapicchi R. 2000. Reversible brain creatine deficiency in two sisters with normal blood creatine level. Ann Neurol 47(4):511–3.

Bickel H. 1954. The effects of a phenylalanine-free and phenylalanine-poor diet in phenylpyruvic oligophrenis. Exp Med Surg 12(1):114–7.

Bickel H, Gerrard J, Hickmans EM. 1953. Influence of phenylalanine intake on phenylketonuria. Lancet 265(6790):812–3.

Bickel H, Gerard J, Hickmans E. 1954. The influence of phenylalanine intake on chemistry and behavior of a phenylketonuria child. Acta Pediatr 43:64–77.

Bielas SL, Gleeson JG. 2004. Cytoskeletal-associated proteins in the migration of cortical neurons. J Neurobiol 58(1):149–59.

Bienvenu T, des Portes V, Saint Martin A, McDonell N, Billuart P, Carrie A, Vinet MC, Couvert P, Toniolo D, Ropers HH, et al. 1998. Non-specific X-linked semidominant mental retardation by mutations in a Rab GDP-dissociation inhibitor. Hum Mol Genet 7(8):1311–5.

Bienvenu T, des Portes V, McDonell N, Carrie A, Zemni R, Couvert P, Ropers HH, Moraine C, van Bokhoven H, Fryns JP, et al. 2000. Missense mutation in PAK3, R67C, causes X-linked nonspecific mental retardation. Am J Med Genet 93(4):294–8.

Bienvenu T, Poirier K, Friocourt G, Bahi N, Beaumont D, Fauchereau F, Ben Jeema L, Zemni R, Vinet MC, Francis F, et al. 2002. ARX, a novel Prd-class-homeobox gene highly expressed in the telencephalon, is mutated in X-linked mental retardation. Hum Mol Genet 11(8):981–91.

Biffi A, De Palma M, Quattrini A, Del Carro U, Amadio S, Visigalli I, Sessa M, Fasano S, Brambilla R, Marchesini S, et al. 2004. Correction of metachromatic leukodystrophy in the mouse model by transplantation of genetically modified hematopoietic stem cells. J Clin Invest 113(8):1118–29.

Billuart P, Bienvenu T, Ronce N, des Portes V, Vinet MC, Zemni R, Roest Crollius H, Carrie A, Fauchereau F, Cherry M, Briault S, Hamel B, Fryns JP, Beldjord C, Kahn A, Moraine C, Chelly J. 1998. Oligophrenin-1 encodes a rhoGAP protein involved in X-linked mental retardation P 1998 Nature 392(6679):923–6.

Binder DK, Scharfman HE. 2004. Brain-derived neurotrophic factor. Growth Factors 22(3):123–31. Review.

Binet A and Simon T. 1905. Methodes nouvelles pour le diagnostic du niveau intellectal des anormaux. L' Anee Psychologique 11:191–244.

Bjornsson HT, Fallin MD, Feinberg AP. 2004. An integrated epigenetic and genetic approach to common human disease. Trends Genet 20(8):350–8.

Blass JP, Avigan J, Uhlendorf BW. 1970. A defect in pyruvate decarboxylase in a patient with an intermittent movement disorder. J Clin Invest 49:423.

Blass JP, Kark AP, Engel WK. 1971. Clinical studies of a patient with pyruvate decarboxylase deficiency. Arch Neurol 25(5):449–60.

Blatt B, Kaplan F. 1976. Photographic essay: Christmas in purgatory, see Blatt B. 1976. In: Rosen M, Clark G, Kivitz M, eds. The History of Mental Retardation, Collected Papers. Baltimore: University Park Press, pp. 345–360.

Blau N, Thony B, Cotton RGH, Hyland K. 2001. Disorders of tetrahydrobiopterin and related amines. In: Scriver CR, Beaudet AL, Sly W, Valle D, eds. The Metabolic and Molecular Bases of Inherited Disease. New York: McGraw-Hill.

Bluml S. 1999. In vivo quantitation of cerebral metabolite concentrations using natural abundance ^{13}C MRS at 1.5 T. J Magn Reson 136(2):219–25.

Bodensteiner JB, Ellis CR, Schaefer GB, 2002. Mental retardation. In: Maria BL, ed. Current Management in Child Neurology. London: BC Decker.

Boeda B, El-Amraoui A, Bahloul A, Goodyear R, Daviet L, Blanchard S, Perfettini I, Fath KR, Shorte S, Reiners J, et al. 2002. Myosin VIIa, harmonin and cadherin 23, three Usher I gene products that cooperate to shape the sensory hair cell bundle. EMBO J 21(24):6689–99.

Boespflug-Tanguy O, Mimault C, Melki J, Cavagna A, Giraud G, Pham Dinh D, Dastugue B, Dautigny A. 1994. Genetic homogeneity of Pelizaeus-Merzbacher disease: tight linkage to the proteolipoprotein locus in 16 affected families. PMD Clinical Group. Am J Hum Genet 55(3):461–7.

Bolton PF, Dennis NR, Browne CE, Thomas NS, Veltman MW, Thompson RJ, Jacobs P. 2001. The phenotypic manifestations of interstitial duplications of proximal 15q with special reference to the autistic spectrum disorders. Am J Med Genet 105(8):675–85.

Bolton PF, Veltman MW, Weisblatt E, Holmes JR, Thomas NS, Youings SA, Thompson RJ, Roberts SE, Dennis NR, Browne CE, Goodson S, Moore V, Brown J. 2004. Chromosome 15q11-13 abnormalities and other medical conditions in individuals with autism spectrum disorders. Psychiatr Genet 14:131–7.

Bonora E, Lamb JA, Barnby G, Sykes N, Moberly T, Beyer KS, Klauck SM, Poustka F, Bacchelli E, Blasi F, et al. 2005. Mutation screening and association analysis of six candidate genes for autism on chromosome 7q. Eur J Hum Genet 13(2):198–207.

Borker A, Yu LC. 2002. Unrelated allogeneic bone marrow transplant in adrenoleukodystrophy using CD34+ stem cell selection. Metab Brain Dis 17(3):139–42.

Bosch AM, Grootenhuis MA, Bakker HD, Heijmans HS, Wijburg FA, Last BF. 2004. Living with classical galactosemia: health-related quality of life consequences. Pediatrics 113(5):423–8.

Botstein D, Risch N. 2003. Discovering genotypes underlying human phenotypes: past successes for mendelian disease, future approaches for complex disease. Nat Genet 33(Suppl):228–37.

Bourgeois BF, Prensky AL, Palkes HS, Talent BK, Busch SG. 1983. Intelligence in epilepsy: a prospective study in children. Ann Neurol 14(4):438–44.

Boussinggault JB. 1825. Goitre prophylaxis. Annales de chimie et de physique. 40.

Boveri T. 1902. Uber mehrpolige mitosen als mittel zur analyse des zellkerns. Verh Phys Med Gesellsch. 35:67–90.

Bozoky Z, Alexa A, Tompa P, Friedrich P. 2004. Multiple interactions of the "transducer" govern its function in calpain activation by Ca2+. Biochem J

Brady RO, Kanfer JN, Mock MB, Fredrickson DS. 1966. The metabolism of sphingomyelin. II. Evidence of an enzymatic deficiency in Niemann-Pick disease. Proc Natl Acad Sci USA 55(2):366–9.

Braverman N, Lin P, Moebius FF, Obie C, Moser A, Glossmann H, Wilcox WR, Rimoin DL, Smith M, Kratz L, et al. 1999. Mutations in the gene encoding 3beta-hydroxysteroid-delta8,delta 7-isomerase cause X-linked dominant Conradi-Hunermann syndrome. Nat Genet 22(3):291–4.

Brenner S, Jacob F, Meselson M. 1961. An unstable intermediate carrying information from genes to ribosomes for protein synthesis Nature 190:576–81.

Brenner S. 1961. RNA, ribosomes, and protein synthesis. Cold Spring Harb Symp Quant Biol 26:101–10.

Briggs SD, Xiao T, Sun ZW, Caldwell JA, Shabanowitz J, Hunt DF, Allis CD, Strahl BD. 2002. Gene silencing: trans-histone regulatory pathway in chromatin. Nature 418(6897):498.

Brock DJ, Sutcliffe RG. 1972. Alpha-fetoprotein in the antenatal diagnosis of anencephaly and spina bifida. Lancet 2(7770):197–9.

Brown FR 3rd, McAdams AJ, Cummins JW, Konkol R, Singh I, Moser AB, Moser HW. 1982. Cerebro-hepato-renal (Zellweger) syndrome and neonatal adreno-leukodystrophy: similarities in phenotype and accumulation of very long chain fatty acids. Johns Hopkins Med J 151(6):344–51.

Brown CJ, Greally JM. 2003. A stain upon the silence: genes escaping X inactivation. Trends Genet 19(8):432–8.

Brown SA, Warburton D, Brown LY, Yu CY, Roeder ER, Stengel-Rutkowski S, Hennekam RC, Muenke M. 1998. Holoprosencephaly due to mutations in ZIC2, a homologue of Drosophila odd-paired. Nat Genet 20(2):180–3.

Brown SD. 1991. XIST and the mapping of the X chromosome inactivation centre. Bioessays 13(11):607–12.

Brownstein Z, Ben-Yosef T, Dagan O, Frydman M, Abeliovich D, Sagi M, Abraham FA, Taitelbaum-Swead R, Shohat M, Hildesheimer M, et al. 2004. The R245X mutation of PCDH15 in Ashkenazi Jewish children diagnosed with nonsyndromic hearing loss foreshadows retinitis pigmentosa. Pediatr Res 55(6):995–1000.

Brunetti-Pierri N, Corso G, Rossi M, Ferrari P, Balli F, Rivasi F, Annunziata I, Ballabio A, Russo AD, Andria G, et al. 2002. Lathosterolosis, a novel multiple-malformation/mental retardation syndrome due to deficiency of 3beta-hydroxysteroid-delta5-desaturase. Am J Hum Genet 71(4):952–8.

Brunig I, Suter A, Knuesel I, Luscher B, Fritschy JM. 2002. GABAergic terminals are required for postsynaptic clustering of dystrophin but not of GABA(A) receptors and gephyrin. J Neurosci 22(12):4805–13.

Brusilow S, Horwich A. 2001. Urea cycle enzymes. In: Scriver CR, Beaudet AL, Sly W, Valle, D, eds. The Metabolic and Molecular Bases of Inherited Disease. New York: McGraw-Hill.

Buiting K, Greger V, Brownstein BH, Mohr RM, Voiculescu I, Winterpacht A, Zabel B, Horsthemke B. 1992. A putative gene family in 15q11-13 and 16p11.2: possible implications for Prader-Willi and Angelman syndromes. Proc Natl Acad Sci USA 89(12):5457–61.

Burd L, Cotsonas-Hassler TM, Martsolf JT, Kerbeshian J. 2003a. Recognition and management of fetal alcohol syndrome. Neurotoxicol Teratol 25(6):681–8.

Burd L, Martsolf JT, Klug MG, Kerbeshian J. 2003b. Diagnosis of FAS: a comparison of the Fetal Alcohol Syndrome Diagnostic Checklist and the Institute of Medicine Criteria for Fetal Alcohol Syndrome. Neurotoxicol Teratol 25(6):719–24.

Burd L, Klug MG, Martsolf JT, Kerbeshian J. 2003c. Fetal alcohol syndrome: neuropsychiatric phenomics. Neurotoxicol Teratol 25(6):697–705.

Burri BJ, Sweetman L, Nyhan WL. 1981. Mutant holocarboxylase synthetase: evidence for the enzyme defect in early infantile biotin-responsive multiple carboxylase deficiency. J Clin Invest 68(6):1491–5.

Butler MG, Bittel DC, Kibiryeva N, Talebizadeh Z, Thompson T. 2004. Behavioral differences among subjects with Prader-Willi syndrome and type I or type II deletion and maternal disomy. Pediatrics 113(3 Pt 1):565–73.

Buxbaum JD, Silverman JM, Smith CJ, Kilifarski M, Reichert J, Hollander E, Lawlor BA, Fitzgerald M, Greenberg DA, Davis KL. 2001. Evidence for a susceptibility gene for autism on chromosome 2 and for genetic heterogeneity. Am J Hum Genet 68(6):1514–20.

Cailloux F, Gauthier-Barichard F, Mimault C, Isabelle V, Courtois V, Giraud G, Dastugue B, Boespflug-Tanguy O. 2000. Genotype–phenotype correlation in inherited brain myelination defects due to proteolipid protein gene mutations. Clinical European Network on Brain Dysmyelinating Disease. Eur J Hum Genet 8(11):837–45.

Cantley LC, Neel BG. 1999. New insights into tumor suppression: PTEN suppresses tumor formation by restraining the phosphoinositide 3-kinase/AKT pathway. Proc Natl Acad Sci USA 96(8):4240–5.

Cardoso C, Leventer RJ, Ward HL, Toyo-Oka K, Chung J, Gross A, Martin CL, Allanson J, Pilz DT, Olney AH, et al. 2003. Refinement of a 400-kb critical region allows genotypic differentiation between isolated lissencephaly, Miller-Dieker syndrome, and other phenotypes secondary to deletions of 17p13.3. Am J Hum Genet 72(4):918–30.

Carrie A, Jun L, Bienvenu T, Vinet MC, McDonell N, Couvert P, Zemni R, Cardona A, Van Buggenhout G, Frints S, et al. 1999. A new member of the IL-1 receptor family highly expressed in hippocampus and involved in X-linked mental retardation. Nat Genet 23(1):25–31.

Carvalho LR, Woods KS, Mendonca BB, Marcal N, Zamparini AL, Stifani S, Brickman JM, Arnhold IJ, Dattani MT. 2003. A homozygous mutation in HESX1 is associated with evolving hypopituitarism due to impaired repressor–corepressor interaction. J Clin Invest 112(8):1192–201.

Casanova MF, Buxhoeveden DP, Brown C. 2002. Clinical and macroscopic correlates of minicolumnar pathology in autism. J Child Neurol 17(9):692–5.

Casaubon LK, Melanson M, Lopes-Cendes I, Marineau C, Andermann E, Andermann F, Weissenbach J, Prevost C, Bouchard JP, Mathieu J, et al. 1996. The gene responsible for a severe form of peripheral neuropathy and agenesis of the corpus callosum maps to chromosome 15q. Am J Hum Genet 58(1):28–34.

Caspersson T, Zech L, Johansson C, Modest EJ. 1970. Identification of human chromosomes by DNA-binding fluorescent agents. Chromosoma 30(2):215–27.

Ceccaldi PE, Grohovaz F, Benfenati F, Chieregatti E, Greengard P, Valtorta F. 1995. Dephosphorylated synapsin I anchors synaptic vesicles to actin cytoskeleton: an analysis by videomicroscopy. J Cell Biol 128(5):905–12.

Cederbaum SD, Shaw KN, Valente M. 1977. Hyperargininemia. J Pediatr 90(4):569–73.

Cederbaum SD, Moedjono SJ, Shaw KN, Carter M, Naylor E, Walzer M. 1982. Treatment of hyperargininaemia due to arginase deficiency with a chemically defined diet. J Inherit Metab Dis 5(2):95–9.

Centerwall SA, Centerwall WR. 2000. The discovery of phenylketonuria: the story of a young couple, two retarded children, and a scientist. Pediatrics 105(1 Pt 1):89–103.

Chace DH, Kalas TA, Naylor EW. 2003. Use of tandem mass spectrometry for multianalyte screening of dried blood specimens from newborns. Clin Chem 49(11):1797–817.

Chai JH, Locke DP, Greally JM, Knoll JH, Ohta T, Dunai J, Yavor A, Eichler EE, Nicholls RD. 2003. Identification of four highly conserved genes between breakpoint hotspots BP1 and BP2 of the Prader-Willi/Angelman syndromes deletion region that have undergone evolutionary transposition mediated by flanking duplicons. Am J Hum Genet 73(4):898–925.

Chance B, Williams GR. 1956. The respiratory chain and oxidative phosphorylation. Adv Enzymol Relat Subj Biochem 17:65–134.

Chargaff E. 1950. Chemical specificity of nucleic acids and mechanisms of their enzymatic degradation. Experientia. 6:201–9.

Chechlacz M, Gleeson JG. 2003. Is mental retardation a defect of synapse structure and function? Pediatr Neurol 29(1):11–17.

Chelly J, Tumer Z, Tonnesen T, Petterson A, Ishikawa-Brush Y, Tommerup N, Horn N, Monaco AP. 1993. Isolation of a candidate gene for Menkes disease that encodes a potential heavy metal binding protein. Nat Genet 3(1):14–9.

Chen WG, Chang Q, Lin Y, Meissner A, West AE, Griffith EC, Jaenisch R, Greenberg ME. 2003. Derepression of BDNF transcription involves calcium-dependent phosphorylation of MeCP2. Science 302(5646):885–9.

Chen ZY, Hendriks RW, Jobling MA, Powell JF, Breakefield XO, Sims KB, Craig IW. 1992. Isolation and characterization of a candidate gene for Norrie disease. Nat Genet 1(3):204–8.

Cheon MS, Shim KS, Kim SH, Hara A, Lubec G. 2003. Protein levels of genes encoded on chromosome 21 in fetal Down syndrome brain: challenging the gene dosage effect hypothesis (Part IV). Amino Acids 25(1):41–7.

Chiurazzi P, Neri G, Oostra BA. 2003. Understanding the biological underpinnings of fragile X syndrome. Curr Opin Pediatr 15(6):559–66.

Chiurazzi P, Tabolacci E, Neri G. 2004. X-Linked mental retardation (XLMR): from clinical conditions to cloned genes. Crit Rev Clin Lab Sci 41(2):117–58.

Christensen B, Arbour L, Tran P, Leclerc D, Sabbaghian N, Platt R, Gilfix BM, Rosenblatt DS, Gravel RA, Forbes P, et al. 1999. Genetic polymorphisms in methylenetetrahydrofolate reductase and methionine synthase, folate levels in red blood cells, and risk of neural tube defects. Am J Med Genet 84(2):151–7.

Chuang DT, Shih V. 2001. Maple syrup urine disease. In: Scriver CR, Beaudet AL, Sly W, Valle D, eds. The Metabolic and Molecular Bases of Inherited Diseases. New York: McGraw-Hill.

Claes L, Ceulemans B, Audenaert D, Smets K, Lofgren A, Del-Favero J, Ala-Mello S, Basel-Vanagaite L, Plecko B, Raskin S, et al. 2003. De novo SCN1A mutations are a major cause of severe myoclonic epilepsy of infancy. Hum Mutat 21(6):615–21.

Clark AG. 2003. Finding genes underlying risk of complex disease by linkage disequilibrium mapping. Curr Opin Genet Dev 13(3):296–302.

Clarke JT. 2003. The Maternal Phenylketonuria Project: a summary of progress and challenges for the future. Pediatrics 112(6 Pt 2):1584–7.

Clayton-Smith J, Laan L. 2003. Angelman syndrome: a review of the clinical and genetic aspects. J Med Genet 40(2):87–95.

Clerc P, Avner P. 2003. Multiple elements within the Xic regulate random X inactivation in mice. Semin Cell Dev Biol 14(1):85–92.

Coffee B, Zhang F, Ceman S, Warren ST, Reines D. 2002. Histone modifications depict an aberrantly heterochromatinized *FMR1* gene in fragile X syndrome. Am J Hum Genet 71(4):923–32.

Cohen MM Jr. 2003a. Craniofacial anomalies: clinical and molecular perspectives. Ann Acad Med Singapore 32(2):244–51.

Cohen MM Jr. 2003b. Mental deficiency, alterations in performance, and CNS abnormalities in overgrowth syndromes. Am J Med Genet 117:49–56.

Cohen MM Jr. 2003c. The hedgehog signaling network. Am J Med Genet A 123(1):5–28.

Cohen MM Jr, Shiota K. 2002. Teratogenesis of holoprosencephaly. Am J Med Genet 109(1):1–15.

Cohen-Cory S, Lom B. 2004. Neurotrophic regulation of retinal ganglion cell synaptic connectivity: from axons and dendrites to synapses. Int J Dev Biol 48(8–9):947–56.

Collins RC, Olney JW, Lothman EW. 1983. Metabolic and pathological consequences of focal seizures. Res Publ Assoc Res Nerv Ment Dis 61:87–107.

Cone T. 1979. History of American Pediatrics. Boston: Little, Brown and Co., pp. 155–156.

Copp AJ, Greene ND, Murdoch JN. 2003. The genetic basis of mammalian neurulation. Nat Rev Genet 4(10):784–93.

Cori G, Cori C, Schmidt G. 1939. The role of glucose-1-phosphate in the formation of blood sugar and synthesis of glycogen in the liver. J Biol Chem 129:629–39.

Cormand B, Pihko H, Bayes M, Valanne L, Santavuori P, Talim B, Gershoni-Baruch R, Ahmad A, van Bokhoven H, Brunner HG, Voit T, Topaloglu H, Dobyns WB, Lehesjoki AE. 2001. Clinical and genetic distinction between Walker-Warburg syndrome and muscle-eye-brain disease. Neurology 56(8):1059–69.

Correns C. 1900. [G. Mendel's law concerning the behavior of progeny of varietal hybrids.] in German Ber. Bot. Ges. 18, 158–168 Translated 1950 Genetics 35(52):33–41.

Costa RM, Federov NB, Kogan JH, Murphy GG, Stern J, Ohno M, Kucherlapati R, Jacks T, Silva AJ. 2002. Mechanism for the learning deficits in a mouse model of neurofibromatosis type 1. Nature 415(6871):526–30.

Coupry I, Monnet L, Attia AA, Taine L, Lacombe D, Arveiler B. 2004. Analysis of CBP (CREBBP) gene deletions in Rubinstein-Taybi syndrome patients using real-time quantitative PCR. Hum Mutat 23(3):278–84.

Couvert P, Bienvenu T, Aquaviva C, Poirier K, Moraine C, Gendrot C, Verloes A, Andres C, Le Fevre AC, Souville I, et al. 2001. MECP2 is highly mutated in X-linked mental retardation. Hum Mol Genet 10(9):941–6.

Cremer RJ, Perryman PW, Richards DH. 1958. Influence of light on the hyper-bilirubinaemia of infants. Lancet 1(7030):1094–7.

Crick FH, Barnett L, Brenner S, Watts-Tobin RJ. 1961. General nature of the genetic code for proteins. Nauchni Tr Vissh Med Inst Sofiia 192:1227–32.

Culotta VC, Lin SJ, Schmidt P, Klomp LW, Casareno RL, Gitlin J. 1999. Intracellular pathways of copper trafficking in yeast and humans. Adv Exp Med Biol 448:247–54.

Curl CL, Fenske RA, Kissel JC, Shirai JH, Moate TF, Griffith W, Coronado G, Thompson B. 2002. Evaluation of take-home organophosphorus pesticide exposure among agricultural workers and their children. Environ Health Perspect 110(12):A787–92.

Curry CJ, Stevenson RE, Aughton D, Byrne J, Carey JC, Cassidy S, Cunniff C, Graham JM Jr, Jones MC, Kaback MM, et al. 1997. Evaluation of mental retardation: recommendations of a consensus conference: American College of Medical Genetics. Am J Med Genet 72(4):468–77.

D'Adamo P, Menegon A, Lo Nigro C, Grasso M, Gulisano M, Tamanini F, Bienvenu T, Gedeon AK, Oostra B, Wu SK, et al. 1998. Mutations in GDI1 are responsible for X-linked non-specific mental retardation. Nat Genet 19(2):134–9.

D'Adamo P, Welzl H, Papadimitriou S, Raffaele di Barletta M, Tiveron C, Tatangelo L, Pozzi L, Chapman PF, Knevett SG, Ramsay MF, et al. 2002. Deletion of the mental retardation gene *Gdi1* impairs associative memory and alters social behavior in mice. Hum Mol Genet 11(21):2567–80.

Dahia PL, Marsh DJ, Zheng Z, Zedenius J, Komminoth P, Frisk T, Wallin G, Parsons R, Longy M, Larsson C, et al. 1997. Somatic deletions and mutations in the Cowden disease gene, *PTEN*, in sporadic thyroid tumors. Cancer Res 57(21):4710–3.

Dahl HH. 1998. Getting to the nucleus of mitochondrial disorders: identification of respiratory chain-enzyme genes causing Leigh syndrome. Am J Hum Genet 63(6):1594–7.

Dahmane N, Sanchez P, Gitton Y, Palma V, Sun T, Beyna M, Weiner H, Ruiz i Altaba A. 2001. The Sonic Hedgehog–Gli pathway regulates dorsal brain growth and tumorigenesis. Development 128(24):5201–12.

Danks DM. 1978. Pteridines and phenylketonuria: report of a workshop. Introductory comments. J Inherit Metab Dis 1(2):47–8.

Darrow, Clarence. 1925. The Edwards and The Jukes. American Mercury 6:147–57.

Darrow, Clarence. 1926. The Eugenics cult. American Mercury 8:129–37.

Darvill T, Lonky E, Reihman J, Stewart P, Pagano J. 2000. Prenatal exposure to PCBs and infant performance on the fagan test of infant intelligence. Neurotoxicology 21(6):1029–38.

Dattani MT, Martinez-Barbera JP, Thomas PQ, Brickman JM, Gupta R, Martensson IL, Toresson H, Fox M, Wales JK, Hindmarsh PC, et al. 1998. Mutations in the homeobox gene *HESX1/Hesx1* associated with septo-optic dysplasia in human and mouse. Nat Genet 19(2):125–33.

D'Azzo A, Hoogeveen A, Reuser AJ, Robinson D, Galjaard H. 1982. Molecular defect in combined beta-galactosidase and neuraminidase deficiency in man. Proc Natl Acad Sci USA 79(15):4535–9.

Debrand E, Chureau C, Arnaud D, Avner P, Heard E. 1999. Functional analysis of the DXPas34 locus, a 3' regulator of Xist expression. Mol Cell Biol 19(12):8513–25.

De Duve C. 1963. The lysosome concept. In: Ciba Foundation Symposium on Lysosomes. London: Churchill.

De Duve C, Baudhuin P. 1966. Peroxisomes. Physiol Rev 46:323–57.

de Koning TJ, Snell K, Duran M, Berger R, Poll-The BT, Surtees R. 2003. L-Serine in disease and development. Biochem J 371(Pt 3):653–61.

de Lange C. 1933. Sur un type nouveau de generation (typus Amsteldamensis). Arch Med Engant 36:713.

Deguchi K, Inoue K, Avila WE, Lopez-Terrada D, Antalffy BA, Quattrocchi CC, Sheldon M, Mikoshiba K, D'Arcangelo G, Armstrong DL. 2003. Reelin and disabled-1 expression in developing and mature human cortical neurons. J Neuropathol Exp Neurol 62(6):676–84.

Delprat B, Michel V, Goodyear R, Yamasaki Y, Michalski N, El-Amraoui A, Perfettini I, Legrain P, Richardson G, Hardelin JP, et al. 2005. Myosin XVa and whirlin, two deafness gene products required for hair bundle growth, are located at the stereocilia tips and interact directly. Hum Mol Genet 14(3):401–10.

Denis PS. 1830. Recherches expérimentales sur le sang humain, considéré à l'état sain, faites pour déterminer les modifications auxquelles est sujette dans l'économie la composition de cette humeur, et apprécier les phénomènes physiologiques qui s'y rapportent, mémoire présenté à l'Institut, Académie des Sciences, en 1828 Commercy : C. F. Denis.

Dermitzakis ET, Reymond A, Scamuffa N, Ucla C, Kirkness E, Rossier C, Antonarakis SE. 2003. Evolutionary discrimination of mammalian conserved non-genic sequences (CNGs). Science 302(5647):1033–5.

Desi I, Nagymajtenyi L, Schulz H, Nehez M. 1998. Epidemiological investigations and experimental model studies on exposure of pesticides.Toxicol Lett 96–97:351–9.

DesGeorges J. 2003. Family perceptions of early hearing, detection, and intervention systems: listening to and learning from families. Ment Retard Dev Disabil Res Rev 9(2):89–93.

des Portes V, Beldjord C, Chelly J, Hamel B, Kremer H, Smits A, van Bokhoven H, Ropers HH, Claes S, Fryns JP, et al. 1999. X-Linked nonspecific mental retardation (MRX) linkage studies in 25 unrelated families: the European XLMR Consortium. Am J Med Genet 85(3):263–5.

De Vries BB, Winter R, Schinzel A, van Ravenswaaij-Arts C. 2003. Telomeres: a diagnosis at the end of the chromosomes. J Med Genet 40(6):385–98.

De Vries H, 1900. Sur les unites des caracteres specifiques et leur application a l'etude des hybrids. Rev Gener Botan 12:257–71.

Dewald GW, Buckley DD, Spurbeck JL, Jalal SM. 1992. Cytogenetic guidelines for fragile X studies tested in routine practice. Am J Med Genet 44(6):816–21.

Diadori P, Carmant L. 2002. The neurologic examination. In: Maria BL, ed. Current Management in Child Neurology. London: BC Decker.

Diamond L, Blackfan KD, Baty JM. 1932. Erythroblastosis fetalis and its association with universal edema of the fetus, icterus gravis, neonatorum and anemia of the newborn. J Pediatr 1:269.

Diaz-Meyer N, Day CD, Khatod K, Maher ER, Cooper W, Reik W, Junien C, Graham G, Algar E, Der Kaloustian VM, et al. 2003. Silencing of CDKN1C (p57KIP2) is associated with hypomethylation at KvDMR1 in Beckwith-Wiedemann syndrome. J Med Genet 40(11):797–801.

Dick RB, Steenland K, Krieg EF, Hines CJ. 2001. Evaluation of acute sensory-motor effects and test sensitivity using termiticide workers exposed to chlorpyrifos. Neurotoxicol Teratol 23(4):381–93.

Ding H, Beckers MC, Plaisance S, Marynen P, Collen D, Belayew A. 1998. Characterization of a double homeodomain protein (DUX1) encoded by a cDNA homologous to 3.3 kb dispersed repeated elements. Hum Mol Genet 7(11):1681–94.

Di Palma F, Holme RH, Bryda EC, Belyantseva IA, Pellegrino R, Kachar B, Steel KP, Noben-Trauth K. 2001. Mutations in Cdh23, encoding a new type of cadherin, cause stereocilia disorganization in waltzer, the mouse model for Usher syndrome type 1D. Nat Genet 27(1):103–7.

Dixon-Salazar T, Silhavy JL, Marsh SE, Louie CM, Scott LC, Gururaj A, Al-Gazali L, Al-Tawari AA, Kayserili H, Sztriha L, et al. 2004. Mutations in the *AHI1* gene, encoding jouberin, cause Joubert syndrome with cortical polymicrogyria. Am J Hum Genet 75(6):979–87.

Doll, E. 1936. The Vineland School Maturity Scale. Publication of the training school at Vineland. Dept. of Research Series. 3: April.

Doskeland AP, Flatmark T. 2001. Conjugation of phenylalanine hydroxylase with polyubiquitin chains catalysed by rat liver enzymes. Biochim Biophys Acta 1547(2):379–86.

Douglas J, Hanks S, Temple IK, Davies S, Murray A, Upadhyaya M, Tomkins S, Hughes HE, Cole TR, Rahman N. 2003. NSD1 mutations are the major cause of Sotos syndrome and occur in some cases of Weaver syndrome but are rare in other overgrowth phenotypes. Am J Hum Genet 72(1):132–43.

Dover J, Schneider J, Tawiah-Boateng MA, Wood A, Dean K, Johnston M, Shilatifard A. 2002. Methylation of histone H3 by COMPASS requires ubiquitination of histone H2B by Rad6. J Biol Chem 277(32):28368–71.

Down, John Langdon.1866. Observations on an ethnic classification in idiots. London Hospital Reports 3:25.

Down JL. 1876. On the Education and Training of the Feeble in Mind. London: Lewis.

Down JL. 1887. Mental Affections of Childhood and Youth. London: J. and A. Churchill.

Dravet C. 2000. Severe myoclonic epilepsy in infants and its related syndromes. Epilepsia 41(Suppl 9):7.

Dreyfus M, Regnier P. 2002. The poly(A) tail of mRNAs: bodyguard in eukaryotes, scavenger in bacteria. Cell 111(5):611–3.

Dubourg C, Lazaro L, Pasquier L, Bendavid C, Blayau M, Le Duff F, Durou MR, Odent S, David V. 2004. Molecular screening of *SHH*, *ZIC2*, *SIX3*, and *TGIF* genes in patients with features of holoprosencephaly spectrum: mutation review and genotype–phenotype correlations. Hum Mutat 24(1):43–51.

Duerbeck NB. 1997. Fetal alcohol syndrome. Compr Ther 23(3):179–83.

Dussault JH, Laberge C. 1973. Thyroxine (T4) determination by radioimmunological method in dried blood eluate: new diagnostic method of neonatal hypothyroidism? (in French). Union Med Can 102(10):2062–4.

Dykens EM, Cassidy SB, King BH. 1999. Maladaptive behavior differences in Prader-Willi syndrome due to paternal deletion versus maternal uniparental disomy. Am J Ment Retard 104(1):67–77.

Dykens EM, Sutcliffe JS, Levitt P. 2004. Autism and 15q11-q13 disorders: behavioral, genetic, and pathophysiological issues. Ment Retard Dev Disabil Res Rev 10(4):284–91. Review.

Egan MF, Kojima M, Callicott JH, Goldberg TE, Kolachana BS, Bertolino A, Zaitsev E, Gold B, Goldman D, Dean M, et al. 2003. The BDNF val66met polymorphism affects activity-dependent secretion of BDNF and human memory and hippocampal function. Cell 112(2):257–69.

Eigsti IM, Shapiro T. 2003. A systems neuroscience approach to autism: biological, cognitive, and clinical perspectives. Ment Retard Dev Disabil Res Rev 9(3):205–15. Review.

Eliot TS. 1942. Little Gidding in Four Quartets reprinted 1991 in Poems of TS Eliot 1909–1962. New York, London: Harcourt Brace and Co., p. 208.

Emden G, Lacuer F. 1921. Uber die Chemie des Lactacidogens III. Z Physiol Chem 113:1–9.

Enard W, Khaitovich P, Klose J, Zollner S, Heissig F, Giavalisco P, Nieselt-Struwe K, Muchmore E, Varki A, Ravid R, et al. 2002a. Intra- and interspecific variation in primate gene expression patterns. Science 296(5566):340–3.

Enard W, Przeworski M, Fisher SE, Lai CS, Wiebe V, Kitano T, Monaco AP, Paabo S. 2002b. Molecular evolution of *FOXP2*, a gene involved in speech and language. Nature 418(6900):869–72.

Endo F, Matsuura T, Yanagita K, Matsuda I. 2004. Clinical manifestations of inborn errors of the urea cycle and related metabolic disorders during childhood. J Nutr 134(6 Suppl):1605S–9S; discussion 1630S–2S, 1667S–72S.

Eng C. 2003. *PTEN*: one gene, many syndromes. Hum Mutat 22(3):183–98.

Engelke UF, Liebrand-van Sambeek ML, de Jong JG, Leroy JG, Morava E, Smeitink JA, Wevers RA. 2004. *N*-Acetylated metabolites in urine: proton nuclear magnetic resonance spectroscopic study on patients with inborn errors of metabolism. Clin Chem 50(1):58–66.

Erlandsen H, Patch MG, Gamez A, Straub M, Stevens RC. 2003. Structural studies on phenylalanine hydroxylase and implications toward understanding and treating phenylketonuria. Pediatrics 112(6 Pt 2):1557–65.

Ephrussi B, Beadle GW. 1935. La transplantation des disque imaginaux chez le Drosophile. CR Acad Sci Paris 201:91–6.

Ephrussi B, Beadle GW. 1936. The differentiation of eye pigments in Drosophila as studied by transplantation. Genetics 21:225–7.

Eskes TK. 2002. Folic acid and homocysteine as risk factors for neural tube defects. In: Massaro EJ, Rogers JM, eds. Folate and Human Development. Totowa, NJ: Humana Press.

Evans MJ, Kaufman MH. 1981. Establishment in culture of pluripotential cells from mouse embryos. Nature 292(5819):154–6.

Evans PD, Anderson JR, Vallender EJ, Gilbert SL, Malcom CM, Dorus S, Lahn BT. 2004. Adaptive evolution of ASPM, a major determinant of cerebral cortical size in humans. Hum Mol Genet 13(5):489–94.

Evenhuis HM, Theunissen M, Denkers I, Verschuure H, Kemme H. 2001. Prevalence of visual and hearing impairment in a Dutch institutionalized population with intellectual disability. J Intellect Disabil Res 45(Pt 5):457–64.

Fagge C. 1871. Sporadic cretinism occurring in England. Br Med J 1:279.

Faiella A, Brunelli S, Granata T, D'Incerti L, Cardini R, Lenti C, Battaglia G, Boncinelli E. 1997. A number of schizencephaly patients including 2 brothers are heterozygous for germline mutations in the homeobox gene *EMX2*. Eur J Hum Genet 5(4):186–90.

Fan JQ, Ishii S, Asano N, Suzuki Y. 1999. Accelerated transport and maturation of lysosomal alpha-galactosidase A in Fabry lymphoblasts by an enzyme inhibitor. Nat Med 5(1):112–5.

Fang P, Lev-Lehman E, Tsai TF, Matsuura T, Benton CS, Sutcliffe JS, Christian SL, Kubota T, Halley DJ, Meijers-Heijboer H, et al. 1999. The spectrum of mutations in UBE3A causing Angelman syndrome. Hum Mol Genet 8(1):129–35.

Fazzi E, Signorini SG, Scelsa B, Bova SM, Lanzi G. 2003. Leber's congenital amaurosis: an update. Eur J Paediatr Neurol 7(1):13–22.

Felisari G, Martinelli Boneschi F, Bardoni A, Sironi M, Comi GP, Robotti M, Turconi AC, Lai M, Corrao G, Bresolin N. 2000. Loss of Dp140 dystrophin isoform and intellectual impairment in Duchenne dystrophy. Neurology 55(4):559–64.

Felsenfeld G, Groudine M. 2003. Controlling the double helix. Nature 421(6921):448–53.

Feng Y, Walsh CA. 2004. Mitotic spindle regulation by Nde1 controls cerebral cortical size. Neuron 44(2):279–93.

Feng Y, Olson EC, Stukenberg PT, Flanagan LA, Kirschner MW, Walsh CA. 2000. LIS1 regulates CNS lamination by interacting with mNudE, a central component of the centrosome. Neuron 28(3):665–79.

Fenton WA, Gravel RA, Rosenblatt DS. 2001. Disorders of propionate and methylmalonate Metabolism. In: Scriver CR, Beaudet AL, Sly W, Valle D, eds. The Metabolic and Molecular Bases of Inherited Diseases. New York: McGraw-Hill.

Ferdinandusse S, Denis S, Van Roermund CW, Wanders RJ, Dacremont G. 2004. Identification of the peroxisomal beta-oxidation enzymes involved in the degradation of long-chain dicarboxylic acids. J Lipid Res 45(6):1104–11.

Ferland RJ, Eyaid W, Collura RV, Tully LD, Hill RS, Al-Nouri D, Al-Rumayyan A, Topcu M, Gascon G, Bodell A, et al. 2004. Abnormal cerebellar development and axonal decussation due to mutations in AHI1 in Joubert syndrome. Nat Genet 36(9):1008–13.

Filipek PA. 1996. Neuroimaging in autism: the state of the science 1995. J Autism Dev Disord 26(2):211–5.

Filippi CG, Ulug AM, Deck MD, Zimmerman RD, Heier LA. 2002. Developmental delay in children: assessment with proton MR spectroscopy. AJNR Am J Neuroradiol 23(5):882–8.

Finckh U, Schroder J, Ressler B, Veske A, Gal A. 2000. Spectrum and detection rate of L1CAM mutations in isolated and familial cases with clinically suspected L1-disease. Am J Med Genet 92(1):40–6.

Fire A, Xu S, Montgomery MK, Kostas SA, Driver SE, Mello CC. 1998. Potent and specific genetic interference by double-stranded RNA in *Caenorhabditis elegans*. Nature 391(6669):806–11.

Fischer E. 1894. Einfluss der Konfiguration auf dir Wirkung der Enzyme. Berl Chem Ges 27:2985–93.

Fisher E. 1906. Untersuchungen uber Aminosauren, Polypeptide, und Proteine. Berl Chem Ges 39:530–610.

Fisher SE, Lai CS, Monaco AP. 2003. Deciphering the genetic basis of speech and language disorders. Annu Rev Neurosci 26:57–80.

Flint J, Knight S. 2003. The use of telomere probes to investigate submicroscopic rearrangements associated with mental retardation. Curr Opin Genet Dev 13(3):310–6.

Fol H. 1979. See Fulton J. 1972. Molecules and Life: Historical Essay on the Interplay of Chemistry and Biology. New York: Wiley Interscience, p. 196.

Folger KR, Wong EA, Wahl G, Capecchi MR. 1982. Patterns of integration of DNA microinjected into cultured mammalian cells: evidence for homologous recombination between injected plasmid DNA molecules. Mol Cell Biol 2(11):1372–87.

Folling A. 1934. Phenylpyruvic acid as a metabolic abnormality in connection with imbecility. Z Physiol Chem 227:169–176.

Fombonne E. 2003. Modern views of autism. Can J Psychiatry 48(8):503–5.

Ford CE, Jones KW, Polani PE, De Almeida JC, Briggs JH. 1959. A sex-chromosome anomaly in a case of gonadal dysgenesis (Turner's syndrome). Lancet 1(7075):711–3.

Fortey R. 2004. Earth: an Intimate History. New York: Knopf.

Fourcade S, Savary S, Gondcaille C, Berger J, Netik A, Cadepond F, El Etr M, Molzer B, Bugaut M. 2003. Thyroid hormone induction of the adrenoleukodystrophy-related gene (ABCD2). Mol Pharmacol 63(6):1296–303.

Fox JW, Lamperti ED, Eksioglu YZ, Hong SE, Feng Y, Graham DA, Scheffer IE, Dobyns WB, Hirsch BA, Radtke RA, et al. 1998. Mutations in filamin 1 prevent migration of cerebral cortical neurons in human periventricular heterotopia. Neuron 21(6):1315–25.

Francastel C, Magis W, Groudine M. 2001. Nuclear relocation of a transactivator subunit precedes target gene activation. Proc Natl Acad Sci USA 98(21):12120–5.

Frankenburg WK, Duncan BR, Coffelt RW, Koch R, Coldwell JG, Son CD. 1968. Maternal phenylketonuria: implications for growth and development. J Pediatr 73(4):560–70.

Franklin RE, Gosling RG. 1953. Molecular configuration in sodium thymonucleate. Nature 171:740–741.

Freiman RN, Tjian R. 2003. Regulating the regulators: lysine modifications make their mark. Cell 112(1):11–7.

Freimer N, Sabatti C. 2003. The human phenome project. Nat Genet 34(1):15–21.

Freude K, Hoffmann K, Jensen LR, Delatycki MB, des Portes V, Moser B, Hamel B, van Bokhoven H, Moraine C, Fryns JP, et al. 2004. Mutations in the FTSJ1 gene coding for a novel S-adenosylmethionine-binding protein cause nonsyndromic X-linked mental retardation. Am J Hum Genet 75(2):305–9.

Frints SG, Froyen G, Marynen P, Fryns JP. 2002. X-Linked mental retardation: vanishing boundaries between non-specific (MRX) and syndromic (MRXS) forms. Clin Genet 62(6):423–32.

Frints SG, Jun L, Fryns JP, Devriendt K, Teulingkx R, Van den Berghe L, De Vos B, Borghgraef M, Chelly J, Des Portes V, et al. 2003. Inv(X)(p21.1;q22.1) in a man with mental retardation, short stature, general muscle wasting, and facial dysmorphism: clinical study and mutation analysis of the NXF5 gene. Am J Med Genet 119A(3):367–74.

Fruman DA, Meyers RE, Cantley LC. 1998. Phosphoinositide kinases. Annu Rev Biochem 67:481–507.

Fryns JP, Borghgraef M, Brown TW, Chelly J, Fisch GS, Hamel B, Hanauer A, Lacombe D, Luo L, MacPherson JN, et al. 2000. 9th International workshop on fragile X syndrome and X-linked mental retardation. Am J Med Genet 94(5):345–60.

Fryns JP, de Ravel TJ. 2002. In London Dysmorphology Database, London Neurogenetics Database and Dysmorphology Photo Library on CD-ROM [version 3]. Hum Genet 111(1):113.

Fryns JP, Kleczkowska A, Kubien E, Van den Berghe H. 1995. XYY syndrome and other Y chromosome polysomies. Mental status and psychosocial functioning. Genet Couns 6(3):197–206.

Fujiwara T, Sugawara T, Mazaki-Miyazaki E, Takahashi Y, Fukushima K, Watanabe M, Hara K, Morikawa T, Yagi K, Yamakawa K, et al. 2003. Mutations of sodium channel alpha subunit type 1 (SCN1A) in intractable childhood epilepsies with frequent generalized tonic-clonic seizures. Brain 126(Pt 3):531–46.

Funakoshi M, Goto K, Arahata K. 1998. Epilepsy and mental retardation in a subset of early onset 4q35-facioscapulohumeral muscular dystrophy. Neurology 50(6):1791–4.

Funk C. 1912. On the chemical nature of the substance which cures polyneuritis in birds induced by a diet of polished rice. J Physiol 43:1911–12.

Gabellini D, Green MR, Tupler R. 2002. Inappropriate gene activation in FSHD: a repressor complex binds a chromosomal repeat deleted in dystrophic muscle. Cell 110(3):339–48.

Gabriels J, Beckers MC, Ding H, De Vriese A, Plaisance S, van der Maarel SM, Padberg GW, Frants RR, Hewitt JE, Collen D, et al. 1999. Nucleotide sequence of the partially deleted D4Z4 locus in a patient with FSHD identifies a putative gene within each 3.3 kb element. Gene 236(1):25–32.

Gage FH. 2002. Neurogenesis in the adult brain. J Neurosci 22(3):612–3.

Gage NM, Siegel B, Callen M, Roberts TP. 2003. Cortical sound processing in children with autism disorder: an MEG investigation. Neuroreport 14(16):2047–51.

Gallagher L, Becker K, Kearney G, Dunlop A, Stallings R, Green A, Fitzgerald M, Gill M. 2003. Brief report: A case of autism associated with del(2)(q32.1q32.2) or (q32.2q32.3). J Autism Dev Disord 33(1):105–8.

Galler JR, Ramsey F, Solimano G, Kucharski LT, Harrison R. 1984. The influence of early malnutrition on subsequent behavioral development. IV. Soft neurologic signs. Pediatr Res 18(9):826–32.

Galler JR, Ramsey FC, Morley DS, Archer E, Salt P. 1990. The long-term effects of early kwashiorkor compared with marasmus. IV. Performance on the national high school entrance examination. Pediatr Res 28(3):235–9.

Galler JR, Ramsey FC, Harrison RH, Brooks R, Weiskopf-Bock S. 1998. Infant feeding practices in Barbados predict later growth. J Nutr 128(8):1328–35.

Garcia CC, Blair HJ, Seager M, Coulthard A, Tennant S, Buddles M, Curtis A, Goodship JA. 2004. Identification of a mutation in synapsin I, a synaptic vesicle protein, in a family with epilepsy. J Med Genet 41(3):183–6.

Garrod A. 1908, 1909. Inborn Errors of Metabolism. The Croonian Lectures Delivered before the Royal College of Physicians of London in June 1908. London: Frowde, Hodder, and Stoughton.

Garrod A. 1923. Inborn Errors of Metabolism, 2nd ed. London: Frowde, Hodder, and Stoughton.

Gaughan DJ, Kluijtmans LA, Barbaux S, McMaster D, Young IS, Yarnell JW, Evans A, Whitehead AS. 2001. The methionine synthase reductase (MTRR) A66G polymorphism is a novel genetic determinant of plasma homocysteine concentrations. Atherosclerosis 157(2):451–6.

Gauthier J, Joober R, Mottron L, Laurent S, Fuchs M, De Kimpe V, Rouleau GA. 2003. Mutation screening of FOXP2 in individuals diagnosed with autistic disorder. Am J Med Genet 118A(2):172–5.

Gecz J, Oostra BA, Hockey A, Carbonell P, Turner G, Haan EA, Sutherland GR, Mulley JC. 1997. FMR2 expression in families with FRAXE mental retardation. Hum Mol Genet 6(3):435–41.

Gehring WJ. 1985a. Homeotic genes, the homeo box, and the genetic control of development. Cold Spring Harb Symp Quant Biol 50:243–51.

Gehring WJ. 1985b. Homeotic genes, the homeobox, and the spatial organization of the embryo. Harvey Lect 81:153–72.

Geiman TM, Sankpal UT, Robertson AK, Chen Y, Mazumdar M, Heale JT, Schmiesing JA, Kim W, Yokomori K, Zhao Y, et al. 2004. Isolation and characterization of a novel DNA methyltransferase complex linking DNMT3B with components of the mitotic chromosome condensation machinery. Nucleic Acids Res 32(9):2716–29.

Gerritsen T, Kaveggia E, Waisman HA. 1965. A new type of idiopathic hyperglycinemia with hypo-oxaluria. Pediatrics 36(6):882–91.

Geschwind DH, Boone KB, Miller BL, Swerdloff RS. 2000. Neurobehavioral phenotype of Klinefelter syndrome. Ment Retard Dev Disabil Res Rev 6(2):107–16.

Giardino D, Finelli P, Gottardi G, De Canal G, Della Monica M, Lonardo F, Scarano G, Larizza L. 2003. Narrowing the candidate region of Albright hereditary osteodystrophy-like syndrome by deletion mapping in a patient with an unbalanced cryptic translocation t(2;6)(q37.3;q26). Am J Med Genet A 122(3):261–5.

Gibbons RJ, Picketts DJ, Villard L, Higgs DR. 1995. Mutations in a putative global transcriptional regulator cause X-linked mental retardation with alpha-thalassemia (ATR-X syndrome). Cell 80(6):837–45.

Gibbons RJ, McDowell TL, Raman S, O'Rourke DM, Garrick D, Ayyub H, Higgs DR. 2000. Mutations in ATRX, encoding a SWI/SNF-like protein, cause diverse changes in the pattern of DNA methylation. Nat Genet 24(4):368–71.

Gieselmann V, von Figura K. 1990. Advances in the molecular genetics of metachromatic leukodystrophy. J Inherit Metab Dis 13(4):560–71. Review.

Giles RE, Blanc H, Cann HM, Wallace DC. 1980. Maternal inheritance of human mitochondrial DNA. Proc Natl Acad Sci USA 77(11):6715–9.

Giliberto F, Ferreira V, Dalamon Viviana, Szijan I. 2004. Dystrophin deletions and cognitive impairment in Duchenne/Becker muscular dystrophy. Neurol Res 26:83–7.

Gjetting T, Romstad A, Haavik J, Knappskog PM, Acosta AX, Silva WA Jr, Zago MA, Guldberg P, Guttler F. 2001. A phenylalanine hydroxylase amino acid polymorphism with implications for molecular diagnostics. Mol Genet Metab 73(3):280–4.

Glickman MH, Ciechanover A. 2002. The ubiquitin–proteasome proteolytic pathway: destruction for the sake of construction. Physiol Rev 82(2):373–428.

Goldfischer S, Moore CL, Johnson AB, Spiro AJ, Valsamis MP, Wisniewski HK, Ritch RH, Norton WT, Rapin I, Gartner LM. 1973. Peroxisomal and mitochondrial defects in the cerebro-hepato-renal syndrome. Science 182(107):62–4.

Gomot M, Gendrot C, Verloes A, Raynaud M, David A, Yntema HG, Dessay S, Kalscheuer V, Frints S, Couvert P, et al. 2003. MECP2 gene mutations in non-syndromic X-linked mental retardation: phenotype–genotype correlation. Am J Med Genet A 123(2):129–39.

Gong X, Jia M, Ruan Y, Shuang M, Liu J, Wu S, Guo Y, Yang J, Ling Y, Yang X, et al. 2004. Association between the *FOXP2* gene and autistic disorder in Chinese population. Am J Med Genet B 127(1):113–6.

Good L. 2003. Translation repression by antisense sequences. Cell Mol Life Sci 60(5):854–61. Review.

Goodman CS, Shatz CJ. 1993. Developmental mechanisms that generate precise patterns of neuronal connectivity. Cell 72(Suppl):77–98. Review.

Goodman MN, Silver J, Jacobberger JW. 1993. Establishment and neurite outgrowth properties of neonatal and adult rat olfactory bulb glial cell lines. Brain Res 619(1–2):199–213.

Gordon N. 2001. Canavan disease: a review of recent developments. Eur J Paediatr Neurol 5(2):65–9.

Gottesman II. 1997. Twins: en route to QTLs for cognition. Science 276(5318):1522–3.

Gottesman II, Erlenmeyer-Kimling L. 2001. Family and twin strategies as a head start in defining prodromes and endophenotypes for hypothetical early-interventions in schizophrenia. Schizophr Res 51(1):93–102.

Gould SJ, Raymond GV, Valle D. 2001. The peroxisome Biogenesis Disorders. In: Scriver CR, Beaudet AL, Valle D, Sly WS, eds. The Metabolic Basis of Inherited Disease. New York: McGraw-Hill.

Govek EE, Newey SE, Akerman CJ, Cross JR, Van der Veken L, Van Aelst L. 2004. The X-linked mental retardation protein oligophrenin-1 is required for dendritic spine morphogenesis. Nat Neurosci 7(4):364–72.

Grabowski GA. 2004. Gaucher disease: lessons from a decade of therapy. J Pediatr 144(5 Suppl):S15–9.

Grabowski GA, Andria G, Baldellou A, Campbell PE, Charrow J, Cohen IJ, Harris CM, Kaplan P, Mengel E, Pocovi M, et al. 2004. Pediatric non-neuronopathic Gaucher disease: presentation, diagnosis and assessment. Consensus statements. Eur J Pediatr 163(2):58–66.

Graham T. 1861. Liquid diffusion applied to analysis. Philos Trans Royal Soc 151:183–224.

Granata T, Farina L, Faiella A, Cardini R, D'Incerti L, Boncinelli E, Battaglia G. 1997. Familial schizencephaly associated with EMX2 mutation. Neurology 48(5):1403–6.

Gravel RA, Kaback M, Proia RL, Sandhoff K, Suzuki K, Suzuki Kunihiko, et al. 2001. The GM$_2$ gangliosidoses. In: Scriver CR, Beaudet AL, Sly W, Valle D, eds. The Metabolic and Molecular Bases of Inherited Diseases. New York: McGraw-Hill.

Green AJ, Smith M, Yates JR. 1994. Loss of heterozygosity on chromosome 16p13.3 in hamartomas from tuberous sclerosis patients. Nat Genet 6(2):193–6.

Green DE, Tzagoloff A. 1966. The mitochondrial electron transfer chain. Arch Biochem Biophys 116(1):293–304.

Greenberg DA, Hodge SE, Sowinski J, Nicoll D. 2001. Excess of twins among affected sibling pairs with autism: implications for the etiology of autism. Am J Hum Genet 69(5):1062–7.

Gregg NM. 1941. Congenital cataract following German measles in the mother. Reprint 1991. Aust N Z J Ophthalmol 19(4):267–76.

Griffin JL. 2004. Metabolic profiles to define the genome: can we hear the phenotypes? Philos Trans R Soc Lond B Biol Sci 359(1446):857–71.

Gropman AL, Batshaw ML. 2004. Cognitive outcome in urea cycle disorders. Mol Genet Metab 81(Suppl 1):S58–62.

Grunewald S, Matthijs G, Jaeken J. 2002. Congenital disorders of glycosylation: a review. Pediatr Res 52(5):618–24.

Guerrini R, Moro F, Andermann E, Hughes E, D'Agostino D, Carrozzo R, Bernasconi A, Flinter F, Parmeggiani L, Volzone A, et al. 2003. Nonsyndromic mental retardation and cryptogenic epilepsy in women with doublecortin gene mutations. Ann Neurol 54(1):30–7.

Gueugnon F, Lambert F, Gondcaille C, Fourcade S, Bellenger J, Cadepond F, El Etr M, Savary S, Bugaut M. 2003. Dehydroepiandrosterone induction of the *Abcd2* and *Abcd3* genes encoding peroxisomal ABC transporters: implications for X-linked adrenoleukodystrophy. Adv Exp Med Biol 544:245.

Guillette EA, Meza MM, Aquilar MG, Soto AD, Garcia IE. 1998. An anthropological approach to the evaluation of preschool children exposed to pesticides in Mexico. Environ Health Perspect 106(6):347–53.

Gupta A, Tsai LH, Wynshaw-Boris A. 2002. Life is a journey: a genetic look at neocortical development. Nat Rev Genet 3(5):342–55.

Guthrie R, Susi A. 1963. A simple phenylalanine method for detecting phenylketonuria in large populations of newborn infants. Pediatrics 32:338–43.

Hallgren B. 1959. Retinitis pigmentosa combined with congenital deafness; with vestibulo-cerebellar ataxia and mental abnormality in a proportion of cases: a clinical and genetico-statistical study. Acta Psychiatr Scand 34(Suppl 138):1–101.

Hallmayer J, Glasson EJ, Bower C, Petterson B, Croen L, Grether J, Risch N. 2002. On the twin risk in autism. Am J Hum Genet 71(4):941–6.

Hamel BC, Smits AP, Otten BJ, van den Helm B, Ropers HH, Mariman EC. 1996. Familial X-linked mental retardation and isolated growth hormone deficiency: clinical and molecular findings. Am J Med Genet 64(1):35–41.

Hamel BC, Smits AP, van den Helm B, Smeets DF, Knoers NV, van Roosmalen T, Thoonen GH, Assman-Hulsmans CF, Ropers HH, Mariman EC, et al. 1999. Four families (MRX43, MRX44, MRX45, MRX52) with nonspecific X-linked mental retardation: clinical and psychometric data and results of linkage analysis. Am J Med Genet 85(3):290–304.

Hammerle B, Elizalde C, Galceran J, Becker W, Tejedor FJ. 2003. The MNB/DYRK1A protein kinase: neurobiological functions and Down syndrome implications. J Neural Transm Suppl(67):129–37.

Hamosh A, Maher JF, Bellus GA, Rasmussen SA, Johnston MV. 1998. Long-term use of high-dose benzoate and dextromethorphan for the treatment of nonketotic hyperglycinemia. J Pediatr 132(4):709–13.

Hamosh A, Johnston, MV. 2001. Non-ketotic hyperglycinemia. In: Scriver CR, Beaudet AL, Sly W, Valle D, eds. The Metabolic and Molecular Bases of Inherited Diseases. New York: McGraw-Hill.

Hampton T. 2004. Maternal diabetes and obesity may have lifelong impact on health of offspring. JAMA 292(7):789–90.

Hanein S, Perrault I, Gerber S, Tanguy G, Barbet F, Ducroq D, Calvas P, Dollfus H, Hamel C, Lopponen T, et al. 2004. Leber congenital amaurosis: comprehensive survey of the genetic heterogeneity, refinement of the clinical definition, and genotype–phenotype correlations as a strategy for molecular diagnosis. Hum Mutat 23(4):306–17.

Hannon GJ. 2002. RNA interference. Nature 418(6894):244–51.

Happle R. 1995. X-Linked dominant chondrodysplasia punctata/ichthyosis/cataract syndrome in males. Am J Med Genet 57(3):493.

Hardy G. 1900. A preliminary investigation of the conditions which determine the stability of irreversible hydrosols. Proc R Soc 66:110–25.

Harington C. 1926. Chemistry of thyroxine: isolation of thyroxine from the thyroid gland. Biochem J 20:293.

Harington C, Barger G. 1927. Chemistry of thyroxine III: constitution and synthesis of thyroxine. Biochem J 21:169–181.

Hariri AR, Goldberg TE, Mattay VS, Kolachana BS, Callicott JH, Egan MF, Weinberger DR. 2003. Brain-derived neurotrophic factor val66met polymorphism affects human memory-related hippocampal activity and predicts memory performance. J Neurosci 23(17):6690–4.

Harris H. 1972. Genetic polymorphism. Sci Basis Med Annu Rev:174–93.

Harris H, Hopkinson D, Robson E. 1973. The incidence of rare alleles determining electrophoretic variants: data on 43 enzyme loci in man. Ann Hum Genet 37:237.

Hassold T, Kumlin E, Takaesu N, Leppert M. 1985. Determination of the parental origin of sex-chromosome monosomy using restriction fragment length polymorphisms. Am J Hum Genet 37(5):965–72.

Hatefi Y. 1985. The mitochondrial electron transport and oxidative phosphorylation system. Annu Rev Biochem 54:1015–69.

Hatten ME. 1999. Central nervous system neuronal migration. Annu Rev Neurosci 22:511–39.

Hattori M, Fujiyama A, Taylor TD, Watanabe H, Yada T, Park HS, Toyoda A, Ishii K, Totoki Y, Choi DK, et al. 2000. The DNA sequence of human chromosome 21. Nature 405(6784):311–9.

Hausler MG, Jaeken J, Monch E, Ramaekers VT. 2001. Phenotypic heterogeneity and adverse effects of serine treatment in 3-phosphoglycerate dehydrogenase deficiency: report on two siblings. Neuropediatrics 32(4):191–5.

Havelaar AC, Mancini GM, Beerens CE, Souren RM, Verheijen FW. 1998. Purification of the lysosomal sialic acid transporter. Functional characteristics of a monocarboxylate transporter. J Biol Chem 273(51):34568–74.

He L, Hannon GJ. 2004. MicroRNAs: small RNAs with a big role in gene regulation. Nat Rev Genet 5(7):522–31.

Hendrich B, Bickmore W. 2001. Human diseases with underlying defects in chromatin structure and modification. Hum Mol Genet 10(20):2233–42.

Herbst DS, Miller JR. 1980. Nonspecific X-linked mental retardation II: the frequency in British Columbia. Am J Med Genet 7(4):461–9.

Herman GE. 2003. Disorders of cholesterol biosynthesis: prototypic metabolic malformation syndromes. Hum Mol Genet 12(Spec 1):R75–88.

Hers HG. 1965. Inborn lysosomal diseases. Gastroenterology 48:625–33.

Higgins JJ, Rosen DR, Loveless JM, Clyman JC, Grau MJ. 2000. A gene for non-syndromic mental retardation maps to chromosome 3p25-pter. Neurology 55(3):335–40.

Hitomi T, Mezaki T, Tsujii T, Kinoshita M, Tomimoto H, Ikeda A, Shimohama S, Okazaki T, Uchiyama T, Shibasaki H. 2003. Improvement of central motor conduction after bone marrow transplantation in adrenoleukodystrophy. J Neurol Neurosurg Psychiatry 74(3):373–5.

Hoffman SL, Peltonen L. 2001. The neuronal ceroid lipofuscinoses. In: Scriver CR, Beaudet AL, Sly W, Valle D, eds. The Metabolic and Molecular Bases of Inherited Diseases. New York: McGraw-Hill.

Hoffmann GF, Athanassopoulos S, Burlina AB, Duran M, de Klerk JB, Lehnert W, Leonard JV, Monavari AA, Muller E, Muntau AC, et al. 1996. Clinical course, early diagnosis, treatment, and prevention of disease in glutaryl-CoA dehydrogenase deficiency. Neuropediatrics 27(3):115–23.

Holland AJ, Hon J, Huppert FA, Stevens F. 2000. Incidence and course of dementia in people with Down's syndrome: findings from a population-based study. J Intellect Disabil Res 44(Pt 2):138–46.

Hommes FA, Kuipers JR, Elema JD, Jansen JF, Jonxis JH. 1968. Propionicacidemia, a new inborn error of metabolism. Pediatr Res 2(6):519–24.

Hong SE, Shugart YY, Huang DT, Shahwan SA, Grant PE, Hourihane JO, Martin ND, Walsh CA. 2000. Autosomal recessive lissencephaly with cerebellar hypoplasia is associated with human RELN mutations. Nat Genet 26(1):93–6.

Hoogenraad CC, Akhmanova A, Galjart N, De Zeeuw CI. 2004. LIMK1 and CLIP-115: linking cytoskeletal defects to Williams syndrome. Bioessays 26(2):141–50.

Hoover-Fong JE, Shah S, Van Hove JL, Applegarth D, Toone J, Hamosh A. 2004. Natural history of nonketotic hyperglycinemia in 65 patients. Neurology 63(10):1847–53.

Hopkins FG. 1912. Feeding experiments illustrating the importance of accessory factors in normal dietaries. J Physiol 44:425–460.

Hopwood JJ, Bunge S, Morris CP, Wilson PJ, Steglich C, Beck M, Schwinger E, Gal A. 1993. Molecular basis of mucopolysaccharidosis type II: mutations in the iduronate-2-sulphatase gene. Hum Mutat 2(6):435–42.

Horvath J, Ketelsen UP, Geibel-Zehender A, Boehm N, Olbrich H, Korinthenberg R, Omran H. 2003. Identification of a novel LAMP2 mutation responsible for X-chromosomal dominant Danon disease. Neuropediatrics 34(5):270–3.

Howard HC, Mount DB, Rochefort D, Byun N, Dupre N, Lu J, Fan X, Song L, Riviere JB, Prevost C, et al. 2002. The K-Cl cotransporter KCC3 is mutant in a severe peripheral neuropathy associated with agenesis of the corpus callosum. Nat Genet 32(3):384–92.

Howe SG. 1849. The condition and capacities of idiots in Massachusetts. Am J Insanity 5:374–5.

Howell CY, Bestor TH, Ding F, Latham KE, Mertineit C, Trasler JM, Chaillet JR. 2001. Genomic imprinting disrupted by a maternal effect mutation in the Dnmt1 gene. Cell 104(6):829–38.

Howitz F. 1893. Cited by Vermeulen F. The treatment of myxoedema by feeding with thyroid glands. Br Med J 1:266.

Howell OW, Scharfman HE, Herzog H, Sundstrom LE, Beck-Sickinger A, Gray WP. 2003. Neuropeptide Y is neuroproliferative for post-natal hippocampal precursor cells. J Neurochem 86(3):646–59.

Hsia YE, Scully KJ, Rosenberg LE. 1969. Defective propionate carboxylation in ketotic hyperglycinaemia. Lancet 1:757.

Huang B, Crolla JA, Christian SL, Wolf-Ledbetter ME, Macha ME, Papenhausen PN, Ledbetter DH. 1997. Refined molecular characterization of the breakpoints in small inv dup(15) chromosomes. Hum Genet 99(1):11–7.

Huang N, vom Baur E, Garnier JM, Lerouge T, Vonesch JL, Lutz Y, Chambon P, Losson R. 1998. Two distinct nuclear receptor interaction domains in NSD1, a novel SET protein that exhibits characteristics of both corepressors and coactivators. EMBO J 17(12):3398–412.

Hudson LD. 2003. Pelizaeus-Merzbacher disease and spastic paraplegia type 2: two faces of myelin loss from mutations in the same gene. J Child Neurol 18(9):616–24.

Huppke P, Held M, Hanefeld F, Engel W, Laccone F. 2002. Influence of mutation type and location on phenotype in 123 patients with Rett syndrome. Neuropediatrics 33(2):63–8.

Hurst JA, Baraitser M, Auger E, Graham F, Norell S. 1990. An extended family with a dominantly inherited speech disorder. Dev Med Child Neurol 32(4):352–5.

Hunt GM. 1999. The Casey Holter lecture. Non-selective intervention in newborn babies with open spina bifida: the outcome 30 years on for the complete cohort. Eur J Pediatr Surg 9(Suppl 1):5–8.

Hutchison JH. 1961. Sporadic goitre and cretinism due to the production of an abnormal thyroid protein. Proc R Soc Med 54:533–7.

Huttenlocher PR. 1974. Dendritic development in neocortex of children with mental defect and infantile spasms. Neurology 24(3):203–10.

Hymes J, Wolf B. 1996. Biotinidase and its roles in biotin metabolism. Clin Chim Acta 255(1):1–11.

Iacobazzi V, Pasquali M, Singh R, Matern D, Rinaldo P, Amat di San Filippo C, Palmieri F, Longo N. 2004. Response to therapy in carnitine/acylcarnitine translocase (CACT) deficiency due to a novel missense mutation. Am J Med Genet A 126(2):150–5.

Imai Y, Takahashi R. 2004. How do Parkin mutations result in neurodegeneration? Curr Opin Neurobiol 14(3):384–9.

International Molecular Genetic Study of Autism Consortium. 1998. A full genome screen for autism with evidence for linkage to a region on chromosome 7q. Hum Mol Genet 7(3):571–8.

International Molecular Genetic Study of Autism Consortium (IMGSAC). 2001. A genomewide screen for autism: strong evidence for linkage to chromosomes 2q, 7q, and 16p. Am J Hum Genet 200169(3):570–81.

Ireland WW. 1877. On Idiocy and Imbecility. London: J. and A. Churchill.

Ireland WW. 1898. Mental Affections of Children. London: J. and A. Churchill.

Irons M, Elias ER, Salen G, Tint GS, Batta AK. 1993. Defective cholesterol biosynthesis in Smith-Lemli-Opitz syndrome. Lancet 341(8857):1414.

Irwin SA, Galvez R, Greenough WT. 2000. Dendritic spine structural anomalies in fragile-X mental retardation syndrome. Cereb Cortex 10(10):1038–44.

Irwin SA, Patel B, Idupulapati M, Harris JB, Crisostomo RA, Larsen BP, Kooy F, Willems PJ, Cras P, Kozlowski PB, et al. 2001. Abnormal dendritic spine characteristics in the temporal and visual cortices of patients with fragile-X syndrome: a quantitative examination. Am J Med Genet 98(2):161–7.

Ishihara N, Yamada K, Yamada Y, Miura K, Kato J, Kuwabara N, Hara Y, Kobayashi Y, Hoshino K, Nomura Y, et al. 2004. Clinical and molecular analysis of Mowat-Wilson syndrome associated with ZFHX1B mutations and deletions at 2q22-q24.1. J Med Genet 41(5):387–93.

Jackson A. 1935. The relation of hypothyroidism and mental deficiency. J Psychoasthenics 40:92–5.

Jackson AP, Eastwood H, Bell SM, Adu J, Toomes C, Carr IM, Roberts E, Hampshire DJ, Crow YJ, Mighell AJ, et al. 2002. Identification of microcephalin, a protein implicated in determining the size of the human brain. Am J Hum Genet 71(1):136–42.

Jacobs P, Dalton P, James R, Mosse K, Power M, Robinson D, Skuse D. 1997. Turner syndrome: a cytogenetic and molecular study. Ann Hum Genet 61(Pt 6):471–83.

Jacobs PA, Strong JA. 1959. A case of human intersexuality having a possible XXY sex-determining mechanism. Nature 183(4657):302–3.

Jacobs PA, Baikie AG, Court Brown WM, Forrest H, Roy JR, Stewart JS, Lennox B. 1959. Chromosomal sex in the syndrome of testicular feminisation. Lancet 2:591–2.

Jacobs PA, Harnden DG, Court Brown WM, Goldstein J, Close HG, Macgregor TN, Maclean N, Strong JA. 1960. Abnormalities involving the X chromosome in women. Lancet 1:1213–6.

Jacquemont S, Hagerman RJ, Leehey M, Grigsby J, Zhang L, Brunberg JA, Greco C, Des Portes V, Jardini T, Levine R, et al. 2003. Fragile X premutation tremor/ataxia syndrome: molecular, clinical, and neuroimaging correlates. Am J Hum Genet 72(4):869–78.

Jacquemont S, Farzin F, Hall D, Leehey M, Tassone F, Gane L, Zhang L, Grigsby J, Jardini T, Lewin F, et al. 2004. Aging in individuals with the FMR1 mutation. Am J Ment Retard 109(2):154–64.

Jacques PF, Bostom AG, Williams RR, Ellison RC, Eckfeldt JH, Rosenberg IH, Selhub J, Rozen R. 1996. Relation between folate status, a common mutation in methylenetetrahydrofolate reductase, and plasma homocysteine concentrations. Circulation 93(1):7–9.

Jaeken J, Matthijs G, Barone R, Carchon H. 1997. Carbohydrate deficient glycoprotein (CDG) syndrome type I. J Med Genet 34(1):73–6.

Jaeken J, Matthijs G. 2001. Congenital disorders of glycosylation. Annu Rev Genomics Hum Genet 2:129–51.

Jaeken J. 2003. Komrower lecture. Congenital disorders of glycosylation (CDG): it's all in it! J Inherit Metab Dis 26(2–3):99–118.

Jaeken J. 2004a. Congenital disorders of glycosylation (CDG): update and new developments. J Inherit Metab Dis 27(3):423–6.

Jaeken J, Carchon H. 2004b. Congenital disorders of glycosylation: a booming chapter of pediatrics. Curr Opin Pediatr 16(4):434–9.

Jaeken J. 2000. Disorders of proline and serine metabolism. In: Fernandes J, Saudubray JM, van den Berge G, eds. Inborn Metabolic Diseases. Berlin, Heidelberg, New York: Springer-Verlag.

Jamain S, Quach H, Betancur C, Rastam M, Colineaux C, Gillberg IC, Soderstrom H, Giros B, Leboyer M, Gillberg C, Bourgeron T. 2003. Paris Autism Research International Sibpair Study. Mutations of the X-linked genes encoding neuroligins NLGN3 and NLGN4 are associated with autism. Nat Genet 34(1):27–9.

Jatzkewitz H, Mehl E. 1969. Cerebroside-sulphatase and arylsulphatase A deficiency in metachromatic leukodystrophy (ML). J Neurochem 16(1):19–28.

Jeffery L, Nakielny S. 2004. Components of the DNA methylation system of chromatin control are RNA-binding proteins. J Biol Chem 279(47):49479–87.

Jellinger KA. 2003. Rett Syndrome—an update. J Neural Transm 110(6):681–701.

Jensen LR, Amende M, Gurok U, Moser B, Gimmel V, Tzschach A, Janecke AR, Tariverdian G, Chelly J, Fryns JP, et al. 2005. Mutations in the JARID1C gene, which is involved in transcriptional regulation and chromatin remodeling, cause X-linked mental retardation. Am J Hum Genet 76(2):227–36.

Jenuwein T, Allis CD. 2001. Translating the histone code. Science 293(5532):1074–80.

Jervis GA. 1953. Phenylpyruvic oligophrenia deficiency of phenylalanine-oxidizing system. Proc Soc Exp Biol Med 82(3):514–5.

Ji Y, Walkowicz MJ, Buiting K, Johnson DK, Tarvin RE, Rinchik EM, Horsthemke B, Stubbs L, Nicholls RD. 1999. The ancestral gene for transcribed, low-copy repeats in the Prader-Willi/Angelman region encodes a large protein implicated in protein trafficking, which is deficient in mice with neuromuscular and spermiogenic abnormalities. Hum Mol Genet 8(3):533–42.

Jiang YH, Sahoo T, Michaelis RC, Bercovich D, Bressler J, Kashork CD, Liu Q, Shaffer LG, Schroer RJ, Stockton DW, et al. 2004. A mixed epigenetic/genetic model for oligogenic inheritance of autism with a limited role for UBE3A. Am J Med Genet A 131(1):1–10.

Johnson CA. 2000. Chromatin modification and disease. J Med Genet 37(12):905–15.

Johnston MV. 2004. Clinical disorders of brain plasticity. Brain Dev 26(2):73–80.

Jones K. 1997. Smith's Recognizable Patterns of Human Malformation. Philadelphia: WB Saunders.

Jones KL, Smith DW. 1973. Recognition of the fetal alcohol syndrome in early infancy. Lancet 2(7836):999–1001.

Kaback MM. 2000. Population-based genetic screening for reproductive counseling: the Tay-Sachs disease model. Eur J Pediatr 159(Suppl 3):S192–5.

Kaback M, Zeiger R. 1972. Heterozygote screening in Tay Sachs disease: a prototype community screening program for the prevention of recessive genetic disorders, In Volk B, Aronson S, eds. Sphingolipids, Sphingolipidoses and Allied Disorders. New York: Plenum Press.

Kahler SG, Fahey MC. 2003. Metabolic disorders and mental retardation. Am J Med Genet C 117(1):31–41.

Kaler SG. 1998a. Diagnosis and therapy of Menkes syndrome, a genetic form of copper deficiency. Am J Clin Nutr 67(5 Suppl):1029S–34S.

Kaler SG. 1998b. Metabolic and molecular bases of Menkes disease and occipital horn syndrome. Pediatr Dev Pathol 1(1):85–98.

Kalscheuer VM, Freude K, Musante L, Jensen LR, Yntema HG, Gecz J, Sefiani A, Hoffmann K, Moser B, Haas S, et al. 2003a. Mutations in the polyglutamine binding protein 1 gene cause X-linked mental retardation. Nat Genet 35(4):313–5.

Kalscheuer VM, Tao J, Donnelly A, Hollway G, Schwinger E, Kubart S, Menzel C, Hoeltzenbein M, Tommerup N, Eyre H, et al. 2003b. Disruption of the serine/threonine kinase 9 gene causes severe X-linked infantile spasms and mental retardation. Am J Hum Genet 72(6):1401–11.

Kamiguchi H. 2003. The mechanism of axon growth: what we have learned from the cell adhesion molecule L1. Mol Neurobiol 28(3):219–28.

Kanner L. 1943. Autistic disturbances of affective contact nervous Child 2:217–250.

Kato M, Das S, Petras K, Kitamura K, Morohashi K, Abuelo DN, Barr M, Bonneau D, Brady AF, Carpenter NJ, Cipero KL, Frisone F, Fukuda T, Guerrini R, Iida E, Itoh M, Lewanda AF, Nanba Y, Oka A, Proud VK, Saugier-Veber P, Schelley SL, Selicorni A, Shaner R, Silengo M, Stewart F, Sugiyama N, Toyama J, Toutain A, Vargas AL, Yanazawa M, Zackai EH, Dobyns WB. 2004. Mutations of ARX are associated with striking pleiotropy and consistent genotype-phenotype correlation. Hum Mutat 23(2):147–59.

Kaufmann WE, Moser HW. 2000. Dendritic anomalies in disorders associated with mental retardation. Cereb Cortex 10(10):981–91.

Kaufmann WE, Cortell R, Kau AS, Bukelis I, Tierney E, Gray RM, Cox C, Capone GT, Stanard P. 2004. Autism spectrum disorder in fragile X syndrome: communication, social interaction, and specific behaviors. Am J Med Genet A 129(3):225–34.

Keats BJ, Savas S. 2004. Genetic heterogeneity in Usher syndrome. Am J Med Genet A 130(1):13–6.

Kelley RI, Wilcox WG, Smith M, Kratz LE, Moser A, Rimoin DS. 1999. Abnormal sterol metabolism in patients with Conradi-Hunermann-Happle syndrome and sporadic lethal chondrodysplasia punctata. Am J Med Genet 83(3):213–9.

Kemper TL, Bauman ML. 2002. Neuropathology of infantile autism. Mol Psychiatry 7(Suppl 2):S12–3.

Kempermann G. 2002. Regulation of adult hippocampal neurogenesis—implications for novel theories of major depression. Bipolar Disord 4(1):17–33.

Kendall E. 1915. The isolation in crystalline form of the compound containing iodine, which occurs in the thyroid: its chemical nature and physiologic activity. JAMA 64:2042–3.

Kennedy Robert F. 1965. In: Rosen M, Clark G, Kivitz M, eds. The Importance of Prevention by Gunnar Dybwad in The History of Mental Retardation Collected papers. Baltimore: University Park Press 1976, p. 345.

Kenwrick S, Watkins A, De Angelis E. 2000. Neural cell recognition molecule L1: relating biological complexity to human disease mutations. Hum Mol Genet 9(6):879–86.

Kevles D. 1985. In the Name of Eugenics: Genetics and the Uses of Human Heredity. New York: Knopf.

Khalil AM, Boyar FZ, Driscoll DJ. 2004. Dynamic histone modifications mark sex chromosome inactivation and reactivation during mammalian spermatogenesis. Proc Natl Acad Sci USA 101(47):16583–7.

Khorana HG. 1966. Polynucleotide synthesis and the genetic code. Harvey Lect 62:79–105.

Kilburn KH, Thornton JC. 1995. Protracted neurotoxicity from chlordane sprayed to kill termites. Environ Health Perspect 103(7–8):690–4.

Kim EY, Hong YB, Lai Z, Kim HJ, Cho YH, Brady RO, Jung SC. 2004. Expression and secretion of human glucocerebrosidase mediated by recombinant lentivirus vectors in vitro and in vivo: implications for gene therapy of Gaucher disease. Biochem Biophys Res Commun 318(2):381–90.

King MC, Wilson AC. 1975. Evolution at two levels in humans and chimpanzees. Science 188(4184):107–16.

King SR, Manna PR, Ishii T, Syapin PJ, Ginsberg SD, Wilson K, Walsh LP, Parker KL, Stocco DM, Smith RG, et al. 2002. An essential component in steroid synthesis, the steroidogenic acute regulatory protein, is expressed in discrete regions of the brain. J Neurosci 22(24):10613–20.

Kishino T, Lalande M, Wagstaff J. 1997. UBE3A/E6-AP mutations cause Angelman syndrome. Nat Genet 15(1):70–3.

Kitada T, Asakawa S, Hattori N, Matsumine H, Yamamura Y, Minoshima S, Yokochi M, Mizuno Y, Shimizu N. 1998. Mutations in the parkin gene cause autosomal recessive juvenile parkinsonism. Nature 392(6676):605–8.

Kleefstra T, Yntema HG, Oudakker AR, Banning MJ, Kalscheuer VM, Chelly J,

Moraine C, Ropers HH, Fryns JP, Janssen IM, et al. 2004. Zinc finger 81 (ZNF81) mutations associated with X-linked mental retardation. J Med Genet 41(5):394–9.

Kleijer WJ, Keulemans JL, van der Kraan M, Geilen GG, van der Helm RM, Rafi MA, Luzi P, Wenger DA, Halley DJ, van Diggelen OP. 1997. Prevalent mutations in the *GALC* gene of patients with Krabbe disease of Dutch and other European origin. J Inherit Metab Dis 20(4):587–94.

Kleinjan DA, van Heyningen V. 2003. Turned off by RNA. Nat Genet 34(2):125–6.

Kleinjan DA, van Heyningen V. 2005. Long-range control of gene expression: emerging mechanisms and disruption in disease. Am J Hum Genet 76(1):8–32.

Klose R, Bird A. 2003. Molecular biology. MeCP2 repression goes nonglobal. Science 302(5646):793–5.

Knusel B, Rabin SJ, Hefti F, Kaplan DR. 1994. Regulated neurotrophin receptor responsiveness during neuronal migration and early differentiation. J Neurosci 14(3 Pt 2):1542–54.

Kobayashi H, Hino M, Shimodahira M, Iwakura T, Ishihara T, Ikekubo K, Ogawa Y, Nakao K, Kurahachi H. 2002. Missense mutation of TRPS1 in a family of tricho-rhino-phalangeal syndrome type III. Am J Med Genet 107(1):26–9.

Kobayashi K, Sasaki J, Kondo-Iida E, Fukuda Y, Kinoshita M, Sunada Y, Nakamura Y, Toda T. 2001. Structural organization, complete genomic sequences and mutational analyses of the Fukuyama-type congenital muscular dystrophy gene, *fukutin*. FEBS Lett 489(2–3):192–6.

Koch R, Moats R, Guttler F, Guldberg P, Nelson M Jr. 2000. Blood–brain phenylalanine relationships in persons with phenylketonuria. Pediatrics 106(5):1093–6.

Kodama H, Murata Y, Kobayashi M. 1999. Clinical manifestations and treatment of Menkes disease and its variants. Pediatr Int 41(4):423–9.

Kornfeld S, Sly W. 2001. I cell disease and pseudo-Hurler polydystrophy. In: Scriver CR, Beaudet AL, Sly W, Valle D, eds. The Metabolic and Molecular Bases of Inherited Disease. New York: McGraw-Hill.

Korzus E, Rosenfeld MG, Mayford M. 2004. CBP histone acetyltransferase activity is a critical component of memory consolidation. Neuron 42(6):961–72.

Krakowiak PA, Wassif CA, Kratz L, Cozma D, Kovarova M, Harris G, Grinberg A, Yang Y, Hunter AG, Tsokos M, et al. 2003. Lathosterolosis: an inborn error of human and murine cholesterol synthesis due to lathosterol 5-desaturase deficiency. Hum Mol Genet 12(13):1631–41.

Krantz ID, McCallum J, DeScipio C, Kaur M, Gillis LA, Yaeger D, Jukofsky L, Wasserman N, Bottani A, Morris CA, et al. 2004. Cornelia de Lange syndrome is caused by mutations in NIPBL, the human homolog of *Drosophila* melanogaster Nipped-B. Nat Genet 36(6):631–5.

Krebs H, Henseleit K. 1932. Untersuchungen uber die Harnstoffbildung im Tierkorper. Z Physiol Chem 210:33–66.

Krebs H, Johnson W. 1937. The role of citric acid in intermediate metabolism in animal tissues. Enzymologica 4:148–56.

Kriaucionis S, Bird A. 2003. DNA methylation and Rett syndrome. Hum Mol Genet 12 (Spec 2):R221–7.

Krichevsky AM, King KS, Donahue CP, Khrapko K, Kosik KS. 2003. A microRNA array reveals extensive regulation of microRNAs during brain development. RNA 9(10):1274–81.

Krivit W, Peters C, Shapiro EG. 1999. Bone marrow transplantation as effective treatment of central nervous system disease in globoid cell leukodystrophy, metachromatic leukodystrophy, adrenoleukodystrophy, mannosidosis, fucosidosis, aspartylglucosaminuria, Hurler, Maroteaux-Lamy, and Sly syndromes, and Gaucher disease type III. Curr Opin Neurol 12(2):167–76.

Kubota T, Wakui K, Nakamura T, Ohashi H, Watanabe Y, Yoshino M, Kida T, Okamoto N, Matsumura M, Muroya K, et al. 2002. The proportion of cells with functional X disomy is associated with the severity of mental retardation in mosaic ring X Turner syndrome females. Cytogenet Genome Res 99(1–4):276–84.

Kuntsi J, Skuse D, Elgar K, Morris E, Turner C. 2000. Ring-X chromosomes: their cognitive and behavioural phenotype. Ann Hum Genet 64(Pt 4):295–305.

Kure S, Sato K, Fujii K, Aoki Y, Suzuki Y, Kato S, Matsubara Y. 2004. Wild-type phenylalanine hydroxylase activity is enhanced by tetrahydrobiopterin supplementation in vivo: an implication for therapeutic basis of tetrahydrobiopterin-responsive phenylalanine hydroxylase deficiency. Mol Genet Metab 83(1–2):150–6.

Kurotaki N, Imaizumi K, Harada N, Masuno M, Kondoh T, Nagai T, Ohashi H, Naritomi K, Tsukahara M, Makita Y, et al. 2002. Haploinsufficiency of NSD1 causes Sotos syndrome. Nat Genet 30(4):365–6.

Kurotaki N, Harada N, Shimokawa O, Miyake N, Kawame H, Uetake K, Makita Y, Kondoh T, Ogata T, Hasegawa T, et al. 2003. Fifty microdeletions among 112 cases of Sotos syndrome: low copy repeats possibly mediate the common deletion. Hum Mutat 22(5):378–87.

Kutsche K, Yntema H, Brandt A, Jantke I, Nothwang HG, Orth U, Boavida MG, David D, Chelly J, Fryns JP, et al. 2000. Mutations in ARHGEF6, encoding a guanine nucleotide exchange factor for Rho GTPases, in patients with X-linked mental retardation. Nat Genet 26(2):247–50.

Kutsche K, Ressler B, Katzera HG, Orth U, Gillessen-Kaesbach G, Morlot S, Schwinger E, Gal A. 2002. Characterization of breakpoint sequences of five rearrangements in L1CAM and ABCD1 (ALD) genes. Hum Mutat 19(5):526–35.

Kuzniecky R, Andermann F, Guerrini R. 1993. Congenital bilateral perisylvian syndrome: study of 31 patients. The CBPS Multicenter Collaborative Study. Lancet 341(8845):608–12.

Kvittingen EA, Guldal G, Borsting S, Skalpe IO, Stokke O, Jellum E. 1986. N-Acetylaspartic aciduria in a child with a progressive cerebral atrophy. Clin Chim Acta 158(3):217–27.

Kyllerman M, Skjeldal O, Christensen E, Hagberg G, Holme E, Lonnquist T, Skov L, Rotwelt T, von Dobeln U. 2004. Long-term follow-up, neurological outcome and survival rate in 28 Nordic patients with glutaric aciduria type 1. Eur J Paediatr Neurol 8(3):121–9.

Laccone F, Junemann I, Whatley S, Morgan R, Butler R, Huppke P, Ravine D. 2004. Large deletions of the MECP2 gene detected by gene dosage analysis in patients with Rett syndrome. Hum Mutat 23(3):234–44.

Lachmann RH, te Vruchte D, Lloyd-Evans E, Reinkensmeier G, Sillence DJ, Fernandez-Guillen L, Dwek RA, Butters TD, Cox TM, Platt FM. 2004. Treatment with miglustat reverses the lipid-trafficking defect in Niemann-Pick disease type C. Neurobiol Dis 16(3):654–8.

La Fetra L. 1916. The hospital care of premature infants. Trans Am Pediatr Soc 28:90.

Lai CS, Fisher SE, Hurst JA, Levy ER, Hodgson S, Fox M, Jeremiah S, Povey S, Jamison DC, Green ED, et al. 2000. The SPCH1 region on human 7q31: genomic characterization of the critical interval and localization of translocations associated with speech and language disorder. Am J Hum Genet 67(2):357–68.

Lai CS, Fisher SE, Hurst JA, Vargha-Khadem F, Monaco AP. 2001. A forkhead-domain gene is mutated in a severe speech and language disorder. Nature 413(6855):519–23.

Lamb JA, Parr JR, Bailey AJ, Monaco AP. 2002. Autism: in search of susceptibility genes. Neuromol Med 2(1):11–28.

Lander F, Ronne M. 1995. Frequency of sister chromatic exchange and hematological effects in pesticide-exposed greenhouse sprayers. Scand J Work Environ Health 21(4):283–8.

Landgraf P, Mayerhofer PU, Polanetz R, Roscher AA, Holzinger A. 2003. Targeting of the human adrenoleukodystrophy protein to the peroxisomal membrane by an internal region containing a highly conserved motif. Eur J Cell Biol 82(8):401–10.

Landsteiner K, Weiner AJ. 1940. An agglutinable factor in human blood recognized by immune sera for rhesus blood. Proc Soc Exp Biol Med 43:223.

Lassker U, Zschocke J, Blau N, Santer R. 2002. Tetrahydrobiopterin responsiveness in phenylketonuria. Two new cases and a review of molecular genetic findings. J Inherit Metab Dis 25(1):65–70.

Lau LF, Mammen A, Ehlers MD, Kindler S, Chung WJ, Garner CC, Huganir RL. 1996. Interaction of the N-methyl-D-aspartate receptor complex with a novel synapse-associated protein, SAP102. J Biol Chem 271(35):21622–8.

Lau YF, Lin CC, Kan YW. 1984. Amplification and expression of human alpha-globin genes in Chinese hamster ovary cells. Mol Cell Biol 4(8):1469–75.

Laumonnier F, Ronce N, Hamel BC, Thomas P, Lespinasse J, Raynaud M, Paringaux C, Van Bokhoven H, Kalscheuer V, Fryns JP, et al. 2002. Transcription factor SOX3 is involved in X-linked mental retardation with growth hormone deficiency. Am J Hum Genet 71(6):1450–5.

Laumonnier F, Bonnet-Brilhault F, Gomot M, Blanc R, David A, Moizard MP, Raynaud M, Ronce N, Lemonnier E, Calvas P, et al. 2004. X-Linked mental retardation and autism are associated with a mutation in the NLGN4 gene, a member of the neuroligin family. Am J Hum Genet 74(3):552–7.

Lavorgna G, Dahary D, Lehner B, Sorek R, Sanderson CM, Casari G. 2004. In search of antisense. Trends Biochem Sci 29(2):88–94.

Lawler SD, Sandler M. 1954. Data on linkage in man: elliptocytosis and blood groups iv: families 5,6,7. Ann Eugen 18:328–34.

Laxova R. 1994. Fragile X syndrome. Adv Pediatr 41:305–42.

Lazaro L, Dubourg C, Pasquier L, Le Duff F, Blayau M, Durou MR, de la Pintiere AT, Aguilella C, David V, Odent S. 2004. Phenotypic and molecular variability of the holoprosencephalic spectrum. Am J Med Genet A 129(1):21–4.

Lazarow PB, De Duve C. 1976. A fatty acyl-CoA oxidizing system in rat liver peroxisomes; enhancement by clofibrate, a hypolipidemic drug. Proc Natl Acad Sci USA 73(6):2043–6.

Leder P. 1978. Discontinuous genes. N Engl J Med 298(19):1079–81.

Lejeune J, Gautier M, Turpin R. 1959a. Study of somatic chromosomes from 9 mongoloid children (in French). C R Hebd Seances Acad Sci 248(11):1721–2.

Lejeune J, Turpin R, Gautier M. 1959b. Mongolism; a chromosomal disease (trisomy) (in French). Bull Acad Natl Med 143(11–12):256–65.

Lejeune J, Lafourcade J, Berger R, Vialatte J, Boeswillwald M, Seringe P, Turpin R. 1963. 3 cases of partial deletion of the short arm of a 5 chromosome (in French). C R Hebd Seances Acad Sci 257:3098–102.

Lemmers RJ, de Kievit P, Sandkuijl L, Padberg GW, van Ommen GJ, Frants RR, van der Maarel SM. 2002. Facioscapulohumeral muscular dystrophy is uniquely associated with one of the two variants of the 4q subtelomere. Nat Genet 32(2):235–6.

Lemmers RJ, Van Overveld PG, Sandkuijl LA, Vrieling H, Padberg GW, Frants RR, van der Maarel SM. 2004. Mechanism and timing of mitotic rearrangements in the subtelomeric D4Z4 repeat involved in facioscapulohumeral muscular dystrophy. Am J Hum Genet 75(1):44–53.

Lenke RR, Levy HL. 1980. Maternal phenylketonuria and hyperphenylalaninemia. An international survey of the outcome of untreated and treated pregnancies. N Engl J Med 303(21):1202–8.

Leroy JG, Ho MW, MacBrinn MC, Zielke K, Jacob J, O'Brien JS. 1972. I-cell disease: biochemical studies. Pediatr Res 6(10):752–7.

Levine P, Burnham L, Katzin E, 1941. The role of isoimmunization in the pathogenesis of erythroblastosis fetalis. Am J Obstet Gynecol 42:925.

Li L, Chin LS, Shupliakov O, Brodin L, Sihra TS, Hvalby O, Jensen V, Zheng D, McNamara JO, Greengard P, et al. 1995. Impairment of synaptic vesicle clustering and of synaptic transmission, and increased seizure propensity, in synapsin I-deficient mice. Proc Natl Acad Sci USA 92(20):9235–9.

Li L, Liu F, Salmonsen RA, Turner TK, Litofsky NS, Di Cristofano A, Pandolfi PP, Jones SN, Recht LD, Ross AH. 2002. PTEN in neural precursor cells: regulation of migration, apoptosis, and proliferation. Mol Cell Neurosci 20(1):21–9.

Li L, Liu F, Ross AH. 2003. PTEN regulation of neural development and CNS stem cells. J Cell Biochem 88(1):24–8.

Li M, Shuman C, Fei YL, Cutiongco E, Bender HA, Stevens C, Wilkins-Haug L, Day-Salvatore D, Yong SL, Geraghty MT, et al. 2001. GPC3 mutation analysis in a spectrum of patients with overgrowth expands the phenotype of Simpson-Golabi-Behmel syndrome. Am J Med Genet 102(2):161–8.

Liebig J. 1847. Researches on the Chemistry of Food. Gregory W, trans. London: Taylor and Walton.

Lin H, Sugimoto Y, Ohsaki Y, Ninomiya H, Oka A, Taniguchi M, Ida H, Eto Y, Ogawa S, Matsuzaki Y, et al. 2004. N-Octyl-beta-valienamine up-regulates activity of F213I mutant beta-glucosidase in cultured cells: a potential chemical chaperone therapy for Gaucher disease. Biochim Biophys Acta 1689(3):219–28.

Linden MG, Bender BG, Robinson A. 1995. Sex chromosome tetrasomy and pentasomy. Pediatrics 96(4 Pt 1):672–82.

Lissens W, De Meirleir L, Seneca S, Liebaers I, Brown GK, Brown RM, Ito M, Naito E, Kuroda Y, Kerr DS, et al. 2000. Mutations in the X-linked pyruvate dehydrogenase (E1) alpha subunit gene (PDHA1) in patients with a pyruvate dehydrogenase complex deficiency. Hum Mutat 15(3):209–19.

Liu J, Raine A, Venables PH, Dalais C, Mednick SA. 2003. Malnutrition at age 3 years and lower cognitive ability at age 11 years: independence from psychosocial adversity. Arch Pediatr Adolesc Med 157(6):593–600.

Lockyer L, Rutter M. 1969. A five- to fifteen-year follow-up study of infantile psychosis. Br J Psychiatry 115(525):865–82.

Lodish H, Baltimore D, Darnell J, Zipursky SL, Berk A, Matsudaira P. Darnell J. 1995. Molecular Cell Biology. New York: Scientific American Books.

Lohman K. Schuster P. 1937. Untersuchungen uber die cocarboxylase. Biochem Z 294:188–214.

Lombroso, C. 1873. Sulla microcephalia e sul cretinismo. Rivista Clinica di Bologna fasc. 7 July.

Lord C, Volkmar F. 2002. Genetics of childhood disorders: XLII. Autism, part 1. Diagnosis and assessment in autistic spectrum disorders. J Am Acad Child Adolesc Psychiatry 41(9):1134–6.

Lozoff B, Jimenez E, Hagen J, Mollen E, Wolf AW. 2000. Poorer behavioral and developmental outcome more than 10 years after treatment for iron deficiency in infancy. Pediatrics 105(4):E51.

Lu C, Knutson DE, Fisker-Andersen J, Fenske RA. 2001. Biological monitoring survey of organophosphorus pesticide exposure among pre-school children in the Seattle metropolitan area. Environ Health Perspect 109(3):299–303.

Lubchenco LO, 1983. The developmental outcome of premature infants. In: Smith GF, Vidyasagar D, eds. Critical Reviews and Recent Advances in Neonatal and Perinatal Medicine. Mead Johnson Nutritional Division.

Lucke T, Illsinger S, Aulehla-Scholz C, Sander J, Das AM. 2003. BH4-sensitive hyperphenylalaninemia: new case and review of literature. Pediatr Neurol 28(3):228–30.

Lugenbeel KA, Peier AM, Carson NL, Chudley AE, Nelson DL. 1995. Intragenic loss of function mutations demonstrate the primary role of FMR1 in fragile X syndrome. Nat Genet 10(4):483–5.

Lujan R, Shigemoto R, Lopez-Bendito G. 2005. Glutamate and GABA receptor signalling in the developing brain. Neuroscience 130(3):567–80.

Lukusa Y, Vermmech JR, Holvoet M, Fryns JP, Devriendt K. 2000. Deletion 2q37.3 and autism: molecular cytogenetic mapping of the candidate region for autistic disorder. Genet Couns 15(3):293–301.

Lupski JR. 1998. Genomic disorders: structural features of the genome can lead to DNA rearrangements and human disease traits. Trends Genet 14(10):417–22.

Luzi P, Rafi MA, Wenger DA. 1995. Characterization of the large deletion in the *GALC* gene found in patients with Krabbe disease. Hum Mol Genet 4(12):2335–8.

Mabry CC, Denniston JC, Nelson TL, Son CD. 1963. Maternal phenylketonuria. A cause of mental retardation in children without the metabolic defect. N Engl J Med 269:1404–8.

Madeiros-Neto G, Stanbury J. 1994. Inherited Disorders of the Thyroid System. Boca Raton, FL: CRC Press.

Maestri NE, Brusilow SW, Clissold DB, Bassett SS. 1996. Long-term treatment of girls with ornithine transcarbamylase deficiency. N Engl J Med 335(12):855–9.

Magasanik B, Chargaff E. 1951. Studies on the structure of ribonucleic acids. Biochim Biophys Acta 7(3):396–412.

Magenis RE, Brown MG, Lacy DA, Budden S, LaFranchi S. 1987. Is Angelman syndrome an alternate result of del(15)(q11q13)? Am J Med Genet 28(4):829–38.

Maguire EA, Gadian DG, Johnsrude IS, Good CD, Ashburner J, Frackowiak RS,

Frith CD. 2000. Navigation-related structural change in the hippocampi of taxi drivers. Proc Natl Acad Sci USA 97(8):4398–403.

Malenka RC. 2003. Synaptic plasticity and AMPA receptor trafficking. Ann NY Acad Sci 1003:1–11.

Malm G, Mansson JE, Winiarski J, Mosskin M, Ringden O. 2004. Five-year follow-up of two siblings with aspartylglucosaminuria undergoing allogeneic stem-cell transplantation from unrelated donors. Transplantation 78(3):415–9.

Malzac P, Webber H, Moncla A, Graham JM, Kukolich M, Williams C, Pagon RA, Ramsdell LA, Kishino T, Wagstaff J. 1998. Mutation analysis of UBE3A in Angelman syndrome patients. Am J Hum Genet 62(6):1353–60.

Mandel JL. 2004. Comparative frequency of fragile-X (FMR1) and creatine transporter (SLC6A8) mutations in X-linked mental retardation. Am J Hum Genet 75(4):730–1; author reply 731–2.

Mandel JL, Biancalana V. 2004. Fragile X mental retardation syndrome: from pathogenesis to diagnostic issues. Growth Horm IGF Res 14(Suppl A):S158–65.

Mann RK, Beachy PA. 2000. Cholesterol modification of proteins. Biochim Biophys Acta 1529(1–3):188–202.

Manning BD, Cantley LC. 2003a. Rheb fills a GAP between TSC and TOR. Trends Biochem Sci 28(11):573–6.

Manning BD, Cantley LC. 2003b. United at last: the tuberous sclerosis complex gene products connect the phosphoinositide 3-kinase/Akt pathway to mammalian target of rapamycin (mTOR) signalling. Biochem Soc Trans 31(Pt 3):573–8.

Marriage BJ, Clandinin MT, Macdonald IM, Glerum DM. 2004. Cofactor treatment improves ATP synthetic capacity in patients with oxidative phosphorylation disorders. Mol Genet Metab 81(4):263–72.

Marlin S, Blanchard S, Slim R, Lacombe D, Denoyelle F, Alessandri JL, Calzolari E, Drouin-Garraud V, Ferraz FG, Fourmaintraux A, Philip N, Toublanc JE, Petit C. 1999. Townes-Brocks syndrome: detection of a SALL1 mutation hot spot and evidence for a position effect in one patient. Hum Mutat 14(5):377–86.

Marrs TC. 1993. Organophosphate poisoning. Pharmacol Ther. 58(1):51–66. Review.

Marsh DJ, Dahia PL, Zheng Z, Liaw D, Parsons R, Gorlin RJ, Eng C. 1997. Germline mutations in PTEN are present in Bannayan-Zonana syndrome. Nat Genet 16(4):333–4.

Marshall L, Magoun H. 1998. Discoveries in the Human Brain: Neuroscience Prehistory, Brain Structure, and Function. Totowa, NJ: Humana Press.

Martin CL, Waggoner DJ, Wong A, Uhrig S, Roseberry JA, Hedrick JF, Pack SD, Russell K, Zackai E, Dobyns WB, et al. 2002. "Molecular rulers" for calibrating phenotypic effects of telomere imbalance. J Med Genet 39(10):734–40.

Martin GR. 1981. Isolation of a pluripotent cell line from early mouse embryos cultured in medium conditioned by teratocarcinoma stem cells. Proc Natl Acad Sci USA 78(12):7634–8.

Martinez M. 2001. Restoring the DHA levels in the brains of Zellweger patients. J Mol Neurosci 16(2–3):309–16; discussion 317–21.

Martinowich K, Hattori D, Wu H, Fouse S, He F, Hu Y, Fan G, Sun YE. 2003. DNA methylation-related chromatin remodeling in activity-dependent BDNF gene regulation. Science 302(5646):890–3.

Marygold SJ, Leevers SJ. 2002. Growth signaling: TSC takes its place. Curr Biol 12(22):R785–7.

Masters C, Crane D. 1995. The Peroxisome: A Vital Organelle. Cambridge: Cambridge University Press.

Matalon R, Matalon KM. 2002. Canavan disease prenatal diagnosis and genetic counseling. Obstet Gynecol Clin North Am 29(2):297–304.

Matalon R, Michals K, Sebesta D, Deanching M, Gashkoff P, Casanova J. 1988. Aspartoacylase deficiency and N-acetylaspartic aciduria in patients with Canavan disease. Am J Med Genet 29(2):463–71.

Matalon R, Surendran S, Matalon KM, Tyring S, Quast M, Jinga W, Ezell E, Szucs S. 2003. Future role of large neutral amino acids in transport of phenylalanine into the brain. Pediatrics 112(6 Pt 2):1570–4.

Matalon R, Koch R, Michals-Matalon K, Moseley K, Surendran S, Tyring S, Erlandsen H, Gamez A, Stevens RC, Romstad A, et al. 2004. Biopterin responsive phenylalanine hydroxylase deficiency. Genet Med 6(1):27–32.

Matsuda J, Suzuki O, Oshima A, Yamamoto Y, Noguchi A, Takimoto K, Itoh M, Matsuzaki Y, Yasuda Y, Ogawa S, et al. 2003. Chemical chaperone therapy for brain pathology in GM1-gangliosidosis. Proc Natl Acad Sci USA 100(26):15912–7.

Matsumoto N, Pilz DT, Fantes JA, Kittikamron K, Ledbetter DH. 1998. Isolation of BAC clones spanning the Xq22.3 translocation breakpoint in a lissencephaly patient with a de novo X;2 translocation. J Med Genet 35(10):829–32.

Matsuura T, Sutcliffe JS, Fang P, Galjaard RJ, Jiang YH, Benton CS, Rommens JM, Beaudet AL. 1997. De novo truncating mutations in E6-AP ubiquitin-protein ligase gene (UBE3A) in Angelman syndrome. Nat Genet 15(1):74–7.

Mattick JS. 2003. Challenging the dogma: the hidden layer of non-protein-coding RNAs in complex organisms. Bioessays 25(10):930–9.

Mattson MP, Shea TB. 2003. Folate and homocysteine metabolism in neural plasticity and neurodegenerative disorders. Trends Neurosci 26(3):137–46.

Maxam AM, Gilbert W. 1977. A new method for sequencing DNA. Proc Natl Acad Sci USA 74(2):560–4.

McGirr GE, Clement WE, Watson WC, Hutchison JH, Currie AR. 1959. Goitre due to dyshormonogenesis. J Endocrinol 18(3):Proc Soc Endocr 73rd xxiii–xxiv.

McDonnell RJ, Johnson Z, Delaney V, Dack P. 1999. East Ireland 1980–1994: epidemiology of neural tube defects. J Epidemiol Community Health 53(12):782–8.

McDowell TL, Gibbons RJ, Sutherland H, O'Rourke DM, Bickmore WA, Pombo A, Turley H, Gatter K, Picketts DJ, Buckle VJ, et al. 1999. Localization of a putative transcriptional regulator (ATRX) at pericentromeric heterochromatin and the short arms of acrocentric chromosomes. Proc Natl Acad Sci USA 96(24):13983–8.

McGuinness MC, Lu JF, Zhang HP, Dong GX, Heinzer AK, Watkins PA, Powers J, Smith KD. 2003. Role of ALDP (ABCD1) and mitochondria in X-linked adrenoleukodystrophy. Mol Cell Biol 23(2):744–53.

McManus MT, Sharp PA. 2002. Gene silencing in mammals by small interfering RNAs. Nat Rev Genet 3(10):737–47.

McMurray WC, Rathbun JC, Mohyuddin F, Koegler SJ. 1963. Citrullinuria. Pediatrics 32:347–57.

McQuade L, Christodoulou J, Budarf M, Sachdev R, Wilson M, Emanuel B, Colley A. 1999. Patient with a 22q11.2 deletion with no overlap of the minimal DiGeorge syndrome critical region (MDGCR). Am J Med Genet 86(1):27–33.

Meadows LS, Malhotra J, Loukas A, Thyagarajan V, Kazen-Gillespie KA, Koopman MC, Kriegler S, Isom LL, Ragsdale DS. 2002. Functional and biochemical analysis of a sodium channel beta1 subunit mutation responsible for generalized epilepsy with febrile seizures plus type 1. J Neurosci 22(24):10699–709.

Mefford HC, Trask BJ. 2002. The complex structure and dynamic evolution of human subtelomeres. Nat Rev Genet 3(2):91–102.

Melhuish TA, Wotton D. 2000. The interaction of the carboxyl terminus-binding protein with the Smad corepressor TGIF is disrupted by a holoprosencephaly mutation in TGIF. J Biol Chem 275(50):39762–6.

Meloni I, Muscettola M, Raynaud M, Longo I, Bruttini M, Moizard MP, Gomot M, Chelly J, des Portes V, Fryns JP, et al. 2002. FACL4, encoding fatty acid-CoA ligase 4, is mutated in nonspecific X-linked mental retardation. Nat Genet 30(4):436–40.

Mendel G. 1866. Versuche uber Pflanzenhydriden. Verh. Naturforsch. Ver. Brunn 4:3–47 Translated in 1901 Experiments in plant hybridization J.R. Hortic. Soc. 26:1–32.

Menkes JH, Hurst PL, Craig JM. 1954. A new syndrome: progressive familial infantile cerebral dysfunction associated with an unusual urinary substance. Pediatrics 14(5):462–7.

Merke F. 1984. History and iconography of endemic goitre and cretinism [translated by D.Q. Stephenson] Berne [Switzerland] : H. Huber, first published 1971.

Mermoud JE, Popova B, Peters AH, Jenuwein T, Brockdorff N. 2002. Histone H3 lysine 9 methylation occurs rapidly at the onset of random X chromosome inactivation. Curr Biol 12(3):247–51.

Meyer G. 2001. Human neocortical development: the importance of embryonic and early fetal events. Neuroscientist 7(4):303–14.

Meyerhof O. 1930. Die Chemische Vorgange im Muskel. Berlin: Springer.

Michaelis L, Menten M. 1913. Zur kinetik der Invertinwirkung. Biochem Z 49:339–69.

Millar JK, Wilson-Annan JC, Anderson S, Christie S, Taylor MS, Semple CA, Devon RS, Clair DM, Muir WJ, Blackwood DH, et al. 2000. Disruption of two novel genes by a translocation co-segregating with schizophrenia. Hum Mol Genet 9(9):1415–23.

Milner B, Squire LR, Kandel ER. 1998. Cognitive neuroscience and the study of memory. Neuron 20(3):445–68.

Milunsky JM, Huang XL. 2003. Unmasking Kabuki syndrome: chromosome 8p22-8p23.1 duplication revealed by comparative genomic hybridization and BAC-FISH. Clin Genet 64(6):509–16.

Milunsky JM, Maher TA, Metzenberg AB. 2003. Molecular, biochemical, and phenotypic analysis of a hemizygous male with a severe atypical phenotype for X-linked dominant Conradi-Hunermann-Happle syndrome and a mutation in EBP. Am J Med Genet A 116(3):249–54.

Ming JE, Kaupas ME, Roessler E, Brunner HG, Golabi M, Tekin M, Stratton RF, Sujansky E, Bale SJ, Muenke M. 2002. Mutations in PATCHED-1, the receptor for SONIC HEDGEHOG, are associated with holoprosencephaly. Hum Genet 110(4):297–301.

Minshew NJ, Goldstein G, Siegel DJ. 1997. Neuropsychologic functioning in autism: profile of a complex information processing disorder. J Int Neuropsychol Soc 3(4):303–16.

Minshew NJ, Meyer J, Goldstein G. 2002a. Abstract reasoning in autism: a dissociation between concept formation and concept identification. Neuropsychology 16(3):327–34.

Minshew NJ, Sweeney J, Luna B. 2002b. Autism as a selective disorder of complex information processing and underdevelopment of neocortical systems. Mol Psychiatry 7(Suppl 2):S14–5.

Mitchell TN, Free SL, Williamson KA, Stevens JM, Churchill AJ, Hanson IM, Shorvon SD, Moore AT, van Heyningen V, Sisodiya SM. 2003. Polymicrogyria and absence of pineal gland due to PAX6 mutation. Ann Neurol 53(5):658–63.

Miura K, Kumagai T, Matsumoto A, Iriyama E, Watanabe K, Goto K, Arahata K. 1998. Two cases of chromosome 4q35–linked early onset facioscapulohumeral muscular dystrophy with mental retardation and epilepsy. Neuropediatrics 29(5):239–41.

Mohandas TK, Park JP, Spellman RA, Filiano JJ, Mamourian AC, Hawk AB, Belloni DR, Noll WW, Moeschler JB. 1999. Paternally derived de novo interstitial duplication of proximal 15q in a patient with developmental delay. Am J Med Genet 82(4):294–300.

Mole SE. 2004. The genetic spectrum of human neuronal ceroid-lipofuscinoses. Brain Pathol 14(1):70–6.

Molinari F, Rio M, Meskenaite V, Encha-Razavi F, Auge J, Bacq D, Briault S, Vekemans M, Munnich A, Attie-Bitach T, et al. 2002. Truncating neurotrypsin mutation in autosomal recessive nonsyndromic mental retardation. Science 298(5599):1779–81.

Montessori, M. 1896. In: Scheerenberger RC, 1983. A History of Mental Retardation. Baltimore: Brookes Publishing, pp. 85–87.

Moolenaar SH, Engelke UF, Wevers RA. 2003. Proton nuclear magnetic resonance spectroscopy of body fluids in the field of inborn errors of metabolism. Ann Clin Biochem 40(Pt 1):16–24.

Morreale de Escobar G, Obregon MJ, Escobar del Rey F. 2004. Role of thyroid hormone during early brain development Eur J Endocrin 151(Supp3):U25–37. Review.

Morris CA, Mervis CB. 2000. Williams syndrome and related disorders. Annu Rev Genomics Hum Genet 1:461–84.

Moser HW, Smith K, Watkins P, Powers J, Moser AB, et al. 2001. X-Linked adrenoleukodystrophy. In: Scriver CR, Beaudet AL, Sly W, Valle D, eds. The Metabolic and Molecular Bases of Inherited Diseases. New York: McGraw-Hill.

Moser H, Dubey P, Fatemi A. 2004a. Progress in X-linked adrenoleukodystrophy. Curr Opin Neurol 17(3):263–9.

Moser HW, Fatemi A, Zackowski K, Smith S, Golay X, Muenz L, Raymond G. 2004b. Evaluation of therapy of X-linked adrenoleukodystrophy. Neurochem Res 29(5):1003–16.

Moslinger D, Muhl A, Suormala T, Baumgartner R, Stockler-Ipsiroglu S. 2003. Molecular characterisation and neuropsychological outcome of 21 patients with profound biotinidase deficiency detected by newborn screening and family studies. Eur J Pediatr 162(Suppl 1):S46–9.

Mott F. 1917. The changes in the central nervous system in hypothyroidism. Proc R Soc Med 10:51.

Mountcastle VB. 1997. The columnar organization of the neocortex. Brain 120(Pt 4):701–22.

Mowat DR, Croaker GD, Cass DT, Kerr BA, Chaitow J, Ades LC, Chia NL, Wilson
MJ. 1998. Hirschsprung disease, microcephaly, mental retardation, and
characteristic facial features: delineation of a new syndrome and identification
of a locus at chromosome 2q22-q23. J Med Genet 35(8):617–23.

Mowat DR, Wilson MJ, Goossens M. 2003. Mowat-Wilson syndrome. J Med Genet
40(5):305–10.

Moyses C. 2003. Substrate reduction therapy: clinical evaluation in type 1 Gaucher
disease. Philos Trans R Soc Lond B Biol Sci 358(1433):955–60.

MRC Vitamin Study Research Group. 1991. Prevention of neural tube defects: results
of the Medical Research Council Vitamin Study. Lancet 338(8760):131–7.

Mudd SH, Skovby F, Levy HL, Pettigrew KD, Wilcken B, Pyeritz RE, Andria G,
Boers GH, Bromberg IL, Cerone R, et al. 1985. The natural history of
homocystinuria due to cystathionine beta-synthase deficiency. Am J Hum
Genet 37(1):1–31.

Muenke M, Cohen MM Jr. 2000. Genetic approaches to understanding brain
development: holoprosencephaly as a model. Ment Retard Dev Disabil *Res* Rev
6(1):15–21.

Muller T, Arbeiter K, Aufricht C. 2002. Renal function in meningomyelocele: risk
factors, chronic renal failure, renal replacement therapy and transplantation.
Curr Opin Urol 12(6):479–84. Review.

Mulley JC, Yu S, Loesch DZ, Hay DA, Donnelly A, Gedeon AK, Carbonell P, Lopez
I, Glover G, Gabarron I, et al. 1995. FRAXE and mental retardation. J Med
Genet 32(3):162–9.

Mullis K, Faloona F, Scharf S, Saiki R, Horn G, Erlich H. 1986. Specific enzymatic
amplification of DNA in vitro: the polymerase chain reaction. Cold Spring
Harb Symp Quant Biol 51(Pt 1):263–73.

Muntau AC, Roschinger W, Habich M, Demmelmair H, Hoffmann B, Sommerhoff
CP, Roscher AA. 2002. Tetrahydrobiopterin as an alternative treatment for
mild phenylketonuria. N Engl J Med 347(26):2122–32.

Muntoni F, Torelli S, Ferlini A. 2003. Dystrophin and mutations: one gene, several
proteins, multiple phenotypes. Lancet Neurol 2(12):731–40.

Murphy M, Whiteman D, Stone D, Botting B, Schorah C, Wild J. 2000. Dietary
folate and the prevalence of neural tube defects in the British Isles: the past two
decades. BJOG 107(7):885–9.

Murray G. 1891. Note on the treatment of myxoedema by hypodermic injections of
extract of the thyroid gland of a sheep. Br Med J 2:796.

Nakao M, Matsui S, Yamamoto S, Okumura K, Shirakawa M, Fujita N. 2001.
Regulation of transcription and chromatin by methyl-CpG binding protein
MBD1. Brain Dev 23(Suppl 1):S174–6.

Nan X, Bird A. 2001. The biological functions of the methyl-CpG-binding protein
MeCP2 and its implication in Rett syndrome. Brain Dev 23(Suppl 1):S32–7.

National Institutes of Health Consensus Development Conference Panel. 2001.
National Institutes of Health Consensus Development Conference Statement.
Phenylketonuria: screening and management, October 16–18, 2000. Pediatrics
108(4):972–82.

Nellist M, van Slegtenhorst MA, Goedbloed M, van den Ouweland AM, Halley DJ,
van der Sluijs P. 1999. Characterization of the cytosolic tuberin–hamartin
complex. Tuberin is a cytosolic chaperone for hamartin. J Biol Chem
274(50):35647–52.

Neufeld E, Muenzer J. 2001. The mucopolysaccharidoses. In: Scriver CR, Beaudet AL, Sly W, Valle D, eds. The Metabolic and Molecular Bases of Inherited Diseases. New York: McGraw-Hill.

Newbury DF, Bonora E, Lamb JA, Fisher SE, Lai CS, Baird G, Jannoun L, Slonims V, Stott CM, Merricks MJ, et al. 2002. *FOXP2* is not a major susceptibility gene for autism or specific language impairment. Am J Hum Genet 70(5):1318–27.

Nirenberg MW, Matthaei JH. 1961. The dependence of cell-free protein synthesis in *E. coli* upon naturally occurring or synthetic polyribonucleotides. Proc Natl Acad Sci USA 47:1588–602.

Nolte J. 2001. The Human Brain. St. Louis: Mosby.

Norrlin S, Strinnholm M, Carlsson M, Dahl M. 2003. Factors of significance for mobility in children with myelomeningocele. Acta Paediatr 92(2):204–10.

North K, Hyman S, Barton B. 2002. Cognitive deficits in neurofibromatosis 1. J Child Neurol 17(8):605–12; discussion 627–9, 646–51.

Nottebohm F. 1981. A brain for all seasons: cyclical anatomical changes in song control nuclei of the canary brain. Science 214(4527):1368–70.

Oberholzer VG, Levin B, Burgess EA, Young WF. 1967. Methylmalonic aciduria. An inborn error of metabolism leading to chronic metabolic acidosis. Arch Dis Child 42(225):492–504.

Oberle I, Rousseau F, Heitz D, Kretz C, Devys D, Hanauer A, Boue J, Bertheas MF, Mandel JL. 1991. Instability of a 550–base pair DNA segment and abnormal methylation in fragile X syndrome. Science 252(5010):1097–102.

O'Connor SE, Kwiatkowski DJ, Roberts PS, Wollmann RL, Huttenlocher PR. 2003. A family with seizures and minor features of tuberous sclerosis and a novel TSC2 mutation. Neurology 61(3):409–12.

Ogier de Baulny H, Saudubray JM. 2002. Branched-chain organic acidurias. Semin Neonatol 7(1):65–74.

Ohlsson R, Tycko B, Sapienza C. 1998. Monoallelic expression: "there can only be one." Trends Genet 14(11):435–8.

Ohlsson R, Renkawitz R, Lobanenkov V. 2001. CTCF is a uniquely versatile transcription regulator linked to epigenetics and disease. Trends Genet 17(9):520–7.

Ohta T, Buiting K, Kokkonen H, McCandless S, Heeger S, Leisti H, Driscoll DJ, Cassidy SB, Horsthemke B, Nicholls RD. 1999a. Molecular mechanism of Angelman syndrome in two large families involves an imprinting mutation. Am J Hum Genet 64(2):385–96.

Ohta T, Gray TA, Rogan PK, Buiting K, Gabriel JM, Saitoh S, Muralidhar B, Bilienska B, Krajewska-Walasek M, Driscoll DJ, et al. 1999b. Imprinting-mutation mechanisms in Prader-Willi syndrome. Am J Hum Genet 64(2):397–413.

Okabe A, Kilb W, Shimizu-Okabe C, Hanganu IL, Fukuda A, Luhmann HJ. 2004. Homogenous glycine receptor expression in cortical plate neurons and Cajal-Retzius cells of neonatal rat cerebral cortex. Neuroscience 123(3):715–24.

Okada S, O'Brien JS. 1969. Tay-Sachs disease: generalized absence of a beta-D-N-acetylhexosaminidase component. Science 165(894):698–700.

Okano M, Xie S, Li E. 1998. Cloning and characterization of a family of novel mammalian DNA (cytosine-5) methyltransferases. Nat Genet 19(3):219–20.

Olson LE, Richtsmeier JT, Leszl J, Reeves RH. 2004. A chromosome 21 critical region does not cause specific Down syndrome phenotypes. Science 306(5696):687–90.

Padberg GW, Frants RR, Brouwer OF, Wijmenga C, Bakker E, Sandkuijl LA. 1995. Facioscapulohumeral muscular dystrophy in the Dutch population. Muscle Nerve 2:S81–4.

Painter TS. 1933. A new method for the study of chromosome rearrangements and plotting of chromosome maps. Science 78:585–6.

Pallade G. 1953. An electron microscope study of mitochondrial structure. J Histochem Cytochem 1:188.

Pandor A, Eastham J, Beverley C, Chilcott J, Paisley S. 2004. Clinical effectiveness and cost-effectiveness of neonatal screening for inborn errors of metabolism using tandem mass spectrometry: a systematic review. Health Technol Assess 8(12):iii, 1–121.

Pang KM, Ishidate T, Nakamura K, Shirayama M, Trzepacz C, Schubert CM, Priess JR, Mello CC. 2004. The minibrain kinase homolog, mbk-2, is required for spindle positioning and asymmetric cell division in early C. elegans embryos. Dev Biol 265(1):127–39.

Pardridge WM. 1998. Blood–brain barrier carrier-mediated transport and brain metabolism of amino acids. Neurochem Res 23(5):635–44.

Pass KA, Lane PA, Fernhoff PM, Hinton CF, Panny SR, Parks JS, Pelias MZ, Rhead WJ, Ross SI, Wethers DL, et al. 2000. US newborn screening system guidelines II: follow-up of children, diagnosis, management, and evaluation. Statement of the Council of Regional Networks for Genetic Services (CORN). J Pediatr 137(4 Suppl):S1–46.

Pasteur L. 1861. Experiences et vues nouvelles sur la nature des fermentations. C R Acad Sci 52:1260–1264.

Pastinen T, Sladek R, Gurd S, Sammak A, Ge B, Lepage P, Lavergne K, Villeneuve A, Gaudin T, Brandstrom H, et al. 2004. A survey of genetic and epigenetic variation affecting human gene expression. Physiol Genomics 16(2):184–93.

Patterson MC. 2003. A riddle wrapped in a mystery: understanding Niemann-Pick disease, type C. Neurologist 9(6):301–10.

Patterson MC, Vanier MT, Suzuki K, Morris JA, Carstea E, Neufeld EB, Blanchette-Mackie J, Penteheu P. 2001. Niemann-Pick disease type C. In: Scriver CR, Beaudet AL, Sly W, Valle D, eds. The Metabolic and Molecular Bases of Inherited Diseases. New York: McGraw-Hill.

Pattison L, Crow YJ, Deeble VJ, Jackson AP, Jafri H, Rashid Y, Roberts E, Woods CG. 2000. A fifth locus for primary autosomal recessive microcephaly maps to chromosome 1q31. Am J Hum Genet 67(6):1578–80.

Pattison S, Pankarican M, Rupar CA, Graham FL, Igdoura SA. 2004. Five novel mutations in the lysosomal sialidase gene (NEU1) in type II sialidosis patients and assessment of their impact on enzyme activity and intracellular targeting using adenovirus-mediated expression. Hum Mutat 23(1):32–9.

Pende M, Um SH, Mieulet V, Sticker M, Goss VL, Mestan J, Mueller M, Fumagalli S, Kozma SC, Thomas G. 2004. S6K1–/–/S6K2–/– mice exhibit perinatal lethality and rapamycin-sensitive 5'-terminal oligopyrimidine mRNA translation and reveal a mitogen-activated protein kinase-dependent S6 kinase pathway. Mol Cell Biol 24(8):3112–24.

Pennisi E. 2002. Primate evolution. Gene activity clocks brain's fast evolution. Science 296(5566):233–5.

Penrose L, Quastel JH. 1937. Metabolic studies in phenylketonuria. Biochem J 31:266–74.

Penrose LS. 1946. Phenylketonuria—a problem in eugenics. Lancet 1:949–53. Reprinted 1998 Ann Hum Genet 62:193–202.

Penrose LS. 1954. The Biology of Mental Defect, Revised Edition. London: Sidgwick and Jackson.

Penrose LS. 1972. The Biology of Mental Defect, Fourth Edition. London: Sidgwick and Jackson.

Perrault I, Hanein S, Gerber S, Barbet F, Dufier JL, Munnich A, Rozet JM, Kaplan J. 2003. Evidence of autosomal dominant Leber congenital amaurosis (LCA) underlain by a CRX heterozygous null allele. J Med Genet 40(7):e90.

Pescucci C, Meloni I, Bruttini M, Ariani F, Longo I, Mari F, Canitano R, Hayek G, Zappella M, Renieri A. 2003. Chromosome 2 deletion encompassing the MAP2 gene in a patient with autism and Rett-like features. Clin Genet 64(6):497–501.

Peters C, Steward CG. 2003. Hematopoietic cell transplantation for inherited metabolic diseases: an overview of outcomes and practice guidelines. Bone Marrow Transplant 31(4):229–39.

Peters C, Charnas LR, Tan Y, Ziegler RS, Shapiro EG, DeFor T, Grewal SS, Orchard PJ, Abel SL, Goldman AI, et al. 2004. Cerebral X-linked adrenoleuko-dystrophy: the international hematopoietic cell transplantation experience from 1982 to 1999. Blood 104(3):881–8.

Peters SU, Beaudet AL, Madduri N, Bacino CA. 2004. Autism in Angelman syndrome: implications for autism research. Clin Genet 66(6):530–6.

Petronis A. 2004. The origin of schizophrenia: genetic thesis, epigenetic antithesis, and resolving synthesis. Biol Psychiatry 55(10):965–70.

Piao X, Basel-Vanagaite L, Straussberg R, Grant PE, Pugh EW, Doheny K, Doan B, Hong SE, Shugart YY, Walsh CA. 2002. An autosomal recessive form of bilateral frontoparietal polymicrogyria maps to chromosome 16q12.2-21. Am J Hum Genet 70(4):1028–33.

Pickart CM, Eddins MJ. 2004. Ubiquitin: structures, functions, mechanisms. Biochim Biophys Acta 1695(1–3):55–72.

Pieribone VA, Shupliakov O, Brodin L, Hilfiker-Rothenfluh S, Czernik AJ, Greengard P. 1995. Distinct pools of synaptic vesicles in neurotransmitter release. Nature 375(6531):493–7.

Pietz J, Kreis R, Rupp A, Mayatepek E, Rating D, Boesch C, Bremer HJ. 1999. Large neutral amino acids block phenylalanine transport into brain tissue in patients with phenylketonuria. J Clin Invest 103(8):1169–78.

Pietz J, Lutz T, Zwygart K, Hoffmann GF, Ebinger F, Boesch C, Kreis R. 2003. Phenylalanine can be detected in brain tissue of healthy subjects by ^{1}H magnetic resonance spectroscopy. J Inherit Metab Dis 26(7):683–92.

Pilia G, Hughes-Benzie RM, MacKenzie A, Baybayan P, Chen EY, Huber R, Neri G, Cao A, Forabosco A, Schlessinger D. 1996. Mutations in GPC3, a glypican gene, cause the Simpson-Golabi-Behmel overgrowth syndrome. Nat Genet 12(3):241–7.

Pind S, Slominski E, Mauthe J, Pearlman K, Swoboda KJ, Wilkins JA, Sauder P, Natowicz MR. 2002. V490M, a common mutation in 3-phosphoglycerate dehydrogenase deficiency, causes enzyme deficiency by decreasing the yield of mature enzyme. J Biol Chem 277(9):7136–43.

Pinero D, Jones B, Beard J. 2001. Variations in dietary iron alter behavior in developing rats. J Nutr 131(2):311–8.

Platt FM, Jeyakumar M, Andersson U, Heare T, Dwek RA, Butters TD. 2003. Substrate reduction therapy in mouse models of the glycosphingolipidoses. Philos Trans R Soc Lond B Biol Sci 358(1433):947–54.

Poirier K, Van Esch H, Friocourt G, Saillour Y, Bahi N, Backer S, Souil E, Castelnau-Ptakhine L, Beldjord C, Francis F, Bienvenu T, Chelly J. 2004. Neuroanatomical distribution of ARX in brain and its localisation in GABAergic neurons. Brain Res Mol Brain Res 122(1):35–46.

Poplawski NK, Harrison JR, Norton W, Wiltshire E, Fletcher JM. 2002. Urine amino and organic acids analysis in developmental delay or intellectual disability. J Paediatr Child Health 38(5):475–80.

Poplawski NK. 2003. Investigating intellectual disability: a genetic perspective. J Paediatr Child Health 39(7):492–506.

Porter FD. 2003. Human malformation syndromes due to inborn errors of cholesterol synthesis. Curr Opin Pediatr 15(6):607–13.

Potter EL. 1947. Rh : Its Relation to Congenital Hemolytic Disease & to Intra-Group Transfusion Reactions. Chicago: Year Book Publishers.

Pradhan S, Esteve PO. 2003. Mammalian DNA (cytosine-5) methyltransferases and their expression. Clin Immunol 109(1):6–16.

Proudfoot N, O'Sullivan J. 2002. Polyadenylation: a tail of two complexes. Curr Biol 12(24):R855–7.

Proudfoot NJ, Furger A, Dye MJ. 2002. Integrating mRNA processing with transcription. Cell 108(4):501–12.

Pujana MA, Nadal M, Gratacos M, Peral B, Csiszar K, Gonzalez-Sarmiento R, Sumoy L, Estivill X. 2001. Additional complexity on human chromosome 15q: identification of a set of newly recognized duplicons (LCR15) on 15q11-q13, 15q24, and 15q26. Genome Res 11(1):98–111.

Pujana MA, Nadal M, Guitart M, Armengol L, Gratacos M, Estivill X. 2002. Human chromosome 15q11–q14 regions of rearrangements contain clusters of LCR15 duplicons. Eur J Hum Genet 10(1):26–35.

Purpura DP. 1979. Pathobiology of cortical neurons in metabolic and unclassified amentias. Res Publ Assoc Res Nerv Ment Dis 57:43–68.

The Rain Plague, prod. Grant Mansfield. London: BBC TV Productions, 30 min, 1991.

Ramakers GJ. 2002. Rho proteins, mental retardation and the cellular basis of cognition. Trends Neurosci 25(4):191–9.

Rampler H, Weinhofer I, Netik A, Forss-Petter S, Brown PJ, Oplinger JA, Bugaut M, Berger J. 2003. Evaluation of the therapeutic potential of PPARalpha agonists for X-linked adrenoleukodystrophy. Mol Genet Metab 80(4):398–407.

Rayasam GV, Wendling O, Angrand PO, Mark M, Niederreither K, Song L, Lerouge T, Hager GL, Chambon P, Losson R. 2003. NSD1 is essential for early post-implantation development and has a catalytically active SET domain. EMBO J 22(12):3153–63.

Raynaud M, Ronce N, Ayrault AD, Francannet C, Malpuech G, Moraine C. 1998. X-Linked mental retardation with isolated growth hormone deficiency is mapped to Xq22-Xq27.2 in one family. Am J Med Genet 76(3):255–61.

Relton CL, Wilding CS, Laffling AJ, Jonas PA, Burgess T, Binks K, Tawn EJ, Burn J. 2004a. Low erythrocyte folate status and polymorphic variation in folate-related genes are associated with risk of neural tube defect pregnancy. Mol Genet Metab 81(4):273–81.

Relton CL, Wilding CS, Pearce MS, Laffling AJ, Jonas PA, Lynch SA, Tawn EJ, Burn J. 2004b. Gene–gene interaction in folate-related genes and risk of neural tube defects in a UK population. J Med Genet 41(4):256–60.

Renwick JH, Lawler SD. 1955. Genetical linkage between ABO and nail-patella loci. Ann Hum Genet 19:312–31.

Rhodin J. 1954. Correlation of ultra-structural organization and function in normal and experimental changing convoluted tubule cells of the mouse kidney. Stockholm: Aktiebolaget Godvil.

Riegel M, Baumer A, Jamar M, Delbecque K, Herens C, Verloes A, Schinzel A. 2001. Submicroscopic terminal deletions and duplications in retarded patients with unclassified malformation syndromes. Hum Genet 109(3):286–94.

Rio C, Rieff HI, Qi P, Khurana TS, Corfas G. 1997. Neuregulin and erbB receptors play a critical role in neuronal migration. Neuron 19(1):39–50.

Rio M, Clech L, Amiel J, Faivre L, Lyonnet S, Le Merrer M, Odent S, Lacombe D, Edery P, Brauner R, et al. 2003. Spectrum of NSD1 mutations in Sotos and Weaver syndromes. J Med Genet 40(6):436–40.

Risch N, Spiker D, Lotspeich L, Nouri N, Hinds D, Hallmayer J, Kalaydjieva L, McCague P, Dimiceli S, Pitts T, et al. 1999. A genomic screen of autism: evidence for a multilocus etiology. Am J Hum Genet 65(2):493–507.

Ritvo ER, Freeman BJ, Scheibel AB, Duong T, Robinson H, Guthrie D, Ritvo A. 1986. Lower Purkinje cell counts in the cerebella of four autistic subjects: initial findings of the UCLA-NSAC Autopsy Research Report. Am J Psychiatry 143(7):862–6.

Rizzo C, Boenzi S, Wanders RJ, Duran M, Caruso U, Dionisi-Vici C. 2003. Characteristic acylcarnitine profiles in inherited defects of peroxisome biogenesis: a novel tool for screening diagnosis using tandem mass spectrometry. Pediatr Res 53(6):1013–8.

Rizzoti K, Brunelli S, Carmignac D, Thomas PQ, Robinson IC, Lovell-Badge R. 2004. SOX3 is required during the formation of the hypothalamo–pituitary axis. Nat Genet 36(3):247–55.

Roberts SE, Dennis NR, Browne CE, Willatt L, Woods G, Cross I, Jacobs PA, Thomas S. 2002. Characterisation of interstitial duplications and triplications of chromosome 15q11-q13. Hum Genet 110(3):227–34.

Robinson BH. 1983. Inborn errors of pyruvate metabolism. Biochem Soc Trans 11(6):623–6.

Robinson BH, Taylor J, Sherwood WG. 1980. The genetic heterogeneity of lactic acidosis: occurrence of recognizable inborn errors of metabolism in pediatric population with lactic acidosis. Pediatr Res 14(8):956–62.

Robinson BH, MacKay N, Chun K, Ling M. 1996. Disorders of pyruvate carboxylase and the pyruvate dehydrogenase complex. J Inherit Metab Dis 19(4):452–62.

Robson KJ, Chandra T, MacGillivray RT, Woo SL. 1982. Polysome immunoprecipitation of phenylalanine hydroxylase mRNA from rat liver and cloning of its cDNA. Proc Natl Acad Sci USA 79(15):4701–5.

Roe CR, Sweetman L, Roe DS, David F, Brunengraber H. 2002. Treatment of cardiomyopathy and rhabdomyolysis in long-chain fat oxidation disorders using an anaplerotic odd-chain triglyceride. J Clin Invest 110(2):259–69.

Ropers HH, Hoeltzenbein M, Kalscheuer V, Yntema H, Hamel B, Fryns JP, Chelly J,

Partington M, Gecz J, Moraine C. 2003. Nonsyndromic X-linked mental retardation: where are the missing mutations? Trends Genet 19(6):316–20.

Rosenberg EH, Almeida LS, Kleefstra T, deGrauw RS, Yntema HG, Bahi N, Moraine C, Ropers HH, Fryns JP, deGrauw TJ, et al. 2004. High prevalence of SLC6A8 deficiency in X-linked mental retardation. Am J Hum Genet 75(1):97–105.

Rosenberg LE, Lilljeqvist A, Hsia YE. 1968. Methylmalonic aciduria: metabolic block localization and vitamin B_{12} dependency. Science 162(855):805–7.

Rosenberger G, Jantke I, Gal A, Kutche K. 2003. Interaction of alpha PIX (ARHGEF6) with beta-parvin (PARVB) suggests an involvement of alphaPIX in integrin-mediated signaling. Hum Mol Genet 12(2):155–67.

Rossi E, Piccini F, Zollino M, Neri G, Caselli D, Tenconi R, Castellan C, Carrozzo R, Danesino C, Zuffardi O, et al. 2001. Cryptic telomeric rearrangements in subjects with mental retardation associated with dysmorphism and congenital malformations. J Med Genet 38(6):417–20.

Rouse B, Azen C. 2004. Effect of high maternal blood phenylalanine on offspring congenital anomalies and developmental outcome at ages 4 and 6 years: the importance of strict dietary control preconception and throughout pregnancy. J Pediatr 144(2):235–9.

Roux W. 1883. Uber die Bedeutung der Kerntheilungsfiguren. Liepzig: Engelmann.

Rovet J, Netley C, Bailey J, Keenan M, Stewart D. 1995. Intelligence and achievement in children with extra X aneuploidy: a longitudinal perspective. Am J Med Genet 60(5):356–63.

Royer G, Hanein S, Raclin V, Gigarel N, Rozet JM, Munnich A, Steffann J, Dufier JL, Kaplan J, Bonnefont JP. 2003. *NDP* gene mutations in 14 French families with Norrie disease. Hum Mutat 22(6):499.

Runte M, Huttenhofer A, Gross S, Kiefmann M, Horsthemke B, Buiting K. 2001. The IC-SNURF-SNRPN transcript serves as a host for multiple small nucleolar RNA species and as an antisense RNA for UBE3A. Hum Mol Genet 10(23):2687–700.

Runte M, Kroisel PM, Gillessen-Kaesbach G, Varon R, Horn D, Cohen MY, Wagstaff J, Horsthemke B, Buiting K. 2004. SNURF-SNRPN and UBE3A transcript levels in patients with Angelman syndrome. Hum Genet 114(6):553–61.

Sacconi S, Salviati L, Sue CM, Shanske S, Davidson MM, Bonilla E, Naini AB, De Vivo DC, DiMauro S. 2003. Mutation screening in patients with isolated cytochrome *c* oxidase deficiency. Pediatr Res 53(2):224–30.

Sachs B. 1887. On arrested cerebral development with special reference to its cortical pathology. J Nerv Ment Dis 14:541–553.

Sakisaka T, Itoh T, Miura K, Takenawa T. 1997. Phosphatidylinositol 4,5-bisphosphate phosphatase regulates the rearrangement of actin filaments. Mol Cell Biol 17(7):3841–9.

Samaco RC, Hogart A, Lasalle JM. 2005. Epigenetic overlap in autism-spectrum neurodevelopmental disorders: *MECP2* deficiency causes reduced expression of *UBE3A* and *GABRB3*. Hum Mol Genet 14(4):483–92.

Samango-Sprouse C. 2001. Mental development in polysomy X Klinefelter syndrome (47,XXY;48,XXXY): effects of incomplete X inactivation. Semin Reprod Med 19(2):193–202.

Sampson PD, Streissguth AP, Bookstein FL, Little RE, Clarren SK, Dehaene P, Hanson JW, Graham JM Jr. 1997. Incidence of fetal alcohol syndrome and prevalence of alcohol-related neurodevelopmental disorder. Teratology 56(5):317–26.

Sandhoff K, Kolter T, Harze K. 2001. Sphingolipid activator proteins. In: Scriver CR, Beaudet AL, Sly W, Valle D, eds. The Metabolic and Molecular Bases of Inherited Diseases. New York: McGraw-Hill.

Sanger F. 1952. The arrangement of amino acids in proteins. Adv Protein Chem 7:1–67.

Sanger F, Coulson AR. 1978. The use of thin acrylamide gels for DNA sequencing. FEBS Lett 87(1):107–10.

Sanger F, Nicklen S, Coulson AR. 1977. DNA sequencing with chain-terminating inhibitors. Proc Natl Acad Sci USA 74(12):5463–7.

Sarde CO, Mosser J, Kioschis P, Kretz C, Vicaire S, Aubourg P, Poustka A, Mandel JL. 1994. Genomic organization of the adrenoleukodystrophy gene. Genomics 22(1):13–20.

Savolainen H. 1976. Isolation of the liver N-aspartyl-beta-glucosaminidase in aspartylglucosaminuria. Biochem J 153(3):749–50.

Sawkar AR, Cheng WC, Beutler E, Wong CH, Balch WE, Kelly JW. 2002. Chemical chaperones increase the cellular activity of N370S beta-glucosidase: a therapeutic strategy for Gaucher disease. Proc Natl Acad Sci USA 99(24):15428–33.

Scaglia F, Towbin JA, Craigen WJ, Belmont JW, Smith EO, Neish SR, Ware SM, Hunter JV, Fernbach SD, Vladutiu GD, et al. 2004. Clinical spectrum, morbidity, and mortality in 113 pediatric patients with mitochondrial disease. Pediatrics 114(4):925–31.

Schaefer GB, Bodensteiner JB. 1992. Evaluation of the child with idiopathic mental retardation. Pediatr Clin North Am 39(4):929–43.

Schaefer GB, Bodensteiner JB, Thompson JN Jr, Kimberling WJ, Craft JM. 1998. Volumetric neuroimaging in Usher syndrome: evidence of global involvement. Am J Med Genet 79(1):1–4.

Schantz SL, Widholm JJ. 2001. Cognitive effects of endocrine-disrupting chemicals in animals. Environ Health Perspect 109(12):1197–206.

Scheerenberger R. 1983. A History of Mental Retardation. Baltimore: Brookes Publishing.

Scheffer IE, Berkovic SF. 2003. The genetics of human epilepsy. Trends Pharmacol Sci 24(8):428–33.

Scherer SW, Cheung J, MacDonald JR, Osborne LR, Nakabayashi K, Herbrick JA, Carson AR, Parker-Katiraee L, Skaug J, Khaja R, et al. 2003. Human chromosome 7: DNA sequence and biology. Science 300(5620):767–72.

Schiestl RH, Khogali F, Carls N. 1994. Reversion of the mouse pink-eyed unstable mutation induced by low doses of X-rays. Science 266(5190):1573–6.

Schoumans J, Anderlid BM, Blennow E, Teh BT, Nordenskjold M. 2004. The performance of CGH array for the detection of cryptic constitutional chromosome imbalances. J Med Genet 41(3):198–202.

Schuchman EH, Desnick RJ. 2001. Niemann-Pick disease types A and B: acid sphingomyelinase deficiencies. In: Scriver CR, Beaudet AL, Valle D, Sly WS, eds. The Metabolic Basis of Inherited Disease. New York: McGraw-Hill.

Schuil J, Meire FM, Delleman JW. 1998. Mental retardation in amaurosis congenita of Leber. Neuropediatrics 29(6):294–7.

Schuler AM, Gower BA, Matern D, Rinaldo P, Wood PA. 2004. Influence of dietary fatty acid chain-length on metabolic tolerance in mouse models of inherited defects in mitochondrial fatty acid beta-oxidation. Mol Genet Metab 83(4):322–9.

Schulz A, Dhar S, Rylova S, Dbaibo G, Alroy J, Hagel C, Artacho I, Kohlschutter A, Lin S, Boustany RM. 2004. Impaired cell adhesion and apoptosis in a novel CLN9 Batten disease variant. Ann Neurol 56(3):342–50.

Schwartz DC, Hochstrasser M. 2003. A superfamily of protein tags: ubiquitin, SUMO and related modifiers. Trends Biochem Sci 28(6):321–8.

Scott C, Ioannou YA. 2004. The NPC1 protein: structure implies function. Biochim Biophys Acta 1685(1–3):8–13.

Scriver CR, Ryans S. 2000. Phenylalanine Hydroxylase Deficiency. Gene Reviews, http://www.geneclinics.org/profiles/pku/details.htm.

Scriver CR. 2004. After the genome—the phenome? J Inherit Metab Dis 27(3):305–17.

Scriver CR, Kaufman S. 2001. Hyperphenylalaninemia: phenylalanine hydroxylase deficiency. In: Scriver CR, Beaudet AL, Sly W, Valle D, eds. The Metabolic and Molecular Bases of Inherited Disease. New York: McGraw-Hill.

Seabright M. 1972. Human chromosome banding. Lancet 1(7757):967.

Seguin E. 1866. Idiocy and Its Treatment by Physiological Methods. New York: W. Wood and Co.

Seidenberg M, Beck N, Geisser M, Giordani B, Sackellares JC, Berent S, Dreifuss FE, Boll TJ. 1986. Academic achievement of children with epilepsy. Epilepsia 27(6):753–9.

Senior K. 2002. Lorenzo's oil may help to prevent ALD symptoms. Lancet Neurol 1(8):468.

Sewell AC, Poets CF, Degen I, Stoss H, Pontz BF. 1996. The spectrum of free neuraminic acid storage disease in childhood: clinical, morphological and biochemical observations in three non-Finnish patients. Am J Med Genet 63(1):203–8.

Seyrantepe V, Poupetova H, Froissart R, Zabot MT, Maire I, Pshezhetsky AV. 2003. Molecular pathology of NEU1 gene in sialidosis. Hum Mutat 22(5):343–52.

Shapiro E, Krivit W, Lockman L, Jambaque I, Peters C, Cowan M, Harris R, Blanche S, Bordigoni P, Loes D, Ziegler R, Crittenden M, Ris D, Berg B, Cox C, Moser H, Fischer A, Aubourg P. 2000. Long-term effect of bone-marrow transplantation for childhood-onset cerebral X-linked adrenoleukodystrophy. Lancet 26; 356(9231):713–8.

Shao Y, Wolpert CM, Raiford KL, Menold MM, Donnelly SL, Ravan SA, Bass MP, McClain C, von Wendt L, Vance JM, et al. 2002. Genomic screen and follow-up analysis for autistic disorder. Am J Med Genet 114(1):99–105.

Shao Y, Cuccaro ML, Hauser ER, Raiford KL, Menold MM, Wolpert CM, Ravan SA, Elston L, Decena K, Donnelly SL, et al. 2003. Fine mapping of autistic disorder to chromosome 15q11-q13 by use of phenotypic subtypes. Am J Hum Genet 72(3):539–48.

Shaw-Smith C, Redon R, Rickman L, Rio M, Willatt L, Fiegler H, Firth H, Sanlaville D, Winter R, Colleaux L, et al. 2004. Microarray based comparative genomic hybridisation (array-CGH) detects submicroscopic chromosomal deletions and duplications in patients with learning disability/mental retardation and dysmorphic features. J Med Genet 41(4):241–8.

Shelov SP, ed. 1991. Caring for Your Baby and Young Child: Birth to Age 5. New York: Bantam Books.

Sherr EH. 2003. The *ARX* story (epilepsy, mental retardation, autism, and cerebral malformations): one gene leads to many phenotypes. Curr Opin Pediatr 15(6):567–71.

Shevell MI, Majnemer A, Rosenbaum P, Abrahamowicz M. 2000. Etiologic yield of single domain developmental delay: a prospective study. J Pediatr 137(5):633–7.

Shevell MI, Majnemer A, Rosenbaum P, Abrahamowicz M. 2001. Etiologic determination of childhood developmental delay. Brain Dev 23(4):228–35.

Shevell M, Ashwal S, Donley D, Flint J, Gingold M, Hirtz D, Majnemer A, Noetzel M, Sheth RD. 2003. Practice parameter: evaluation of the child with global developmental delay: report of the Quality Standards Subcommittee of the American Academy of Neurology and The Practice Committee of the Child Neurology Society. Neurology 60(3):367–80.

Shi Y. 2003. Mammalian RNAi for the masses. Trends Genet 19(1):9–12.

Shibayama A, Cook EH Jr, Feng J, Glanzmann C, Yan J, Craddock N, Jones IR, Goldman D, Heston LL, Sommer SS. 2004. MECP2 structural and 3'-UTR variants in schizophrenia, autism and other psychiatric diseases: a possible association with autism. Am J Med Genet B 128(1):50–3.

Shin HT, Chang MW. 2001. Trichorhinophalangeal syndrome, type II (Langer-Giedion syndrome). Dermatol Online J 7(2):8.

Shoffner J. 2001. Oxidative phosphorylation. In: Scriver CR, Beaudet AL, Sly W, Valle D, eds. The Metabolic and Molecular Bases of Inherited Disease. New York: McGraw-Hill.

Shoichet SA, Hoffmann K, Menzel C, Trautmann U, Moser B, Hoeltzenbein M, Echenne B, Partington M, Van Bokhoven H, Moraine C, et al. 2003. Mutations in the *ZNF41* gene are associated with cognitive deficits: identification of a new candidate for X-linked mental retardation. Am J Hum Genet 73(6):1341–54.

Shorter E. 2000. The Kennedy Family and the Story of Mental Retardation. Philadelphia: Temple University Press.

Siderius LE, Hamel BC, van Bokhoven H, de Jager F, van den Helm B, Kremer H, Heineman-de Boer JA, Ropers HH, Mariman EC. 1999. X-Linked mental retardation associated with cleft lip/palate maps to Xp11.3-q21.3. Am J Med Genet 85(3):216–20.

Siemens J, Kazmierczak P, Reynolds A, Sticker M, Littlewood-Evans A, Muller U. 2002. The Usher syndrome proteins cadherin 23 and harmonin form a complex by means of PDZ-domain interactions. Proc Natl Acad Sci USA 99(23):14946–51.

Simpson JL, de la Cruz F, Swerdloff RS, Samango-Sprouse C, Skakkebaek NE, Graham JM Jr, Hassold T, Aylstock M, Meyer-Bahlburg HF, Willard HF, et al. 2003. Klinefelter syndrome: expanding the phenotype and identifying new research directions. Genet Med 5(6):460–8.

Sistermans EA, de Coo RF, van Beerendonk HM, Poll-The BT, Kleijer WJ, van Oost BA. 2000. Mutation detection in the aspartoacylase gene in 17 patients with Canavan disease: four new mutations in the non-Jewish population. Eur J Hum Genet 8(7):557–60.

Slager RE, Newton TL, Vlangos CN, Finucane B, Elsea SH. 2003. Mutations in RAI1 associated with Smith-Magenis syndrome. Nat Genet 33(4):466–8.

Smeets E, Schollen E, Moog U, Matthijs G, Herbergs J, Smeets H, Curfs L, Schrander-

Stumpel C, Fryns JP. 2003. Rett syndrome in adolescent and adult females: clinical and molecular genetic findings. Am J Med Genet A 122(3):227–33.

Smith DW, Lemli L, Opitz JM. 1964. a newly recognized syndrome of multiple congenital Anomalies. J Pediatr 64:210–7.

Smith I, Lloyd J. 1974. Atypical phenylketonuria accompanied by a severe progressive neurological illness unresponsive to dietary treatment. Arch Dis Child 49(3):245.

Smith M, Escamilla JR, Filipek P, Bocian ME, Modahl C, Flodman P, Spence M. 2001. Molecular genetic delineation of 2q37.3 deletion in autism and osteodystrophy: report of a case and of new markers for deletion screening by PCR. Cytogenet Cell Genet 94(1–2):15–22.

Smith M, Filipek PA, Wu C, Bocian M, Hakim S, Modahl C, Spence MA. 2000. Analysis of a 1-megabase deletion in 15q22-q23 in an autistic patient: identification of candidate genes for autism and of homologous DNA segments in 15q22-q23 and 15q11-q13. Am J Med Genet 96(6):765–70.

Smith M, Woodroffe A, Smith R, Holguin S, Martinez J, Filipek PA, Modahl C, Moore B, Bocian ME, Mays L, et al. 2002. Molecular genetic delineation of a deletion of chromosome 13q12→q13 in a patient with autism and auditory processing deficits. Cytogenet Genome Res 98(4):233–9.

Smithells RW, Sheppard S, Schorah CJ. 1976. Vitamin dificiencies and neural tube defects. Arch Dis Child 51(12):944–50.

Smithells RW, Sheppard S, Schorah CJ, Seller MJ, Nevin NC, Harris R, Read AP, Fielding DW.1981. Apparent prevention of neural tube defects by periconceptional vitamin supplementation. Arch Dis Child 56(12):911–8.

Sogayar MC, Camargo AA, Bettoni F, Carraro DM, et al. 2004. A transcript finishing initiative for closing gaps in the human transcriptome. Genome Res 14(7):1413–23.

Solot CB, Gerdes M, Kirschner RE, McDonald-McGinn DM, Moss E, Woodin M, Aleman D, Zackai EH, Wang PP. 2001. Communication issues in 22q11.2 deletion syndrome: children at risk. Genet Med 3(1):67–71.

Song ZM, Undie AS, Koh PO, Fang YY, Zhang L, Dracheva S, Sealfon SC, Lidow MS. 2002. D_1 dopamine receptor regulation of microtubule-associated protein-2 phosphorylation in developing cerebral cortical neurons. J Neurosci 22(14):6092–105.

Staba SL, Escolar ML, Poe M, Kim Y, Martin PL, Szabolcs P, Allison-Thacker J, Wood S, Wenger DA, Rubinstein P, et al. 2004. Cord-blood transplants from unrelated donors in patients with Hurler's syndrome. N Engl J Med 350(19):1960–9.

Stanbury J, Hetzel B. 1980. Endemic Goiter and Endemic Cretinism: Iodine Nutrition in Health and Disease. New York: Wiley.

Steegers-Theunissen RP, Boers GH, Trijbels FJ, Eskes TK. 1991. Neural-tube defects and derangement of homocysteine metabolism. N Engl J Med 324(3):199–200.

Steenland K, Dick RB, Howell RJ, Chrislip DW, Hines CJ, Reid TM, Lehman E, Laber P, Krieg EF Jr, Knott C. 2000. Neurologic function among termiticide applicators exposed to chlorpyrifos. Environ Health Perspect 108(4):293–300.

Steinberg S, Chen L, Wei L, Moser A, Moser H, Cutting G, Braverman N. 2004. The PEX gene screen: molecular diagnosis of peroxisome biogenesis disorders in the Zellweger syndrome spectrum. Mol Genet Metab 83(3):252–63.

Stevenson RE, Schroer RJ, Skinner C, Fender D, Simensen RJ. 1997. Autism and macrocephaly. Lancet 349(9067):1744–5.

Stokke O, Eldjarn L, Norum K, Steen-Johnsen J, Halvorsen S. 1967. Methylmalonic acidemia: a new inborn error of metabolism which may cause fatal acidosis in the newborn period. Scand J Clin Invest 20:213.

Stoll C. 2001. Problems in the diagnosis of fragile X syndrome in young children are still present. Am J Med Genet 100(2):110–5.

Stone DM, Hynes M, Armanini M, Swanson TA, Gu Q, Johnson RL, Scott MP, Pennica D, Goddard A, Phillips H, et al. 1996. The tumour-suppressor gene patched encodes a candidate receptor for Sonic hedgehog. Nature 384(6605):129–34.

Strachan T, Read AP. 1999. Human Molecular Genetics. New York: Wiley-Liss.

Strauss KA, Puffenberger EG, Robinson DL, Morton DH. 2003. Type I glutaric aciduria, part 1: natural history of 77 patients. Am J Med Genet C 121(1):38–52.

Stromme P, Mangelsdorf ME, Scheffer IE, Gecz J. 2002. Infantile spasms, dystonia, and other X-linked phenotypes caused by mutations in Aristaless related homeobox gene, *ARX*. Brain Dev 24(5):266–8.

Stroustrup Smith A, Grable I, Levine D. 2004. Case 66: caudal regression syndrome in the fetus of a diabetic mother. Radiology 230(1):229–33.

Sturtevant AH. 1965. A History of Genetics. New York: Harper and Row.

Sudhof TC. 2004. The synaptic vesicle cycle. Annu Rev Neurosci 27:509–47.

Sun ZW, Allis CD. 2002. Ubiquitination of histone H2B regulates H3 methylation and gene silencing in yeast. Nature 418(6893):104–8.

Sutherland GR, Baker E. 1986a. Effects of nucleotides on expression of the folate sensitive fragile sites. Am J Med Genet 23(1–2):409–17.

Sutherland GR, Baker E. 1986b. Induction of fragile sites in fibroblasts. Am J Hum Genet 38(4):573–5.

Sutherland GR, Gecz J, Mulley JC. 2002. Fragile X and other causes of X-linked mental retardation. In: Rimoin DL, O'Connor JM, Pyeritz RE, Korf BR, eds. Emery and Rimoin's Principles and Practice of Medical Genetics. New York: Churchill Livingstone.

Sutton WS. 1902. On the morphology of the chromosome group in *Brachystola magna* Biol Bull 4:24–49. See Sutton quote on p. 37 in Sturtevant AH. A History of Genetics.

Suzuki Y, Sakuraba H, Hayashi K, Suzuki K, Imahori K. 1981. Beta-galactosidase-neuraminidase deficiency: restoration of beta-galactosidase activity by protease inhibitors. J Biochem (Tokyo) 90(1):271–3.

Suzuki Y, Oshima A. 1993. A beta-galactosidase gene mutation identified in both Morquio B disease and infantile GM1 gangliosidosis. Hum Genet 91(4):407–15.

Suzuki Y, Oshima, A, Nanba E. 2001. Beta galactosidase deficiency: GM_1 gangliosidosis and Morquio B disease. In: Scriver CR, Beaudet AL, Valle D, Sly WS, eds. The Metabolic Basis of Inherited Disease. New York: McGraw Hill.

Svedberg T. 1937. The ultra-centrifuge and the study of high molecular weight compounds. Nature 139:1051–1062.

Svennerholm L, Vanier MT, Mansson JE. 1980. Krabbe disease: a galacto-sylsphingosine (psychosine) lipidosis. J Lipid Res 21(1):53–64.

Sweatt JD, Weeber EJ. 2003a. Genetics of childhood disorders: LII. Learning and memory. Part 5: Human cognitive disorders and the ras/ERK/CREB pathway. J Am Acad Child Adolesc Psychiatry 42(7):873–6.

Sweatt JD, Weeber EJ, Lombroso PJ. 2003b. Genetics of childhood disorders: LI. Learning and memory. Part 4: Human cognitive disorders and the ras/ERK/CREB pathway. J Am Acad Child Adolesc Psychiatry 42(6):741–4.

Sweetman L, Bates SP, Hull D, Nyhan WL. 1977. Propionyl-CoA carboxylase deficiency in a patient with biotin-responsive 3-methylcrotonylglycinuria. Pediatr Res 11(11):1144–7.

Tanaka K, Budd MA, Efron ML, Isselbacher KJ. 1966. Isovaleric acidemia: a new genetic defect of leucine metabolism. Proc Natl Acad Sci USA 56(1):236–42.

Taneja PR, Pandya A, Foley DL, Nicely LV, Arnos KS. 2004. Attitudes of deaf individuals towards genetic testing. Am J Med Genet A 130(1):17–21.

Taniguchi K, Kobayashi K, Saito K, Yamanouchi H, Ohnuma A, Hayashi YK, Manya H, Jin DK, Lee M, Parano E, et al. 2003. Worldwide distribution and broader clinical spectrum of muscle–eye–brain disease. Hum Mol Genet 12(5):527–34.

Tarpey P, Parnau J, Blow M, Woffendin H, Bignell G, Cox C, Cox J, Davies H, Edkins S, Holden S, et al. 2004. Mutations in the *DLG3* gene cause non-syndromic X-linked mental retardation. Am J Hum Genet 75(2):318–24.

Tassabehji M, Metcalfe K, Karmiloff-Smith A, Carette MJ, Grant J, Dennis N, Reardon W, Splitt M, Read AP, Donnai D. 1999. Williams syndrome: use of chromosomal microdeletions as a tool to dissect cognitive and physical phenotypes. Am J Hum Genet 64(1):118–25.

Tay W. 1881. Symmetrical changes in the region of the yellow spot in each eye of an infant. Trans Opthalmol Soc 1:55–57.

Tayebi N, Stubblefield BK, Park JK, Orvisky E, Walker JM, LaMarca ME, Sidransky E. 2003. Reciprocal and nonreciprocal recombination at the glucocerebrosidase gene region: implications for complexity in Gaucher disease. Am J Hum Genet 72(3):519–34.

Temin H. Baltimore D. 1972. RNA directed DNAQ synthesis and RNA tumor viruses Advan Virus Res 17:129–86.

Tessier-Lavigne M. 1994. Axon guidance by diffusible repellants and attractants. Curr Opin Genet Dev 4(4):596–601.

Thomas GH. 2001. Disorders of glycoprotein degradation: alpha mannosidosis, beta mannosidosis, fucosidosis and sialidosis. In: Scriver CR, Beaudet AL, Valle D, Sly WS, eds. The Metabolic Basis of Inherited Disease. New York: McGraw-Hill.

Thomas JA, Johnson J, Peterson Kraai TL, Wilson R, Tartaglia N, LeRoux J, Beischel L, McGavran L, Hagerman RJ. 2003. Genetic and clinical characterization of patients with an interstitial duplication 15q11-q13, emphasizing behavioral phenotype and response to treatment. Am J Med Genet A 119(2):111–20.

Tian H, Jeong J, Harfe BD, Tabin CJ, McMahon AP. 2005. Mouse Disp1 is required in sonic hedgehog–expressing cells for paracrine activity of the cholesterol-modified ligand. Development 132(1):133–42.

Tjio J, Levan A. 1956. The chromosome number in man. Hereditas 42:1–6.

Toda T, Kobayashi K. 1999. Fukuyama-type congenital muscular dystrophy: the first human disease to be caused by an ancient retrotransposal integration. J Mol Med 77(12):816–23.

Toda T, Kobayashi K, Kondo-Iida E, Sasaki J, Nakamura Y. 2000. The Fukuyama congenital muscular dystrophy story. Neuromuscul Disord 10(3):153–9.

Todd JA. 2001. Human genetics. Tackling common disease. Nature 411(6837):537–9.

Tolmie JL. 2002. Clinical genetics of neural tube defects and other congenital central nervous system malformations. In: Rimoin DL, Connor JM, Pyeritz RE, Korf BR, eds. Emery and Rimoin's Principles and Practice of Medical Genetics. New York, London, Toronto: Churchill Livingstone, pp 2976–3011.

Tomblin JB, Pandich J. 1999. Lessons from children with specific language impairment. Trends Cogn Sci 3(8):283–5.

Tonkin ET, Smith M, Eichhorn P, Jones S, Imamwerdi B, Lindsay S, Jackson M, Wang TJ, Ireland M, Burn J, et al. 2004. A giant novel gene undergoing extensive alternative splicing is severed by a Cornelia de Lange–associated translocation breakpoint at 3q26.3. Hum Genet 115(2):139–48.

Toyo-oka K, Shionoya A, Gambello MJ, Cardoso C, Leventer R, Ward HL, Ayala R, Tsai LH, Dobyns W, Ledbetter D, et al. 2003. 14-3-3Epsilon is important for neuronal migration by binding to NUDEL: a molecular explanation for Miller-Dieker syndrome. Nat Genet 34(3):274–85.

Trefz FK, Aulela-Scholz C, Blau N. 2001. Successful treatment of phenylketonuria with tetrahydrobiopterin. Eur J Pediatr 160(5):315.

Tropak MB, Reid SP, Guiral M, Withers SG, Mahuran D. 2004. Pharmacological enhancement of beta-hexosaminidase activity in fibroblasts from adult Tay-Sachs and Sandhoff patients. J Biol Chem 279(14):13478–87.

Tucker KL. 2001. Methylated cytosine and the brain: a new base for neuroscience. Neuron 30(3):649–52.

Tufarelli C, Stanley JA, Garrick D, Sharpe JA, Ayyub H, Wood WG, Higgs DR. 2003. Transcription of antisense RNA leading to gene silencing and methylation as a novel cause of human genetic disease. Nat Genet 34(2):157–65.

Tumer Z, Birk Moller L, Horn N. 2003. Screening of 383 unrelated patients affected with Menkes disease and finding of 57 gross deletions in ATP7A. Hum Mutat 22(6):457–64.

Tupler R, Gabellini D. 2004. Molecular basis of facioscapulohumeral muscular dystrophy. Cell Mol Life Sci 61(5):557–66.

Turkmen S, Gillessen-Kaesbach G, Meinecke P, Albrecht B, Neumann LM, Hesse V, Palanduz S, Balg S, Majewski F, Fuchs S, et al. 2003. Mutations in NSD1 are responsible for Sotos syndrome, but are not a frequent finding in other overgrowth phenotypes. Eur J Hum Genet 11(11):858–65.

Tyler WJ, Perrett SP, Pozzo-Miller LD. 2002. The role of neurotrophins in neurotransmitter release. Neuroscientist 8(6):524–31.

Van den Veyver IB, Zoghbi HY. 2002. Genetic basis of Rett syndrome. Ment Retard Dev Disabil Res Rev 8(2):82–6.

van der Put NM, Steegers-Theunissen RP, Frosst P, Trijbels FJ, Eskes TK, van den Heuvel LP, Mariman EC, den Heyer M, Rozen R, Blom HJ. 1995. Mutated methylenetetrahydrofolate reductase as a risk factor for spina bifida. Lancet 346(8982):1070–1.

van Praag H, Christie BR, Sejnowski TJ, Gage FH. 1999. Running enhances neurogenesis, learning, and long-term potentiation in mice. Proc Natl Acad Sci USA 96(23):13427–31.

Van Wagenen B. 1914. Surgical sterilization as a eugenics measure. J Psychoasthenics 18:185–96.

Varki A, Kornfeld S. 1981. Purification and characterization of rat liver alpha-N-acetylglucosaminyl phosphodiesterase. J Biol Chem 256(19):9937–43.

Varki AP, Reitman ML, Kornfeld S. 1981. Identification of a variant of mucolipidosis III (pseudo-Hurler polydystrophy): a catalytically active N-acetylglucosaminylphosphotransferase that fails to phosphorylate lysosomal enzymes. Proc Natl Acad Sci USA 78(12):7773–7.

Vasconcellos E, Wyllie E, Sullivan S, Stanford L, Bulacio J, Kotagal P, Bingaman W.

2001. Mental retardation in pediatric candidates for epilepsy surgery: the role of early seizure onset. Epilepsia 42(2):268–74.

Veltman MW, Thompson RJ, Roberts SE, Thomas NS, Whittington J, Bolton PF. 2004. Prader-Willi syndrome—a study comparing deletion and uniparental disomy cases with reference to autism spectrum disorders. Eur Child Adolesc Psychiatry 13(1):42–50.

Venter PA, Christianson AL, Hutamo CM, Makhura MP, Gericke GS. 1995. Congenital anomalies in rural black South African neonates—a silent epidemic? S Afr Med J 85(1):15–20.

Venturin M, Guarnieri P, Natacci F, Stabile M, Tenconi R, Clementi M, Hernandez C, Thompson P, Upadhyaya M, Larizza L, et al. 2004. Mental retardation and cardiovascular malformations in NF1 microdeleted patients point to candidate genes in 17q11.2. J Med Genet 41(1):35–41.

Verheijen FW, Verbeek E, Aula N, Beerens CE, Havelaar AC, Joosse M, Peltonen L, Aula P, Galjaard H, van der Spek PJ, et al. 1999. A new gene, encoding an anion transporter, is mutated in sialic acid storage diseases. Nat Genet 23(4):462–5.

Verkerk AJ, Pieretti M, Sutcliffe JS, Fu YH, Kuhl DP, Pizzuti A, Reiner O, Richards S, Victoria MF, Zhang FP, et al. 1991. Identification of a gene (*FMR-1*) containing a CGG repeat coincident with a breakpoint cluster region exhibiting length variation in fragile X syndrome. Cell 65(5):905–14.

Vilain A, Apiou F, Vogt N, Dutrillaux B, Malfoy B. 1996. Assignment of the gene for methyl-CpG-binding protein 2 (MECP2) to human chromosome band Xq28 by in situ hybridization. Cytogenet Cell Genet 74(4):293–4.

Villard L, Nguyen K, Cardoso C, Martin CL, Weiss AM, Sifry-Platt M, Grix AW, Graham JM Jr, Winter RM, Leventer RJ, et al. 2002. A locus for bilateral perisylvian polymicrogyria maps to Xq28. Am J Hum Genet 70(4):1003–8.

Vincent I, Bu B, Erickson RP. 2003. Understanding Niemann-Pick type C disease: a fat problem. Curr Opin Neurol 16(2):155–61.

Vlangos CN, Yim DK, Elsea SH. 2003. Refinement of the Smith-Magenis syndrome critical region to approximately 950kb and assessment of 17p11.2 deletions. Are all deletions created equally? Mol Genet Metab 79(2):134–41.

von Bohlen und Halbach O, Dermietzel R. 2002. Neurotransmitters and Neuromodulators: Handbook of Receptors and Biological Effects. Weinheim: Wiley-VCH.

von Figura K, Gieselmann V, Jaeken J. 2001. Metachromatic leukodystrophy. In: Scriver CR, Beaudet AL, Sly W, Valle D, eds. The Metabolic and Molecular Bases of Inherited Diseases. New York: McGraw-Hill.

Vreugdenhil HJ, Lanting CI, Mulder PG, Boersma ER, Weisglas-Kuperus N. 2002. Effects of prenatal PCB and dioxin background exposure on cognitive and motor abilities in Dutch children at school age. J Pediatr 140(1):48–56.

Vulpe C, Levinson B, Whitney S, Packman S, Gitschier J. 1993. Isolation of a candidate gene for Menkes disease and evidence that it encodes a copper-transporting ATPase. Nat Genet 3(1):7–13.

Wajner M, Latini A, Wyse AT, Dutra-Filho CS. 2004. The role of oxidative damage in the neuropathology of organic acidurias: insights from animal studies. J Inherit Metab Dis 27(4):427–48.

Wald NJ, Cuckle H, Brock JH, Peto R, Polani PE, Woodford FP. 1977. Maternal serum-alpha-fetoprotein measurement in antenatal screening for anencephaly and spina bifida in early pregnancy. Report of U.K. collaborative study on alpha-fetoprotein in relation to neural-tube defects. Lancet 1(8026):1323–32.

Wallerstein H. 1946. Treatment of severe erythroblastosis fetalis by simultaneous removal and replacement of the blood of the newborn infant. Science 103:583.

Wallis DE, Muenke M. 1999. Molecular mechanisms of holoprosencephaly. Mol Genet Metab 68(2):126–38.

Wallis DE, Roessler E, Hehr U, Nanni L, Wiltshire T, Richieri-Costa A, Gillessen-Kaesbach G, Zackai EH, Rommens J, Muenke M. 1999. Mutations in the homeodomain of the human SIX3 gene cause holoprosencephaly. Nat Genet 22(2):196–8.

Wanders RJ. 2004. Metabolic and molecular basis of peroxisomal disorders: a review. Am J Med Genet A 126(4):355–75.

Wandstrat AE, Schwartz S. 2000. Isolation and molecular analysis of inv dup(15) and construction of a physical map of a common breakpoint in order to elucidate their mechanism of formation. Chromosoma 109(7):498–505.

Warwick MM, Doody GA, Lawrie SM, Kestelman JN, Best JJ, Johnstone EC. 1999. Volumetric magnetic resonance imaging study of the brain in subjects with sex chromosome aneuploidies. J Neurol Neurosurg Psychiatry 66(5):628–32.

Waters PJ, Parniak MA, Akerman BR, Jones AO, Scriver CR. 1999. Missense mutations in the phenylalanine hydroxylase gene (PAH) can cause accelerated proteolytic turnover of PAH enzyme: a mechanism underlying phenylketonuria. J Inherit Metab Dis 22(3):208–12.

Watson JD, Crick FH. 1953. Molecular structure of nucleic acids; a structure for deoxyribose nucleic acid. Nature 171(4356):737–8.

Weatherall D. 2004. 2003 William Allan Award address. The thalassemias: the role of molecular genetics in an evolving global health problem. Am J Hum Genet 74(3):385–92.

Webb T. 1991. Molecular genetics of fragile X: a cytogenetics viewpoint. Report of the Fifth International Symposium on X Linked Mental Retardation, Strasbourg, France, 12 to 16 August 1991 (organiser Dr J-L Mandel). J Med Genet 28(12):814–7.

Weber P, Scholl S, Baumgartner ER. 2004. Outcome in patients with profound biotinidase deficiency: relevance of newborn screening. Dev Med Child Neurol 46(7):481–4.

Weeber EJ, Sweatt JD. 2002. Molecular neurobiology of human cognition. Neuron 33(6):845–8.

Weglage J, Pietsch M, Feldmann R, Koch HG, Zschocke J, Hoffmann G, Muntau-Heger A, Denecke J, Guldberg P, Guttler F, et al. 2001a. Normal clinical outcome in untreated subjects with mild hyperphenylalaninemia. Pediatr Res 49(4):532–6.

Weglage J, Wiedermann D, Denecke J, Feldmann R, Koch HG, Ullrich K, Harms E, Moller HE. 2001b. Individual blood–brain barrier phenylalanine transport determines clinical outcome in phenylketonuria. Ann Neurol 50(4):463–7.

Weinhofer I, Forss-Petter S, Zigman M, Berger J. 2002. Cholesterol regulates ABCD2 expression: implications for the therapy of X-linked adrenoleukodystrophy. Hum Mol Genet 11(22):2701–8.

Weintraub H, Groudine M. 1976. Chromosomal subunits in active genes have an altered conformation. Science 193(4256):848–56.

Weiss MC, Green H. 1967. Human-mouse hybrid cell lines containing partial complements of human chromosomes and functioning human genes. Proc Natl Acad Sci USA 58(3):1104–11.

Weisskopf MG, Hu H, Mulkern RV, White R, Aro A, Oliveira S, Wright RO. 2004. Cognitive deficits and magnetic resonance spectroscopy in adult monozygotic twins with lead poisoning. Environ Health Perspect 112(5):620–5.

Weksberg R, Shuman C, Caluseriu O, Smith AC, Fei YL, Nishikawa J, Stockley TL, Best L, Chitayat D, Olney A, et al. 2002. Discordant KCNQ1OT1 imprinting in sets of monozygotic twins discordant for Beckwith-Wiedemann syndrome. Hum Mol Genet 11(11):1317–25.

Weller S, Gartner J. 2001. Genetic and clinical aspects of X-linked hydrocephalus (L1 disease): mutations in the *L1CAM* gene. Hum Mutat 18(1):1–12.

Weller S, Gould SJ, Valle D. 2003. Peroxisome biogenesis disorders. Annu Rev Genomics Hum Genet 4:165–211.

Wenger DA, Rafi MA, Luzi P, Datto J, Costantino-Ceccarini E. 2000. Krabbe disease: genetic aspects and progress toward therapy. Mol Genet Metab 70(1):1–9.

Wenger D, Suzuki K, Suzuki Y, Suzuki, Kinuko. 2001. Galactosylceramide Lipidosis: Krabbe disease. In: Scriver CR, Beaudet AL, Sly W, Valle D, eds. The Metabolic and Molecular Bases of Inherited Diseases. New York: McGraw-Hill.

Werner-Felmayer G, Golderer G, Werner ER. 2002. Tetrahydrobiopterin biosynthesis, utilization and pharmacological effects. Curr Drug Metab 3(2):159–73.

Wijmenga C, Sandkuijl LA, Moerer P, van der Boorn N, Bodrug SE, Ray PN, Brouwer OF, Murray JC, van Ommen GJ, Padberg GW, et al. 1992. Genetic linkage map of facioscapulohumeral muscular dystrophy and five polymorphic loci on chromosome 4q35-qter. Am J Hum Genet 51(2):411–5.

Willard HF. 2001. The sex chromosomes and X inactivation. In: Scriver CR, Beaudet AL, Sly W, Valle D, eds. The Metabolic and Molecular Bases of Inherited Disease. New York: McGraw-Hill.

Willemsen R, Oostra BA, Bassell GJ, Dictenberg J. 2004. The fragile X syndrome: from molecular genetics to neurobiology. Ment Retard Dev Disabil Res Rev 10(1):60–7.

Williams CA, Frias JL. 1982. The Angelman ("happy puppet") syndrome. Am J Med Genet 11(4):453–60.

Winchester BG. 2001. Lysosomal membrane proteins. Eur J Paediatr Neurol 5(Suppl A):11–9.

Winrow CJ, Hemming ML, Allen DM, Quistad GB, Casida JE, Barlow C. 2003. Loss of neuropathy target esterase in mice links organophosphate exposure to hyperactivity. Nat Genet 33(4):477–85.

Wolf B. 2001. Disorders of biotin metabolism. In: Scriver CR, Beaudet AL, Valle D, Sly WS, eds. The Metabolic Basis of Inherited Disease. New York: McGraw-Hill.

Wolpert CM, Menold MM, Bass MP, Qumsiyeh MB, Donnelly SL, Ravan SA, Vance JM, Gilbert JR, Abramson RK, Wright HH, et al. 2000. Three probands with autistic disorder and isodicentric chromosome 15. Am J Med Genet 96(3):365–72.

Woo SL, Lidsky AS, Guttler F, Chandra T, Robson KJ. 1983. Cloned human phenylalanine hydroxylase gene allows prenatal diagnosis and carrier detection of classical phenylketonuria. Nature 306(5939):151–5.

Woodward K, Malcolm S. 1999. Proteolipid protein gene: Pelizaeus-Merzbacher disease in humans and neurodegeneration in mice. Trends Genet 15(4):125–8.

Woodward K, Kendall E, Vetrie D, Malcolm S. 1998. Pelizaeus-Merzbacher disease: identification of Xq22 proteolipid-protein duplications and characterization of breakpoints by interphase FISH. Am J Hum Genet 63(1):207–17.

World Health Organizations. World Health Report 2001. Mental retardation http:// www.who.intl/mediacentre/factsheets/fs265/en/

Xu Q, Wang Y, Dabdoub A, Smallwood PM, Williams J, Woods C, Kelley MW, Jiang L, Tasman W, Zhang K, et al. 2004. Vascular development in the retina and inner ear: control by Norrin and Frizzled-4, a high-affinity ligand–receptor pair. Cell 116(6):883–95.

Yagi H, Furutani Y, Hamada H, Sasaki T, Asakawa S, Minoshima S, Ichida F, Joo K, Kimura M, Imamura S, et al. 2003. Role of TBX1 in human del22q11.2 syndrome. Lancet 362(9393):1366–73.

Yamagishi A, Tomatsu S, Fukuda S, Uchiyama A, Shimozawa N, Suzuki Y, Kondo N, Sukegawa K, Orii T. 1996. Mucopolysaccharidosis type I: identification of common mutations that cause Hurler and Scheie syndromes in Japanese populations. Hum Mutat 7(1):23–9.

Yan H, Yuan W, Velculescu VE, Vogelstein B, Kinzler KW. 2002. Allelic variation in human gene expression. Science 297(5584):1143.

Yamasaki K, Joh K, Ohta T, Masuzaki H, Ishimaru T, Mukai T, Niikawa N, Ogawa M, Wagstaff J, Kishino T. 2003. Neurons but not glial cells show reciprocal imprinting of sense and antisense transcripts of Ube3a. Hum Mol Genet 12(8):837–47.

Yntema HG, Hamel BC, Smits AP, van Roosmalen T, van den Helm B, Kremer H, Ropers HH, Smeets DF, van Bokhoven H. 1998. Localisation of a gene for non-specific X linked mental retardation (MRX46) to Xq25-q26. J Med Genet 35(10):801–5.

Yntema HG, van den Helm B, Kissing J, van Duijnhoven G, Poppelaars F, Chelly J, Moraine C, Fryns JP, Hamel BC, Heilbronner H, et al. 1999a. A novel ribosomal S6-kinase (RSK4; RPS6KA6) is commonly deleted in patients with complex X-linked mental retardation. Genomics 62(3):332–43.

Yntema HG, van den Helm B, Knoers NV, Smits AP, van Roosmalen T, Smeets DF, Mariman EC, van der Burgt I, van Bokhoven H, Ropers HH, et al. 1999b. X-Linked mental retardation: evidence for a recent mutation in a five-generation family (MRX65) linked to the pericentromeric region. Am J Med Genet 85(3):305–8.

Yntema HG, Poppelaars FA, Derksen E, Oudakker AR, van Roosmalen T, Jacobs A, Obbema H, Brunner HG, Hamel BC, van Bokhoven H. 2002. Expanding phenotype of XNP mutations: mild to moderate mental retardation. Am J Med Genet 110(3):243–7.

Yogalingam G, Hopwood JJ. 2001. Molecular genetics of mucopolysaccharidosis type IIIA and IIIB: diagnostic, clinical, and biological implications. Hum Mutat 18(4):264–81.

Yoshida A, Kobayashi K, Manya H, Taniguchi K, Kano H, Mizuno M, Inazu T, Mitsuhashi H, Takahashi S, Takeuchi M, Herrmann R, Straub V, Talim B, Voit T, Topaloglu H, Toda T, Endo T. 2001. Muscular dystrophy and neuronal migration disorder caused by mutations in a glycosyltransferase, POMGnT1. Dev Cell 1(5):717–24.

Young ID, Harper PS, Archer IM, Newcombe RG. 1982a. A clinical and genetic study of Hunter's syndrome. 1. Heterogeneity. J Med Genet 19(6):401–7.

Young ID, Harper PS, Newcombe RG, Archer IM. 1982b. A clinical and genetic study of Hunter's syndrome. 2. Differences between the mild and severe forms. J Med Genet 19(6):408–11.

Yu S, Pritchard M, Kremer E, Lynch M, Nancarrow J, Baker E, Holman K, Mulley JC, Warren ST, Schlessinger D, et al. 1991. Fragile X genotype characterized by an unstable region of DNA. Science 252(5010):1179–81.

Yuste R, Bonhoeffer T. 2004. Genesis of dendritic spines: insights from ultrastructural and imaging studies. Nat Rev Neurosci 5(1):24–34.

Zamenhof S. 1952. Purification and analysis of the transforming principle of hemophilus influenza. Bull NY Acad Med 28(5):349–50.

Zemni R, Bienvenu T, Vinet MC, Sefiani A, Carrie A, Billuart P, McDonell N, Couvert P, Francis F, Chafey P, et al. 2000. A new gene involved in X-linked mental retardation identified by analysis of an X;2 balanced translocation. Nat Genet 24(2):167–70.

Zetterberg H. 2004. Methylenetetrahydrofolate reductase and transcobalamin genetic polymorphisms in human spontaneous abortion: biological and clinical implications. Reprod Biol Endocrinol 2(1):7.

Zhao X, Ueba T, Christie BR, Barkho B, McConnell MJ, Nakashima K, Lein ES, Eadie BD, Willhoite AR, Muotri AR, et al. 2003. Mice lacking methyl-CpG binding protein 1 have deficits in adult neurogenesis and hippocampal function. Proc Natl Acad Sci USA 100(11):6777–82.

Zigman AF, Lavine JE, Jones MC, Boland CR, Carethers JM. 1997. Localization of the Bannayan-Riley-Ruvalcaba syndrome gene to chromosome 10q23. Gastroenterology 113(5):1433–7.

Zinder ND, Lederberg J. 1952. Genetic exchange in salmonella. J Bacteriol 64(5):679–99.

Zoghbi HY. 2003. Postnatal neurodevelopmental disorders: meeting at the synapse? Science 302(5646):826–30.

Zweier C, Temple IK, Beemer F, Zackai E, Lerman-Sagie T, Weschke B, Anderson CE, Rauch A. 2003. Characterisation of deletions of the ZFHX1B region and genotype–phenotype analysis in Mowat-Wilson syndrome. J Med Genet 40(8):601–5.

Index